USMLE
FINAL REVIEW
STEP 2&3

Rachelle R. Doom, MD

DEDICATION

This book is dedicated to my wonderful family and friends that have been such a major support in my journey through medicine. I hope this book is a gift to many students that use it for their final review for their exams. Above all, I thank God for making all my medical dreams come true.

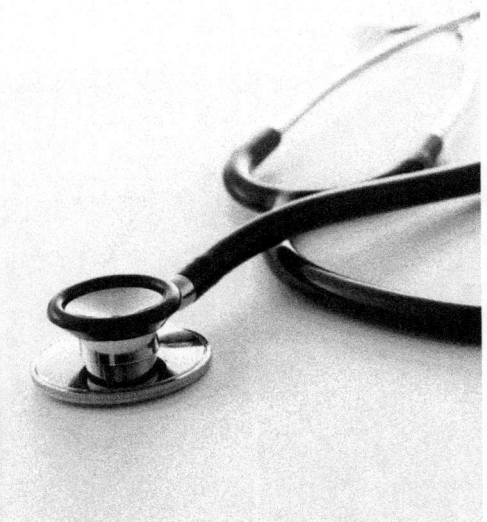

This book is designed to review high-yield key points that will be on your USMLE exams. To reach your maximum performance on your exam; review one chapter and test your knowledge on that subject before reviewing the next chapter. In the last two chapters you will find an invaluable checklist for taking a history and physical exam, which will be extremely useful in your third and fourth year rotations.

CONTENTS

CONTENTS

ACKNOWLEDGMENTS

The author would like to acknowledge the wonderful physicians at San Joaquin General Hospital in French Camp, California. **Deepak Shrivastava MD,** has been an outstanding mentor and has given me invaluable guidance throughout my medical journey. It has been both an honor and a pleasure to work with **Sheela Kapre MD, Usman Ali MD, James Saffier MD, Syung Min Jung MD, Mohsen Saadat DO, Vincent Lo MD, and Ramiro Zuniga MD.** Working with **Theodore G Rose, Jr, MD** at Alameda County Medical Center was an amazing privilege. Last, but certainly not least, **Jefry L. Biehler MD** at Miami Children's Hospital, Miami, Florida, taught me the meaning of, "caring for the children." I will never forget how each of these physicians has truly inspired me with their passion for medicine and their dedication to their patients.

1 CHAPTER
CARDIOVASCULAR

Cardiology

1) Electrocardiogram		2) Gallops
Normal- **Up** QRS in Lead I and II **L-Axis-** Up Lead I, Down II. **R-Axis-** Down Lead I, and II. **LBBB "WiLLiaM"** **W** QRS V1–V2 **M** V3–V6 **RBBB "MaRRoW"** **M** QRS V1–V2 **W** V3–V6	**Atrioventricular (AV) block** PR >200msec or P w/no QRS. **Congenital Long QT** (Jervell-Lange Nielson) Si/Sx- ↓ **hearing, FH** sudden cardiac death. Dx- EKG shows **QTc > 440ms.** Tx- **beta-blockers**.	• **S3 Gallop** **Dilated** cardiomyopathy, **SYSTOLIC dysfunction** ↓ **EF <50%** (floppy ventricle). "Aka CHF" (pulm edema, tachy, hypotension) Tx-diuretics, **ACEI** (↓mortality in CHF).
3) Gallops	**4) Murmurs**	
• **S4 Gallop** **Stiff** ventricle, **DIASTOLIC dysfunction**. Cx- HTN (most common) Tx- **beta-blockers, CCBs.** **RIGHT** side murmur ↑ **inspiration.** **LEFT** side murmur ↑ **expiration.**	**SYSTOLIC Murmurs** • **Aortic stenosis** • **Mitral regurgitation** (↑expiration) most common cause is **mitral prolapse** (midsystolic **CLICK,** best heard at **apex** radiating to **axilla,** atypical **chest pain, squatting** ↓murmur). • **Tricuspid regurgitation** (↑inspiration)	**DIASTOLIC Murmurs** (diastolic murmurs should always be investigated) • Aortic regurgitation (**EARLY diastolic** decrescendo) • **Mitral stenosis** (**Mid**-diastolic, low-pitch murmur, ↑S1).

Cardiology

5) Aortic Stenosis

Cx- age-related **calcification, bicuspid aortic** valve, rheumatic fever. Si/Sx- syncopal episodes, **dyspnea** (most common), chest pain (↑**O2 demand**), ACS: Angina, CHF, Syncope. **Pulsus parvus et tardus** (WEAK, delated **carotid** upstroke).	Si/Sx- systolic murmur at **2nd right intercostal** to **carotids,** murmur ↑**expiration** (left sided heart murmurs). Improve with valsalva (↓preload) this is opposite with HOCM (louder with ↓preload). Dx- echo, **cardiac catheterization and angiography** (most accurate diagnosis).	Tx- asymp pts reduce preload with **thiazides** or loop diuretics. All **symp** pts with aortic stenosis require **valve replacement**.

6) Mitral Stenosis / 7) Aortic Regurgitation

6) Mitral Stenosis		7) Aortic Regurgitation
Cx- **rheumatic fever** (more common in developing countries). Si/Sx- dyspnea on exertion, SOB, **cough, hemoptysis. Opening SNAP, mid-late** diastolic, low-pitch murmur at **APEX,** ↑**S1**. Affected women become **symptomatic during pregnancy** (↑blood vol).	Comp: **atrial fibrillation** (due to left atrial dilation). Dx- echo, R/O **Atrial Myxoma** (mid-diastolic rumbling murmur at apex). Tx- **balloon valvotomy** for mild SOB, severe regurgitation proceed with **valve replacement**.	Cx: **"CREAM"** C- Congenital R- Rheumatic damage E- Endocarditis **A- Aortic dissection** A- Aortic root dilations **M- Marfan's syndrome** Si/Sx- bounding pulses with "**WIDE pulse pressure**" (wide difference between systolic-diastolic BP). **Early diastolic murmur** heard at the left sternal border. Symptoms are worst while lying supine and **while lying on left side.**

Cardiology

8) Aortic Regurgitation

Si/Sx	Dx- **ECHO**	
• **De Musset's** sign (head bob)	Tx- stable and asymp give meds: **diuretics** (↓preload), **ACEI** (↓afterload), **nifedipine** (↓afterload), hydralazine, digoxin, or CCBs.	**Clinical PEARL: Marfan's syndrome** (mutation of **fibrillin-1**) can cause aortic regurgitation from **aortic root dilation** (diastolic murmur). Other symps: **mitral valve prolapse,** blue sclera, **upward dislocation of lens** (ectopia lentis), whole body is LONG.
• **Corrigan's** sign (water-hammer pulse)		
• **Duroziez's** sign (femoral bruit)	Pts with **symps, aortic valve** replacement.	
• **Austin flint murmur** (diastolic rumble)		

9) Heart Blocks
(AV block)

First-degree PR>200m/sec Tx-none **Second-degree** • **MOBITZ I** (Wenckebach) **Progress PR until drop beat.** Tx- none	**Second-degree** • **MOBITZ II** Unexpected **drop beat without change PR**. Tx- symps give **atropine**, if pt does not improve **pacemaker**.	**Third-degree** No relationship between P and QRS. Tx- **pacemaker**. If pt has 3rd degree block and symp **bradycardia** give **IV atropine** first before pacemaker and see if pt improves. Risk factor- inferior wall MI, or post coronary intervention of <24hrs.

Cardiology

10) Supra-Ventricular Tachy

• **Atrial flutter** (variable AV node conduction). Si/Sx- asymp, palpitations, syncope. Dx-ECG shows **"SAWTOOTH" (300bpm).** Dx- EKG Tx- anticoagulation, **rate control,** cardiovert if AMS/unstable.	• **Multifocal Atrial Tachycardia** Cx- **COPD,** hypoxemia. Si/Sx-asymp. Dx- ECG shows **>3 or more UNIQUE P-waves** morphologies rate >100. Obtain **O2 saturation** r/o hypoxia. Tx- underlying cx, and **rate control;** verapamil or beta-blocker.	**Tx all SVT: Carotid massage** (1st-line), **valsalva maneuver,** or immersion in **COLD water** (↑vagal tone, ↓conduction through AV node) then **adenosine,** followed by verapamil or diltiazem. **Clinical PEARL: Premature atrial beats (PAB)** are benign and need no follow up or tx.

11) Atrial Fibrillation

Cx- pulm disease, ischemia, anemia, ethanol, sepsis, thyrotoxicosis. Risk factors: hyperthyroidism, cocaine, metabolic, **rheumatic fever.** Si/Sx- asymp, SOB, chest pain. Dx-ECG shows absent P waves, **"IRREGULAR, IRREGULAR" rate,** and narrow QRS complex. HR >140beats/minute.	Tx- **ABCD A- Anticoagulate** (aspirin for lone AF, warfarin if CHADS2 score>2) **B- Beta-blockers** (control rate) **C-** Cardiovert/calcium blocker **D-** Digoxin **Clinical PEARL: Digoxin toxicity** Si/Sx- diarrhea, **nausea, vomiting, anorexia,** fatigue, HA, dizziness, AMS, **yellow-green** distortion to colors, bradycardia. **Atrial tachycardia** with **AV block.** Risk factor: **hypokalemia, verapamil** (↓renal clearance of digoxin).	Tx- if pt is **unstable** (AMS, chest pain, hypotension) **SYNCHRONOUS cardioversion** (asynchronous cardioversion in pulseless arrest (V-fib, or PVT). **Stroke Risk** use **CHAD2 score:** • **Age >75 (1)** • **HTN (1)** • **DM (1)** • **CHF (1)** • **Prior stroke (2)** (0= low risk give **aspirin,** 1-2= med risk, >2= high risk anticoagulation with **warfarin** or dabigatran).

Cardiology

12) AVNRT	13) AVRT	14) Sick Sinus Syndrome
AtrioVentricular Nodal Reentry Tachycardia Cx-**P wave buried in QRS.** Si/Sx- SOB, angina, syncope, palpitations, lightheadedness. Dx-ECG Tx- **adenosine,** if unstable cardiovert.	AtrioVentricular Reciprocating Tachycardia Assoc- **Wolff-Parkinson-White.** Si/Sx- SOB, angina, syncope, palpitations, lightheadedness. Dx- ECG Tx- **adenosine,** if unstable cardiovert. **Procainamide** for WPW (avoid rate control because this will ↓AV nodal).	**Abnormal supraventricular impulse=>** leads to bradyarrhythmias and supraventricular tachy. Si/Sx- tachycardia or bradycardia, chest pain, dyspnea, risk of TIA. Dx- ECG Tx- **pacemaker placement.**
15) PVC		
Premature Ventricular Contraction; ectopic beats, **ventricular foci.** Cx- hypoxia, electrolyte abn, hyperthyroidism. Si/Sx- asymp, palpitations.	Dx- ECG shows **widened QRS** >120msec**, bizarre morphology,** and compensatory pause. If syncope or palpitations do **24-hr Holter monitoring.**	Tx- underlying cause, if no symps **observation.** If symps give **beta-blocker.** Avoid tobacco, alcohol, caffeine and stress.

Cardiology

16) Ventricular Tachycardia (VT)		17) Ventricular Fibrillation (VF)
Si/Sx- asymp, palpitations.

Comp- **V-fib.**

Dx- ECG shows **3+ consecutive PVCs.**

Tx- **cardioversion** and antiarrhythmics; **amiodarone (1st-line).** | Tx
Can also use **procainamide or lidocaine** (AE: risk of asystole).

Clinical PEARL: Amiodarone AE: **LFTs, PFTs, TFTs** (hypo- or hyperthyroid), corneal deposits, **BLUE-GRAY skin** discoloration). | Cx- **reentrant** ventricular arrhythmia.

Si/Sx- syncope, palpitations, may lack BP, and/or lack pulse.

Assoc- **MI** (V-fib is the most common cx of death in acute MI).

Dx- ECG show **erratic wide-complex.**

Tx- **electrical cardioversion** (defibrillation) primary importance. Time of defibrillation is strongly correlated to survival. |
| **18) Torsades de Pointes** | | |
| Polymorphic ventricular tachycardia; ECG shows **TWIST around isoelectric line.**

Cx- long QT syndrome, meds; sotalol, **hypokalemia, hypomagnesemia.** | Si/Sx- dizziness, syncope, palpitations, sudden cardiac death.

Dx- ECG shows "twisting of the points" **VT rate 150-250bpm.** | Tx- IV adm of **magnesium sulfate** (MgSO4), correct K+.

If **unstable** immediate **unsynchronized cardioversion.**

If refractory to medical tx temporary pacemaker. |

Cardiology

19) Peripheral Arterial Disease		
Cx- **atherosclerotic** plaque. Risk factors: age (>70yo), DM, smoking, HTN, hyperlipidemia. Si/Sx- **intermittent claudication;** leg **pain while walking, relieved with rest.** Pt may also have erectile dysfunction.	Dx- **ankle-brachial index (ABI);** ankle and brachial systolic BP. Evidence of atherosclerosis, rest pain usually occurs at **ABI<0.4.** If pt has normal ABI do **exercise testing** and preexercise and **postexercise ABI.**	Dx- **Doppler U/S** to eval for stenosis and occlusion. **Arteriography** for surgical eval. Tx- **ASA, cilostazol,** possibly angioplasty and stent. Arterial bypass or amputation if tx fails. Avoid beta-blockers (vasoconstriction).
20) Buerger Disease	**21) Coronary Artery Disease**	
Thromboangiitis Obliterans Cx- **SMOKING** Si/Sx- **intermittent claudication,** ulcers, normal proximal pulses, **migratory thrombophlebitis,** in someone that smokes. Dx- normal ABI, **angiography shows "corkscrew"** vessels. Tx- **STOP smoking.**	**Coronary Artery Disease (CAD) risks:** • Age • Male • FH • Hyperlipidemia • DM • HTN • Obesity • Smoking	**Acute Coronary Syndromes (ACS):** spectrum syndromes that cx plaque disruption or vasospasm => MI. Dx- EKG, when **EKG** is difficult to interpret and pt is **suspected ACS** order **ECHO.**

Cardiology

22) Acute Coronary Syndrome (ACS)		
Tx- recommended ACS **discharge meds**: • **Aspirin** (all pts) • **Clopidogrel** (post MI for 9-12mos, or after stent placement)	• **Beta-blockers;** metoprolol or carvedilol. (all pts) • **ACEI** (ACS in CHF) • **Statins** (all pts) • **Nitrates** (all pts should be prescribed short-acting nitrates. Can give Isosorbide for continuous or frequent chest pain).	• **Warfarin** (only ACS pts that are **high risk** for systemic thromboembolism because of A-fib, mural thrombus, or CHF). **Clinical PEARL: Dihydropyridine calcium blockers (nifedipine)** worsen ischemia => peripheral vasodilation and **reflex tachycardia,** C/I in ACS.
23) Angina Pectoris (symps of CAD)		
Si/Sx **Classic triad:** • Substernal **chest pain** ($\uparrow$O2 demand) • Provoked by **exertion** • Relieved by **rest or nitrates.** Dx- If pt has normal EKG, then order **exercise test** to look for **ST depression** that reverses. Should withhold **beta-blockers and digoxin** (anti-ischemic meds) before stress test.	Dx **Exercise thallium** (coronary vessel disease shows hypoperfusion). **or** **Stress echo** (wall dysmotility and hypokinesia) are done when EKG is unreadable or there is previous ischemia (LBBB, digoxin use, pacemaker in place, LVH, abn EKG).	Tx • **ASA** • **Beta-blockers** • **O$_2$** • **Nitroglycerin** ($\downarrow$pulm edema, $\downarrow$preload **vasodilation,** $\downarrow$afterload by arterial dilation), • **Morphine** • **CCBs** (ditiazem, verapamil) • **ACEIs** **Clinical PEARL:** $\downarrow$**MORTALITY;** ASA, Beta-Blocker.

Cardiology

24) Unstable Angina & NSTEMI	25) TIMI Score	26) STEMI
• **Unstable Angina**: New onset **chest pain at REST**. • **NSTEMI**: Myocardial necrosis, with no ST changes on EKG, but marked ↑**Trop T,** ↑**Trop I** (lasts for 7-10days), or ↑**CK-MB** (for 1-2days). Tx- nitrates, **ASA, clopidogrel, beta-blocker, ACEI, statin,** CCBs (2nd-line).	**Risk of thrombolysis** in myocardial infarction (1pt for each risk factor): • **>65yrs** • **>3 CAD risk factors** (FH, DM, smoking, HTN, ↑cholesterol) • **CAD** (stenosis >50%) • **ASA** in past 7 days • **Severe angina** • **ST deviation**>0.5mm • **+Cardiac markers** **Risk score-** total pts (0–7).	Si/Sx- pain radiates to back, both scapulaes, and **pain radiates to ARMS** is strongly suggestive of MI. Dx ST-elevations or new LBBB, with ↑**CK-MB** (stays elevated for 1-2days), +troponin-I (stays elevated for 7-10days) most sensitive.

27) STEMI		
ST-elevations: **Lead II, III, aVF:** Inferior MI **(RCA)**. Tx- **fluid resuscitation, "AVOID Nitrates."** **Lead V1-V4:** Anterior MI **(LAD)**. **Lead I, aVL, V5-V6:** Lateral MI **(LAD or circumflex)**.	Tx **ASA, clopidogrel** (also post PCI), **beta-blockers, ACEI** (↓ventricular remodeling), **statin,** morphine, nitrates, and O₂. ↓**Mortality:** ASA, Beta-blockers, ACEIs, and statin. **Clinical PEARL: Nitrates** reduce pain in acute MI by **venodilation** (↓preload) => ↓myocardial O2 demand.	Tx • **PCI** (percutaneous coronary intervention) within **90min** of STEMI (door-to-balloon time). • **Fibrinolytics** "door-to-needle" time **30min** is goal. • **Thrombolysis (alteplase)** with in <**12hrs** of STEMI. **Long-term prognosis** is most influenced by time that lapses before **coronary blood flow is restored**.

Cardiology

28) STEMI		29) Variant Angina (Prinzmetal's)
Tx Indications for **CABG:** • If **left main coronary artery** stenosis • **Three-vessel** disease • **Two-vessel** disease with DM **Clinical PEARL:** • **Dihydropyridine** calcium blockers; **nifedipine** worsen ischemia => peripheral vasodilation and reflex tachycardia, C/I is STEMI. • **NON-Dihydropyridine**; **diltiazem** and **verapamil** are SAFE in STEMI.	**POST-MI Risks:** • **Papillary muscle rupture** (mitral regurgitation 3-7 days post-MI). • **Interventricular free wall rupture** (3-5days post MI). Si/Sx- holosystolic murmur at left sternal border. Left-to-right shunt; ↑RV pressure, ↑RA pressure, and ↑pulm artery pressure. O2 saturation RA<RV. • **Pericarditis** (dressler's syndrome) • **Ventricular aneurysm** (persistent ST elevations on ECG).	Focal coronary vasospasm. Risk factor- smoking (greatest risk factor). Si/Sx- **"angina-like"** symptoms that occur at rest, classically **AWAKENS pt from sleep.** Pts are younger, healthy women. Assoc- **Raynaud disease**. Dx- ECG may show transient ischemia **ST-segment elevations**. Tx- pt typically respond to **nitrates** and **CCBs.**

30) Indications for CABG	31) Hyper-cholesterolemia	32) ATPIII Guide for Risk
"DUST" **D- Depressed** ventricular function. **U-Unable** perform PCI (percutaneous coronary intervention) **S- Stenosis** of left main coronary artery. **T- Triple-** vessel disease (or two vessel disease with DM).	• **Total cholesterol** >200 mg/dL • **LDL > 130** mg/dL • **Triglycerides** >500 mg/dL • **HDL <40** mg/dL **Clinical PEARL: Tangier dz- ↓HDL** (alpha-lipoprotein def) Si/Sx- polyneuropathy, lymphadenopathy, hepato-splenomegaly, **orange-yellow tonsillar hyperplasia.**	Guide for Hypercholesterolemia • **0–1 Risk factor: Goal LDL<160.** (>160 tx lifestyle changes, >190 tx statin) • **2+ Risk factors: Goal LDL<130.** (>130 tx lifestyle changes, >160 tx statin) • **CAD or diabetes: Goal LDL <100.** (>100 tx lifestyle changes, >130 tx statin) **Risk factors-** age, male, hyperlipidemia, DM, HTN, obesity, FH, smoking.
33) Lipid-Lowering Agents		34) Causes of Pericarditis
• **Statins** (HMG-CoA reductase inh, ↓CoQ10) Tx- **↓LDL, ↓Trig.** AE- ↑CPK, **myalgias, ↑LFTs,** ↑BUN/Cr. • **Fibrates** (lipoprotein lipase stim) Gemfibrozil, feno**fibrate.** Tx- **↓Trig, ↑HDL,** hyper-triglyceridemia (palmar xanthomas).	• **Ezetimibe (zetia)** (cholesterol absorption inhibitors) Tx- **↓LDL** • **Niacin** (↓fatty acid release from adipose tissue) Tx- **↓LDL, ↑HDL** AE- **FLUSHING,** pruritis (prostaglandin-induced vasodilatation) • **Cholestyramine, colestipol, colesevelam** (binds bile acids=> ↓bile acid stores and ↓LDL) Tx- **↓LDL**	**"CARDIAC RIND"** **C-** Collagen vascular **A-** Aortic dissection **D-** Drugs **I-** Infections **(TB)** **A-** Acute renal failure **C-** Cardiac (MI) **R-** Rheumatic fever **I-** Injury **N-** Neoplasms **D-** Dressler's syndrome

Cardiology

35) PERICarditis	36) Causes of Secondary HTN	37) Fibromuscular Dysplasia
Si/Sx- PERIC; P- Pulsus paradoxus (systolic ↓BP >10 on inspiration) E- ECG changes R- Rub I- ↑JVP C-Chest pain, relieved by leaning forward. Dx- EKG shows DIFFUSE ST-Elevations. Sharp 'x' and 'y' descents on central venous tracing. Tx- NSAIDs (1st-line), steroids if NSAIDs are not effective.	CHAPS C- Cushing's syndrome Si/Sx- HTN, acne, bruising, fatigue, cataracts, osteopenia, proximal muscle weakness. Dx-↑Cortisol, ↓K+, ↑Na+, ↑Glu. H- Hyper-aldosteronism (Conn's syndrome) A- Aortic coarctation P- Pheochromocytoma S- Stenosis of renal artery (fibromuscular dysplasia)	Renal artery stenosis; is responsible for 20% of all cases of renal HTN. Si/Sx- HA, HTN, renal hum or "renal BRUIT" in costovertebral angle. Dx- angiogram shows "string of beads" pattern to renal artery. Tx- percutaneous angioplasty with stent placement (1st-line).
38) HTN		
Si/Sx- asymp, HA. Dx- BP >140/90 on three separate appointments. Tx- ABCD A- ACEIs/ARBs B- Beta-blockers C- CCBs D- Diuretics (thiazide)	Also, "WEIGHT LOSS" is the most beneficial lifestyle modification, with BMI goal of 18.5-24.9kg/m2. (smoking has little effect on ↓BP)	Clinical PEARL: Malignant HTN (BP >200/140) Si/Sx- papilledema, oliguria, LVH. Dx- ophthamoscopy shows papilledema (confirms diagnosis).

Cardiology

39) Anti-hypertensives

• **Diuretics** (thiazide, loop, K+ sparing) AE- **hypokalemia** (except K+ sparing)	• **CCBs** -**Dihydropyridines** (nife**dipine**, felo**dipine**, amlo**dipine**) AE- flush, headache, **peripheral edema,** C/I- in STEMI (reflex tachycardia).	• **ACEIs** (capto**pril**, enala**pril**, fosino**pril**, benaze**pril**, lisino**pril**) AE- **COUGH** ($\uparrow$kinin), rash, hyperkalemia.
• **Beta-blockers** (propran**olol**, metopr**olol**, nad**olol**, aten**olol**, tim**olol**, carvedilol, labetalol) AE-**bronchospasm**	-**Non-Dihydropyridine** (**diltiazem, verapamil**) SAFE in STEMI. AE- $\downarrow$contractility.	• **ARBs** (lo**sartan**, val**sartan**, irbe**sartan**) Block aldosterone. AE- **NO COUGH**, rash, hyperkalemia.
• **Adrenergic Agonists** (methyldopa, clonidine) AE-**rebound HTN** from withdrawal of medication.	• **Vasodilators** -**Hydralazine** (relax smooth muscles, works on arteries and arterioles, $\downarrow$afterload) AE- HA, lupus. -**Minoxidil** AE: hirsutism.	• **Alpha1 blockers** (**prazosin**, te**razosin**, phenoxybenzamine) AE- **orthostatic hypotension** (drop systolic $\downarrow$BP >20 from lying down to standing).

Cardiology

40) Anti-HTN Specifics		
• CHF Tx- **beta-blocker, ACEIs** or **ARBs,** and/or diuretics (including **spironolactone**) • **Diabetes with proteinuria** Tx- **ACEIs** or **ARBs**	• **Systolic HTN** Tx- **diuretics,** long-acting CCBs (Dihyd: nife**dipine,** felo**dipine,** amlo**dipine**) • **MI** Tx- **beta-blockers** (not in acute symptoms), ACEIs.	• **Osteoporosis** Tx- **thiazide** diuretics. • **BPH** Tx- alpha1 blockers (**prazosin,** te**razosin,** phenoxybenzamine). • **Benign Essential Tremor** Tx- propran**olol** (beta-blocker)

41) CHF		
Congestive Heart Failure (CHF) Assoc- **chronic HTN, previous MI** both predispose to CHF. Si/Sx- dyspnea on exertion, **orthopnea, paroxysmal nocturnal dyspnea,** JVD.	Si/Sx- wheezing (cardiac asthma), tachypnea, bibasilar crackles in lung bases. ↑Hepato-jugular reflex (suggests heart edema). Comp- **pleural effusion** (dullness to percussion, ↓BS over effusion).	Dx- ↑**BNP >100pg/mL,** ↑**PCWP, ABG;** hypoxia, hypocapnia, respiratory alkalosis, **echo** (confirms diagnosis). Systolic HF (↓EF): ↓**Cardiac index,** ↑**TPR,** ↑**LVEDV.** **Hyponatremia** is a bad prognostic factor.

Cardiology

42) CHF Management

Acute CHF Tx:	Chronic CHF Tx:	ALL ↓mortality:
"LMNOP"	• **Diuretics** (1ˢᵗLine)	**ACEI, beta-blockers,** and **spironolactone.**
L- Lasix		
M- Morphine	• **Beta-blockers**	
N- Nitrates (most rapidly acting)	(carvedilol, metoprolol)	**Digoxin and furosemide** ↓ **hospitalizations** (do not improve survival).
O- Oxygen	• **ACEIs**	
P- Position (upright)		
	• **Spironolactone**	
Beta-blockers: NOT in decompensated CHF but started once stable.	**(eplerenone** alternative no gynecomastia).	

43) NYHA Class CHF	44) Classification CHF Stages	
Class I **NO limitations** or symp with activity.	• **Stage A:** **High RISK factors;** HTN, smoking, alcohol abuse, hyperlipidemia, obesity, lack of exercise. Tx- **ACEIs**	• **Stage C:** Heart disease + **symp** **CHF.** Tx- **ACEIs,** **beta-blocker, diuretics,** and salt restriction.
Class II **Slight limitation** with activity, comfortable at rest.		
Class III **Marked limitations** with activity, **comfortable ONLY AT REST.**	• **Stage B:** **Structural heart disease** (MI), but no symps of CHF. Tx- **ACEIs and beta-blockers.**	• **Stage D:** **Marked symps** of CHF at REST. Tx- **heart transplantation.**
Class IV Confined to no activity, **symps while at REST.**		

Cardiology

45) Types of Diuretics		
• LOOPS (furosemide, ethacrynic acid, bumetanide, torsemide) "Loops Loss Ca" AE- ototoxicity, ↓Ca, ↓K, gout.	• THIAZIDE (1st-line) (chlorothiazide, chlorthalidone, HCTZ) AE- ↓K, ↑Glu, ↑Ca, ↑lipidemia, ↑uricemia.	• K+ SPARING (spironolactone, triamterene, amiloride) AE- ↑K, gynecomastia, hirsutism, sexual dysfunction.
46) Types of Diuretics	**47) Pericardial Effusion**	**48) Pericardial Tamponade**
• Carbonic Anhydrase Inhibitors (acetazolamide) AE- neuropathy, sulfa allergy. • Mannitol AE- pulmonary edema, dehydration, C/I in anuria and CHF.	Cx- idiopathic, post-MI, uremia, malignancy, hypothyroidism. Risk factor- cardiac tamponade. Si/Sx- SOB, difficult to palpate point of max impulse. Dx- CXR shows "WATER BOTTLE" shaped cardiac silhouette. Tx- pericardiocentesis.	Si/Sx- syncope, BECK's triad: • Distant heart sounds • JVD (↑CVP and Kussmaul's sign; ↑JVD on inspiration) • Hypotension Dx- ECG reveals "electrical alternans" (amplitude of QRS alternates as heart moves in fluid-filled pericardial sac), echocardiogram. Tx- emergent pericardiocentesis.

Cardiology

49) Abdominal Aortic Aneurysm		
Cx- **atherosclerosis** Si/Sx-asymp, **PULSATILE abd mass or abd bruits**. If AAA ruptures pts may have referred **lower back pain and ↓BP**. Risk factors: >60yo, smokers, men. Dx- **abdominal U/S**. **Screening** via abd U/S should be done in male **smokers age 65-75yo**.	Tx- surgical >**5.5cm** (abd), >6cm (thoracic). **Smoking cessation** has the greatest likelihood of slowing AAA progression. Comp- **colonic ischemia**, spinal cord ischemia (weakness, bowel/bladder dysfunction).	**Clinical PEARL:** **Ruptured AAA** Si/Sx- acute onset of **back pain,** profound **hypotension, syncope, hematuria.** Possibly pulsatile abd mass at umbilicus. Tx- **emergent surgical repair** (mortality 50%).
50) Aortic Dissection		
Tear in the intima => blood into media. Cx- **HTN** (most common) Assoc- **Marfan's syndrome**. Si/Sx- HTN, **sudden tearing pain** in anterior chest, or **interscapular BACK pain.** **Early diastolic murmur** (dissection causes aortic regurgitation).	Si/Sx- variation in pulse or **BP between RIGHT and LEFT ARMS** >30mmHg). Neurologic deficits if spinal arteries are involved. Dx- CXR shows **widening of the mediastinum.** ECG to r/o MI. **Transesophageal echocardiography (TEE)**, but control HTN first with **labetalol.**	Dx- **CT angiography** (gold standard). Tx- **labetalol** (beta-blocker) to control BP. • **Ascending** aortic dissection **"surgical emergency."** • **Descending** aortic dissection manage **BP and HR.**

Cardiology

51) Deep Venous Thrombosis (DVT)		
Cx **Virchow's triad:** • **Hemostasis** (ex- long flight or in bed for a long time) • **Trauma** (endothelial damage) • **Hypercoagulability** (ex- malignancy, pregnancy, OCP)	Si/Sx- **Homan's sign** (calf tenderness with dorsiflexion). Dx- Neg d-dimer r/o PE. If +d-dimer order **doppler U/S; spiral CT** (C/I in renal failure or contrast allergy). If cannot do spiral CT order **V/Q scan** to r/o PE.	Tx- IV unfractionated **heparin** or SQ low-molecular-weight heparin followed by PO **warfarin** for 3-6mos. **IVC filter** in pts that are unable to have anticoagulation.

52) Acute Ischemia 6 P's		
Cx- **Emboli** from the heart (80%), thrombosis, or trauma. Risk factor- **atrial fibrillation**. Prevention: **Anticoagulation with warfarin** in pts with atrial fibrillation.	Si/Sx- stroke and limb ischemia. **6 P's of acute ischemia** P- Pain P- Pallor P- Pulselessness P- Paralysis P- Paresthesia P- Poikilthermia	Dx- **angiography** shows abrupt cutoff of aterial blood flow. **Echo** to r/o thrombus in left ventricle. Tx- **IV heparin** immediately upon suspicion. Surgical **embolectomy** or **intra-arterial fibrinolysis.**

Cardiology

53) Dilated Cardiomyopathy		
Dilated ventricles and diffuse hypokinesia, **SYSTOLIC** dysfunction ($\downarrow$EF). Cx- wet beriberi, pheochromocytoma, acromegaly. • Drugs; **alcohol,** doxorubicin, AZT, **cocaine.** • Infxs; **coxsackie B virus** (hx URI), **chagas' disease** (protozoal, trypanosoma cruzi. Assoc- megacolon, megaesophagus)	Si/Sx **CHF** symp; dyspnea on exertion, **orthopnea, paroxysmal nocturnal dyspnea, pulm edema (rales),** tachycardia, hypotension. Pts may also have **JVD, S3 gallop** (dilated), mitral and tricuspid regurgitation. Comp- pleural effusion (dullness to percussion at lung bases).	Dx- **CXR** shows balloon-heart. **ECG** shows nonspecific ST-T changes, **LBBB common. ECHO** (diagnostic). Tx- underlying etiology, CHF symp; **diuretics, ACEIs, beta-blockers, aldosterone antagonist.**
54) Hypertrophic Cardiomyopathy		**55) Restrictive Cardiomyopathy**
DIASTOLIC dysfunction (filling impaired); **septal hypertrophy** and **systolic anterior motion** (SAM) of mitral valve. Cx- **HOCM** (AD) (hypertrophic obstructive cardiomyopathy). Si/Sx- asymp, syncope, dyspnea, angina, palpitations, or **sudden death in young, healthy athlete.** S4 gallop (stiff), **systolic crescendo-decrescendo** murmur along the **left sternal border without** carotid radiation.	Si/Sx- $\uparrow$murmur valsalva ($\downarrow$preload). Dx- CXR may show left atrial enlargement. **ECG shows LVH. Echo** (diagnostic) shows thick left ventricular wall. **HOCM** due a **transthoracic echo** followed by **Holter** (continuous ECG). Tx- **beta-blocker (1st-line,** $\uparrow$preload) CCBs (2nd-line). **HOCM- asymp** avoid strenuous sports activities, with **symps implantable cardiac defibrillator.**	$\downarrow$Elasticity of myocardium=> impaired **DIASTOLIC filling.** Cx- sarcoidosis, amyloidosis, hemochromatosis, radiation. Si/Sx- JVD, peripheral edema, **S4 gallop** (stiff ventricular wall). Dx- CXR, MRI, cardiac cath, ECG may show LBBB, **Echo** (diagnostic). Tx- **diuretics** for fluid overload.

2 CHAPTER
DERMATOLOGY

Dermatology

1) Urticaria (Hives)		
Type I Hypersensitivity; superficial edema from histamine and prostaglandins. Cx- food, virus, insect bite, drugs; NSAIDs, ACEIs, contrast media, aspirin.	Si/Sx- **itchy bumps to anaphylaxis.** Typical lesions are reddish and widespread. Pts may have **tongue swelling, angioedema,** GI symps, and/or fever.	Dx- clinical. Tx- **antihistamines** (diphenhydramine; benadryl). If severe anaphylaxis **IM epinephrine** (1st-line).
2) Drug Eruption	**3) Erythema Multiforme**	
High suspicion in HOSPITALIZED pts that develope a **RASH**. Si/Sx- **7–14 days after exposure,** widespread, symmetrical, and pruritic. **Drugs** can cause ALL four hypersensitivity reactions. Dx- clinical impression. Tx- **antihistamines** (diphenhydramine; benadryl).	Cx- predisposing infx is **HERPES simplex** (most common), mycoplasma, fungal disease, and drugs. Si/Sx- **TARGET appearance,** start on erythematous macules => **centrally clear** often on **PALMS and SOLES**. Severe Erythema Multiforme => can lead to **TEN or Stevens-Johnson Syndrome.**	Dx- clinical, some pts may have a history of recurrent **libial herpes.** Tx- corticosteroids are of **no benefit.** Pts with HSV, use **acyclovir.** **Acyclovir AE: Crystalline nephropathy**; renal tubular obstruction. Avoid nephropathy by giving adequate amount hydration.

Dermatology

4) SJS and TEN		5) Erythema Nodosum
Stevens Johnson Syndrome/ Toxic Epidermal Necrolysis (life-threatening exfoliation). • SJS <10% BSA • TEN >30% BSA Cx- viral infx, malignancies, **allergic reaction to MEDS**; sulfonamides, NSAIDs, phenytoin. Si/Sx- **mucosal erosions.** Pt may have started a **NEW drug** that has caused the reaction.	Dx- +Nikolsky's sign. • **SJS:** degeneration of **basal layer** epidermis. • **TEN: full-thickness** of epidermal necrosis. **TEN vs. SSSS** • **TEN** full-thickness (**adult**). • **SSSS** (staph scalded skin syndrome) **Superficial** damage exfoliative, fever, also has +Nikolsky's sign (<6yr). Tx- same as for burn victims; **topical silver sulfadiazine** and **mafenide, IV fluids,** narcotic analgesia.	Chronic inflam disease; Sarcoidosis, Crohn's, UC, Behcet's (oral and genital ulcers), SLE. Si/Sx- **painful, erythematous nodules on "LOWER LEGS,"** turn brown or gray, **fever, joint pain.** Dx- clinical, **False+ VDRL** (seen in SLE). Tx- treat underlying disease.
6) Pemphigus Vularis		**7) Bullous Pemphigoid**
Life-threatening **autoimmune** condition; **intra-epidermal blisters =>** widespread, painful erosion of **SKIN and MUCOUS** membranes. Assoc- **middle-aged (40–60yo).** Si/Sx- **MOUTH ulcers,** and skin erosions, with crusting, weeping, **and secondary infections.**	Dx- + **Nikolsky's sign,** biopsy shows **acantholysis** (intraepidermal **splitting** of keratinocytes) in blister. Confirm diagnosis with immunofluorescence and ELISA showing **ANTI-DESMOGLEIN antibodies.** Tx- systemic **corticosteroids.** For steroid sparing can use mycophenolate mofetil, azathioprine. Can also use rituximab and IVIG.	Si/Sx- acquired **BLISTERING disease** => lead separation at epidermal BM, **blisters are stable.** Assoc- **60–80yo.** Dx- **NEG Nikosky's sign.** Subepidermal blister, **IgG and C3 at dermal-epidermal** junction. Tx- systemic and/or topical **corticosteroids.**

Dermatology

8) A-Atopic Dermatitis (Eczema)		9) Contact Dermatitis
Assoc: **A-ASTHMA, A-ALLERGIC** rhinitis.	• **Adults-** dry, fissured skin on **hands** with **lichenification.**	Type IV Hypersensitivity
Si/Sx- **"ITCH that RASHES."** Pruritus=> **lichenification** (thick epidermis).	Dx- clinically Tx- **moisturizers, nondrying soaps,** avoid triggers. Topical corticosteroids.	Cx- **poison ivy, poison oak, NICKEL** jewelry, diaper dermatitis, soaps, detergents, cosmetics, and rubber with latex, **poison sumas** (woody shrub, may be found in firewood).
• **Infants-** pruritic, weeping patches on **face, scalp, extensor surfaces,** but sparing the diaper region (classic symps).	**Clinical PEARL: Eczema Herpeticum** Cx- **HSV** Si/Sx- numerous **vesicles** superimposed infx on healing **atopic dermatitis.** Tx- **acyclovir**	Si/Sx- intense **pruritus and rash;** tiny blisters and crusts.
• **Child-** pruritic, dry, **SCALY** patches on **neck and flexural areas.**		
10) Contact Dermatitis	11) Seborrheic Dermatitis	
Dx- clinical, **Patch test** (causative allergen).	Cx- **pityrosporum ovale** (fungal infx).	Tx- **HIV** pts are resistant to tx.
Tx- avoid allergen. Use **topical** or systemic **corticosteroids,** and/or zinc oxide ointment.	Assoc- **Parkinson disease, HIV,** infants.	• **Infants: "Diaper Rash,"** with yellow scale, or **"Cradle Cap"** scalp.
Clinical PEARL: • **Strawberry hemangioma** Benign, strawberry appearing, **vascular tumor** appear **first wk** of life and regress by 5-8yo. • **Cherry hemangioma** Small red cutaneous papules seen with aging.	Si/Sx- **"OILY skin"** areas like scalp, central face, midchest. **WAXY scales** with underlying erythema. Dx-clinical. Tx- - topical antifungal or corticosteroids. **Selenium sulfide** or **zinc pyrithione** shampoos for scalp.	• **Child/adults:** red, scaly patches on **EARS** and **eyebrows.** • **HIV/AIDS and PARKINSON'S:** severe seborrheic dermatitis.

Dermatology

12) Psoriasis (T-cell inflam)		13) Impetigo
Assoc- seronegative arthritis, HLA-B27+. Si/Sx- **patches** and **"SILVERY scales,"** on **extensor surfaces. Onycholysis** (lift nail plate), **Koebner's phenomenon** (lesions from trauma), **psoriatic arthritis "SAUSAGE" digits.**	Dx- **Auspitz sign** (bleed scale scraped), **Munro's microabscess** (neutrophils in stratum corneum). Tx- **topical steroids,** methotrexate in severe. NSAIDs for arthritis.	Cx- group A strep **(GAS)** and **staph.** Si/Sx-weeping, **"HONEY-colored crust"** on face, small **patch on CHEEK.** Can be large, stable blisters => that can lead to **SSSS.** **Clinical PEARL: Strep Impetigo** risk of developing **post-streptococcal glomerulonephritis.**
14) Impetigo	**15) Erythrasma**	
Dx-clinical Tx- topical **mupirocin (1st-line)** or oral penicillin. **Clinical PEARL: Erysipelas** Cx- group A strep (strep pyogenes). Si/Sx- small **red patch on cheek=> painful** plaque. Tx- penicillin	Cx- **corynebacterium minutissimum.** Si/Sx- itchy rash, sharply demarcated, **"RED-BROWN" patches** in **major skin folds,** digital web spaces. Assoc- **DIABETICS**	Dx- **Wood's light exam; coral-red fluorescence** of lesion; **coproporphyrin III deposition** in stratum corneum. Gram +, filamentous rods. Tx- **ERYTHRomycin** for ERYTHRasma.

Dermatology

16) Scarlet Fever "S's"	17) Cellulitis	
Cx- **S. Pyogens (GAS)** Si/Sx • **S- Severe FEVER** • **S-Strawberry** tongue • **S- Sunburn** with **goosebumps**. • **S- Salmonella typhi "rose Spots"** (pink trunk), with + gallbladder disease. Dx- clinical Tx- **cholecystectomy** (for salmonella typhi gallbladder disease).	Infection of **DEEP subcutaneous tissue** of the skin. Cx- group A strep **(GAS),** staph or **MRSA**. Si/Sx- **red, swollen, hot, tender skin** with fever and chills.	Dx- clinical, BCx. Tx- 7–10 days oral **dicloxacillin**. For cellulitis with systemic signs use **IV nafcillin or cefazolin** (1st-line).
18) Herpes Simplex Virus (HSV)		
• **HSV-1** (oral) • **HSV-2** (genital) Si/Sx- **PAINFUL VESICULAR eruption** in **oral** lesions or **genital** lesions, with erythema swelling.	**Clinical PEARL: Herpetic whitlow** Si/Sx- lesion on pulp of **finger/digit** from direct contact of **oral herpes**. Ex- direct contact with infx orotracheal secretions, like dentist.	Dx- **multinucleated Giant cells** on **TZANCK smear.** Tx- **acyclovir** (ointment, oral, or IV), valacy**clovir**, or famci**clovir** (2nd-line).

Dermatology

19) Dermatitis HERPetiformis	20) Varicella-Zoster Virus (VZV)	
Cx- **NON-herpes** virus infx (looks like herpes). Assoc- **CELIAC disease.** Si/Sx- "appearance is like herpes," **pruritic papules on elbows, knees, buttocks**, scalp, and neck. Dx- **granular IgA** in dermal papillae. Tx- **DAPSONE (1st-line)** and gluten-free diet.	• **Varicella Virus** Resp droplet or direct contact. Si/Sx- Chickenpoxs; **dewdrop rose petal, "all STAGES"** of lesions over **entire body,** but **palms and soles are spared.** Adults can have systemic **pneumonia and encephalitis.** If pt has not had vaccine, **varicella vaccine** can be given if it is within first **3-5 days of exposure.**	• **Zoster Virus** Si/Sx- **dermatomal** distribution with intense local pain. Older pts can develop **postherpetic neuralgia.** Dx- clinical Tx- **self-limited,** prevention with **vaccine.** Adults give **acyclovir,** pain control for postherpetic neuralgia.

Dermatology

21) Molluscus Contagiosum		22) Verrucae (HPV warts)
Skin-skin transmission and by sexual contact. Cx- **poxvirus** Assoc- young children, pts on chemotherapy, corticosteroid use, and **HIV/AIDS pts** (cellular immuno-deficiency). Si/Sx- firm, dome-shaped, **flesh-colored, tiny waxy papules,** with **"CENTRAL umbilication"** on face, extremities, trunk, and genitalia.	Si/Sx- lesions in **AIDS pts** are very **large on FACE.** Dx- **Giemsa and Wright's stain** show large inclusion or **"Molluscus bodies."** Tx- trichloroacetic acid, freeze or may resolve spontaneously in mos-yrs.	Cx- **HPV** (esp 16, 18) Si/Sx- **"WARTS"** on hands or genital warts. **Condylomata acuminata** (anogenital warts) **"Cauliflower-like;"** verrucous, papilliform lesions. Dx- clinical, **acetowhitening** helps visualize lesions.
23) Verrucae (HPV warts)	24) Folliculitis	
Tx- cryotherapy or curettage. Genital warts **podophyllin,** imiquimod, trichloroacetic acid. Screening: **HPV of cervix** must be monitored for cancer.	Hair follicle inflam. Cx- **staph, strep,** gram negs, yeast (candida, pityrosporum). Si/Sx- tiny pustules at hair follicle. • **Furuncle** (deeper, abscess) • **Carbuncle** (adjacent follicles)	**"Hot tub folliculitis"** Cx- **pseudomonas** aeruginosa. Dx- clinical, CT possible for abscess. Tx- **topical antibiotics,** if severe systemic abxs.

Dermatology

25) Ludwig's Angina	26) Necrotizing Fascitis	
Infected tooth => **bilateral cellulitis** submaxillary and sublingual spaces. Si/Sx- fever, **red warm mouth,** dysphagia (difficulty swallowing), drooling, risk of **asphyxiation (suffocation).** Tx- **abxs, protection of airway,** urgent maxillo-facial surgery with **incision and drainage.**	Cx- S. pyogenes (GAS) or clostridium perfringens. Si/Sx- **sudden pain and swelling** after **recent surgery or trauma**. Dx- XR or CT may show **"AIR in tissue,"** biopsy edge of lesion (diagnostic).	Tx- **surgical debridement. Penicillin** or clindamycin for strep. **Metronidazole** or 3rd cephalosporin for anerobic coverage. **Clinical PEARL:** Pts on **metronidazole** should avoid alcohol due to risk of disulfiram-like reaction.

27) Acne Vulgaris		
Cx- Propionibacterium **ACNES.** Assoc- adolescents. Si/Sx- comedo **(blackhead or whitehead),** inflam pustule => scar if picking at papules.	Dx- clinical. Tx: • Mild use topical **tretinoin** (Retin-A), adapalene or **benzoyl peroxide.** • Topical abxs, **erythromycin** if there is inflammation.	• Severe use **oral ISOTRETINOIN** greatly improves symps. Used in pts that have **nodulocystic** form and **scars.** **Isotretinoin** AE: **tetratogenic** and pts should be given a **preg test** before use.

Dermatology

28) Pilonidal Cysts	29) Tinea Versicolor (fungal)	
Cx- **Bacteroides**. Si/Sx- tender, warm, indurated **abscess** in **sacrococcygeal** region. Comp- **perianal fistulas**. Dx- CT scan. Tx- **incision and drainage** of abscess under local anesthesia followed by sterile packing.	Cx- **Malassezia furfur** (fungal infx) part normal skin flora. Si/Sx- small, scaly patch, that **varies in COLOR (hypo- or hyperpigmented) that do "NOT TAN"** on chest and/or back (due to azelaic acid produced by hyphal).	Dx- clinical, **potassium hydroxide (KOH)** preparation shows: **"Spaghetti and Meatballs"** pattern of hyphae and spores. Tx- topical **selenium sulfide** daily for 1wk. Can also use **ketoconazole** shampoo.
30) Candidiasis		
Cx- **C. albicans** Assoc- diabetes, antibiotic use, steroid use, HIV with CD4<50/microL. Si/Sx • **ORAL- painless white plaques** that **"CAN scrape OFF."** Pts may develop esophagitis; substernal burning, painful swallowing.	Si/Sx • **SKIN- circular, pink,** erythematous macules near skin folds. Dx- clinical, **KOH** preparation visible **hyphae.** Tx- oral **fluconazole, nystatin; "Swish and Swallow,"** or topical nystatin.	If pt does not respond to tx in 3-5 days perform **esophagoscopy with cytology**, biopsy and culture for specific etiology. **Clinical PEARL: Leukoplakia** Si/Sx- **Hard to remove** white patches in oral mucosa. May lead to **squamous cell carcinoma (SCC).** Risk factors: smoking, alcohol.

Dermatology

31) Dermatophyte Infections (fungal)		
Dermatophytes is a fungal infx that lives in **keratin (skin, nail, and hair).** Cx- Microsporum (**pets** are reservoir), tricho**phyton**, and epidermo**phyton**.	• **Tinea Corporis** (body) Si/Sx-rash on **TRUNK** that is **scaly boarders,** pruritic with **sharp, irregular boarder,** often with **CENTRAL clearing.** Assoc- infected **PETS**.	• **Tinea pedia** "Athlete's foot." • **Tinea Cruris** "Jock itch" (groin, sparing the scrotum). • **Tinea Capitis** "**Ringworm**" scaly scalp (similar to seborrheic dermatitis).
32) Dermatophyte Infections (fungal)	**33) Lice** (parasitic)	
Dx- **KOH** shows **HYPHAE.** Tx- topical antifungal; **terbinafine,** systemic; **griseofulvin.** **Tinea CAPITIS** need; **ORAL griseofulvin** for 6-12wks. **Selenium sulfide** shampoo is also helpful.	Lice (parasitic) spread by contact and secrete toxins => lead to **pruritus.** Cx- head, body, and pubic **louse.** Assoc- poor hygiene, crowded living.	Si/Sx- **severe pruritus,** childhood classroom epidemics, **bites turn BLUE.** Dx- visually see lice. Tx- topical **P-Permethrin** or **P-Pyrethrin** (P-Parasite).

Dermatology

34) Scabies (parasitic)	35) Decubitus Ulcers (pressure)	
Female digs into corneum and lays eggs. female **burrowing=> pruritus.** Cx- **Sarcoptes scabies** Si/Sx- **pruritus** at night and after hot showers affecting hands, axillae, genital. Dx- clinical, may have family with pruritus. Tx- topical **5% Permethrin** neck down or oral **ivermectin.**	Cx- bedridden patient. Si/Sx **Grades** I: Redness **II:** Ulceration **III:** Beneath skin **IV:** Deep into muscle, tendon, or even bone. Dx- clinical appearance.	Tx- **routinely move pt every two hours,** pressure reducing devices (air/foam mattresses), **wound care,** and possibly surgical debridement if severe.
36) Venous Stasis Ulcers	**37) Arterial Insufficiency**	**38) Neuropathic Ulcers**
Cx-valve incompetence. Si/Sx- **xerosis** (dry skin), edema, **stasis dermatitis, medial MALLEOLUS ulcers.** Dx- clinical Tx- leg elevation, compression stockings or **Unna boots.**	Assoc: **atherosclerosis** Si/Sx **"PainFUL"** ulcer on **HEEL and/or TIPS of TOES.** Dx- clinical Tx- underlying disease.	Assoc: **diabetic neuropathy**. Si/Sx **"PainLESS"** ulcers on **UNDERSIDE** of foot and toes. Dx- clinical Tx- underlying disease.

Dermatology

39) Gangrene		40) Acanthosis Nigricans
• **DRY** Cx- **atherosclerosis** Assoc- DM, smoking Si/Sx- cold, aching with **blue-black** appearance. • **WET** Cx-**bacterial infx** Si/Sx- swollen, bruised and may have **blistered with pus.**	• **GAS** Cx- **clostridium perfringens** Si/Sx- skin pale=> dark red, producing gas **"medical emergency."** Dx- clinical Tx- abxs, surgical **debridement** with amputation if needed. **Gas gangrene** give **hyperbaric O$_2$** toxic to **C. perfingens** (anaerobic).	Hyperkeratotic and **hyperpigmented skin.** Assoc- **DM, obesity** Si/Sx- thickening and hyperpigmentation of skin of flexural areas. **"VELVETY" appearance** in nape of neck, axillary, and genital area. Dx- clinical. Tx- typically not treated, but can use **topical retinoids.**
41) Lichen Planus "P" Disease		
Si/Sx- **ITCHY RASH on skin or mouth.** **"P" Disease** **P-PUZZLING** P-Planar P-Purple P-Pruritic P-Perioral P-Persistent P-Polygonal P-koebner's Phenomenon (lesions at site of trauma)	Chronic inflammatory dermatosis. Assoc- HCV Si/Sx- pruritic, **FLAT-topped, polygonal papules** of skin and **mucous** membrane. • **Wickham's Striae (White Stripes)** on mucous membrane. • **Koebner's phenomena** (lesions at site of trauma).	Dx- **T-lymphocytes** at **epidermal-dermal juction** which damages the basal layer. Tx- most resolve spontaneously. Can use topical or systemic **corticosteroids. Tretinoin** gel for oral mucosa.

Dermatology

42) Vitiligo		43) Pityriasis Rosea
Autoimmune **destruction of melanocytes** => depigmentation that involves the acral and peri-orficial areas. Assoc: **Autoimmune** diseases; DM, **pernicious anemia** (anti-parietal cells, anti-intrinsic factor), thyroid dz.	Si/Sx- sharply demarcated **DEPIGMENTED** macules and/or patches on face, hands, or genitalia. Dx- histology shows **ABSENTS of melanocytes** (from destruction of melanocytes). Tx- topical or systemic **psoralens,** sunscreen, chemical bleach.	Assoc- **human herpes virus (HHV 6 or 7)**. Si/Sx- "HERALD **patch"** => days to weeks later pruritic, **pink, scaly** acute dermatitis with **cigarette paper** apperance and **"CHRISTMAS tree" pattern** on back. Dx- clinical, KOH r/o fungus. Tx- none, heal without tx in 2–3wks.
44) Rosacea	45) Seborrheic Keratosis= StucK	46) Actinic Keratosis
Si/Sx- red/erythema facial "FLUSHING." **Telangiectasia** over cheeks, nose, and chin. Flushing precipitated by **heat, emotion,** and/or **hot drinks.** Assoc- **rhinophyma** (sebaceous gland hyperplasia of nose), **ocular keratitis.** Dx- clinical Tx- topical **metronidazole** (1st-line) or topical corticosteroids.	Si/Sx- **waxy brown** papules and plaques, **"STUCK-ON"** appearance. Dx- clinical, histology show benign hyperplasia of **epidermal cells with horn pseudocysts.** Tx- cryotherapy or curettage.	Precursor **SCC in situ.** (squamous cell carcinoma) Cx- sunlight Si/Sx- several lesions that are **thick and "CRUSTED"** on **sun-exposed areas;** arms and face. Mole may grow into a **"HORN shape."** Dx- clinical, biopsy shows **atypia.** Tx- cryosurgery, topical **imiquimod,** or topical 5-FU.

Dermatology

47) Basal-Cell Carcinoma

SKIN cancer (most common type), rarely mets. Cx- UV light, arsenic, **inherited BC nevus syndrome.** Si/Sx- **"FLESHY,"** telangiectatic nodule with **varying** degrees of **pigmentations.** Most common tumor of **"EYELID"** (rarely found on lips).	Dx- **excisional biopsy** with narrow margins; invasive clusters of **"SPINDLE cells"** surrounded by **palisaded basal cells.** **Clinical PEARL: Chalazion** Si/Sx- painful swelling on **eyelid margin** => nodular rubbery lesion. Dx- persistent chalazion requires **biopsy** to r/o basal-cell carcinoma.	Tx- curettage, cryotherapy, excision or **Moh's surgery** (narrow surgical margins, with high cure rate). • <1mm lesion depth: excised with 1cm tumor free margin. • >1mm depth: should have **sentinel lymph node** study.

48) Nevus Sebaceus | 49) Squamous Cell Carcinoma |

48) Nevus Sebaceus	49) Squamous Cell Carcinoma	
Congenital lesion with elements of **skin** and predominantly **sebaceous glands.** Si/Sx- **yellow-orange, raised,** oval plaque on head or neck. Comp- epithelial skin tumors, secondary malignancy, esp **basal cell carcinoma** (BCC). Dx- clinical, diagnosis confirmed by biopsy. Tx- **remove lesion,** can be excised before adolescence.	Arising from **Actinic Keratoses (AK).** Cx- **UV light (sunlight)** is the most important **risk factor,** radiation, chemical carcinogens. Si/Sx- crusting and **ULCERATING lesion** of erythematous plaque. Pt may have non-healing, **ULCER** in vermilion zone of **lower LIP.**	Dx- **biopsy** with graded histology; invasive cords of squamous cells with **keratin PEARLS.** R/O **keratoacanthoma** (benign epithelial tumor, that looks like SCC). Tx- surgical excision, **high metastatic potential**.

Dermatology

50) Types of Melanoma		
• **Lentigo maligna** Si/Sx- sun on **FACE**. • **Superficial spread** (most common >75%) Si/Sx- **primarily FLAT** lesion with **nonuniform** color, **asymmetry**, and nondistinct borders, **trunk** on men, **legs** on women.	• **Nodular** Si/Sx- rapid **vertical** growth. • **Amelanotic** Si/Sx- without pigment • **Acral lentiginous** Si/Sx- **hands/feet**	Most common **life-threatening** skin cancer. Risk factors: Immunosuppression (highest risk factor), **intense sun exposure,** congenital melanocytic nevi, ↑# nevi, **familial atypical mole and melanoma (FAM-M).**
51) Melanoma		
Si/Sx- **irregular** pigment, contour, and borders. Pt reports changes in size, shape, contour, and color. Dx- **ABCDEs** A- **Asymmetric** B- **Border** irregular C- **Color** irregular D- **Diameter** >6mm E- **Evolution** (changing)	Dx Changes in **mole size or shape** is the strongest risk factor for malignancy. Prevention: **Sun avoidance** and wearing protective clothing are the best methods of photo-protection.	Dx **Excisional biopsy, Breslow's** thickness (depth), **Clark's** level (depth). **TNM Stages:** **Stage 0-** melanoma in situ (Clark level I) **Stage I-** primary **Stage II-** local or regional metastasis **Stage III-** distant mets
52) Melanoma	**53) Kaposi's Sarcoma**	
Tx- **excision with margins,** surveillance for relapse. **Clinical PEARL: Metastatic Melanoma** "fascinating disease" Si/Sx- **lie dormant for 15-25yrs** even after primary tumor has been removed. **Spreads to unimaginable** places like the **eye, or brain** causing bleeding.	Cx- **HHV-8** (kaposi's sarcoma herpesvirus; KSHV). Assoc- **HIV/AIDS** Si/Sx- **purple papules and plaques** with multicentric vascular macules.	Dx- clinical, biopsy (confirms); **spindle cells +HHV-8 staining**. Tx- **HAART therapy** improves disease.

Dermatology

54) Myocosis Fungoides		55) Hypersensitivity Reactions- Type I
"NOT a fungus infx." Cx- cutaneous **T-cell lymphoma**. Si/Sx- pruritic, **psoriatic-like plaques. SEZARY'S syndrome**; sezary cells in blood, erythroderma, and lymph.	Dx- clinical, biopsy with histology for chronic disease and shows **Sezary, or Lutzner cells.** Tx- **photopheresis** in most cases. Early stages **topical steroids**, retinoids, or PUVA. Severe cases use **systemic** interferon or retinoids.	• **Type I** "First and Fast" Cx- **anaphylactic, atopic.** Mech- **IgE** cross-links on mast cells and basophils => release histamine.
56) Hypersensitivity Reactions- Type I	**57) Hypersensitivity Reactions- Type II**	**58) Hypersensitivity Reactions- Type III**
Ex- **anaphylaxis, asthma,** urticarial drug reactions, latex allergy. Si/Sx- labored breathing, tachycardia, hypotension, stridor and wheezing. Tx- **IM epinephrine** (1st-line) for anaphylaxis. **Clinical PEARL: Epinephrine** Alpha1 agonist; vasoconstricts=> ↑BP. Beta2 agonist; relax bronchial smooth m.	"Cy-2-toxic" Mech: **IgM and IgG** bind enemy cell => lysis or phyagocytosis. Ex- **autonomic hemolytic anemia,** rheumatic fever, **Goodpasture's** syndrome, **Rh disease** (erythroblastosis fetalis).	"3 antigen-antibody complex" Mech: **Antigen-antibody complexes =>** neutrophils release lysosomal enzymes. Ex- SLE, RA, immune glomerulonephritis, polyarteritis nodosa (PAN), **serum sickness, arthus reaction** (interdermal injection antigen).

Dermatology

59) Hypersensitivity Reactions- Type III		60) Hypersensitivity Reactions- Type IV
• Serum Sickness Cx- penicillin, amoxicillin, cefaclor, and TMP-SMX. Si/Sx- fever, urticaria, arthralgias **two weeks after starting offending agent,** in setting of viral illness.	• Polyarteritis Nodosa (PAN) Si/Sx- arthritis, abd pain, CNS changes, skin nodules/ulcers. **"NO LUNG"** involvement. Dx- **peripheral lesion biopsy.**	4th last delayed Mech: **CELL mediated T lymphocytes** that are sensitized encounter antigen. Ex- TB skin test, **transplant rejection** (GVHD), and contact dermatitis **(poison ivy, poison oak).**

3 CHAPTER
EMERGENCY MEDICINE

EmergencyMed		
1) First Survey of Trauma "ABCDE"		
A- Airway Consider intubation, cricothyroidotomy, and/or C-spine. **Clinical PEARL: Intubation Risk** Risk of intubating into right mainstem bronchus=> leading to ↓ **breath sounds on left side.** Pulling back on endotracheal tube so tip is between carina and vocal cords to solve this problem.	**B- Breathing** Consider airway obstruction, tension pneumothorax, cardiac tamponade, hemothorax, **Pulmonary contusion** (worsened by intravascular volume expansion=> ↓pO2)	**C- Circulation** Put pressure on wounds, start IV, give isotonic fluids **3:1 ratio;** fluid to blood loss. **D- Disability** Check for CNS dysfunction, Glasgow coma scale. **E- Exposure** Disrobe pt and assess injuries and pts temp.
2) Blunt Abdominal Trauma (BAT)		
Cx- MVA, gunshot wound. **RISK of the following:** • **Splenic laceration** Si/Sx- abdominal pain, hypotension, **left shoulder pain** hours after trauma. • **Pulm contusion** Si/Sx-SOB, hypoxia. Dx- CXR shows patchy alveolar infiltrates. • **Aortic contusion** • **Bladder DOME ruputre** Si/Sx-full, distended bladder.	**RISK of the following:** • **Urethral injury** Si/Sx-inability to void, **high riding prostate,** scrotal hematoma, palpable **distended bladder.** Dx- **retrograde urethrogram.** Dx and Tx • **Stable pt- CT scan.** To r/o splenic laceration order abd CT with IV contrast. • **Peritoneal irritation** Rigid, tender abd=> acute abdomen=> **laparotomy.**	Dx and Tx • **Internal bleeding** **"UNSTABLE"** pt=> emergent **U/S scan;** best inital test is **FAST** (focused assessment with sonography for trauma). If FAST is inconclusive order **DPL (diagnostic peritoneal lavage).** Positive findings on **FAST or DPL** require **emergent exploratory laparotomy.**

EmergencyMed		
3) Blunt CHEST Trauma		
• **Bronchial Rupture**	• **Esophageal Rupture**	• **Hemothorax**
Cx-MVA, chest trauma Si/Sx- **persistent pneumothorax** despite chest tube placement and pneumo-mediastinum. Dx- CT, bronchoscopy. Tx- surgery	Cx- following **endoscopy, Boerhaave** syndrome (recurrent retching alone). Si/Sx- SOB, burning substernal chest pain after every meal, and radiating to the back. Dx- CXR shows **pleural effusion, pneumomediastinum,** and/or pneumothorax. Order **water-soluble contrast esophagram.** Tx- **surgery** with primary closure of esophagus and drainage of mediastinum within 6hrs of presentation.	Cx- laceration of lung parenchyma, damage to intercostal artery, or internal mammary artery. Si/Sx-**hypotensive,** tachycardic and **tachypneic after IV fluids** and supplemental O2. Possibly tracheal deviation, ↓breath sounds and dullness to percussion to the side involved. Tx- **needle thoracostomy**.
4) Glasgow Coma Scale (GCS)		
"**4 Eyes** (see), **Jackson-5** (verbal), **V6 Engine** (motor)" **4 EYES open** 4 spontaneously 3 on command 2 open to pain 1 no response	**VERBAL** "Jackson 5" 5 alert, oriented 4 confused 3 inappropriate 2 incomprehensive 1 no response **Glasgow Coma Scale (GCS)-** endotracheal intubation is warranted with **GCS<8.**	**MOTOR** "V6 Engine" 6 follows direction 5 localize pain 4 withdraws to pain **3 decorticate (flexed)** **2 decerebrate (extended)** 1 no response

EmergencyMed

5) Second Survey of Trauma	6) H's & T's cause Cardiac Arrest	
"FAST" Focused Abdominal Sonography Trauma scan to look at: **Morrison's pouch** (kidney and liver), splenorenal recess, **pouch of douglas** (posterior bladder), pericardium. • **CXR**- for ALL thoracic traumas. • **C-spine CT**- in pts with neck pain or neurologic findings.	**H's:** • **Hypovolemia** ($\downarrow$blood vol) • **Hypoxia** ($\downarrow O_2$) • **Hydrogen ions** (acidosis) • **Hyper- or Hypokalemia** • **Hypothermia** ($\downarrow$body temp) • **Hyper- or Hypoglycemia**	**T's:** • **Tension pneumothorax** • **Thrombosis** (MI) • **Thromboembolism** (PE) • **Tamponade** • **Tablets/Toxins** • **Trauma** (Pulseless Electrical Activity, **PEA**) Tx- in cardiac arrest and/or PEA start **immediate CPR** with chest compressions, followed by **Asynchronous cardioversion**.

Quick Quiz:
• Pt has neck pain and neurologic findings, what is next best step?

• Pt was in a MVA and now has pulseless electrical activity. What is next best step?

• What are the H's and T's that can cause cardiac arrest?

EmergencyMed

7) Drug Overdose and Tx		
• **Acetaminophen** (obtain levels at 4hrs) Dx- ↑**AST**, ↑**ALT**, hepatocellular pattern of injury. Tx- **N-acetylcysteine** (adm within 8hrs).	• **Carbon Monoxide** Dx-carboxyhemoglobin Tx- **O₂**	• **Heparin** Tx- **protamine sulfate**
	• **IRON salts** Si/Sx- colicky abd pain, GI bleeding. Ex- child sees **iron pills as candy**. Tx- **deferoxamine** (binds ferric iron=> urinary excretion)	• **Lead** Tx- **penicillamine**
• **Beta-blockers** Tx- atropine, IV fluids, **glucagon** (↑contractility).		• **Opioids** Tx- **naloxone,** for long term addiction can give **methadone**.
• **Barbiturates** Tx- supportive care, charcoal, urine alkalinization, if needed dialysis.	• **Methanol** AE: **vision loss,** optic disc hyperemia. Tx- **fomepizole,** Ca gluconate, EtOH.	• **Salicylates** Tx- charcoal, urine alkalinization.
• **Benzodiazepines** Tx- **flumazenil**	**Ethylene glycol** AE: kidney damage; **envelope-shaped** calcium **oxalate crystals.** Tx- **fomepizole,** Ca gluconate, EtOH.	• **Warfarin** Tx- **Vit K, FFP.**
• **Methemoglobin** Tx- methylene blue		• **Alcohol** Tx- **benzodiazepines, thiamine,** folate, and multivitamin.
		• **Digitalis** Tx- anti-digitalis Fab.

8) Drug Overdose Tx	9) Drug-induced SLE	10) Inhibition of P-450
• **Narcan (Naloxone)** Tx- **Opiates overdose** of heroin or morphine. Si/Sx- pts with life threatening overdose causing **CNS and/or respiratory depression.**	• **Procainamide** • **Hydralazine** • **Isoniazid (INH)** • **Penicillamine** • **Chlorpromazine** • **Methyldopa** • **Quinidine**	These drugs will **inhibit P-450 and** ↑**drug level in body** of other drugs. • **Cimetidine** • **Ketoconazole** • **INH** • **Grapefruit** • **Erythromycin** • **Sulfonamides**

Quick Quiz:

• Pt is homeless and a known alcoholic. A U/A is done and is found to have oxalate crystals in urine. What is the next best step?

EmergencyMed

11) Aspects of PAIN	12) Acute Appendicitis	
"OPQRST" O- Onset P- Precipitating Q- Quality R- Radiating S- Symptoms T- **Temporal** course/ treatment	Si/Sx- abd pain, fever, and nausea/vomiting. Initial pain is **peri-umbilical** (**visceral,** referred)=> becomes **RLQ pain** (somatic). • **McBurney's point** 1/3 from iliac spine to umbilicus. • **Psoas sign** Passive extension of hip causes RLQ pain. • **Obturator sign** Internal rotation flexed hip RLQ pain.	• **Rovsing's sign** Deep palpation LLQ lead RLQ pain. Dx- clinical Tx- **appendectomy.** Comp: • **Perforation** (within 72hrs of symp onset) Tx-emergent laparotomy. • **Pelvic abscess** Si/Sx- RLQ pain for **>5days.** Pts may have perforation with abscess formation. Tx- IV hydration, abxs, bowel rest, and appendectomy.
13) RULE of 9's for %BSA		**14) Thermal Inhalation Injury**
9% head 9% arms (each) 18% chest 18% back 18% legs (each) 1% perineum **PARKLAND formula First 24hrs = (4) x (pt's weight in kg) x (% BSA)** Give 50% fluid in **first 8 hrs**; second half in following **16 hrs.**	Comp: • **Marjolin's Ulcer;** Squamous-cell carcinoma (SCC). Si/Sx- **ulcer** arising within **burn wounds.** Dx- biopsy all chronic wounds that are failing to heal to r/o malignancy. • **Circumferential Eschar** Tx- **escharotomy** • **Hypovolemic Shock** (leading to sepsis and septic shock). Cx- burn wound **infxs** or pulm **infxs.**	**Carbon monoxide** (CO) poisoning ($\downarrow$oxygen delivery to the tissue). Cx- smoke inhalation, automobile exhaust. Si/Sx- HA, nausea, dizziness, AMS, dyspnea. Pt may have a hx of being in a **burning building.** Dx- **>10% Carboxyhemoglobin,** polycythemia ($\uparrow$RBCs), anion gap **metabolic acidosis** ($\uparrow$lactic acid from anaerobic metabolism). Tx-100% O2 facemask, early **intubation.**

EmergencyMed		
15) Vitamin Deficiency		
• **Vit A deficiency** Si/Sx- **NIGHT BLINDNESS,** photophobia, **DRY SKIN,** xerosis conjunctiva, xerosis cornea, **bitot spots** (dry-gray plaques on bulbar conjunctiva).	• **Vit B1 deficiency (thiamine)** Si/Sx- **Beriberi;** polyneuritis, dilated cardio, CHF, edema. **Wernicke-Korsakoff syndrome** (confusion, ataxia).	• **Vit B2 deficiency (riboflavin)** Si/Sx- **angular stomatitis** (inflam mouth), **cheilosis** (lesion mouth), corneal vascularization.
16) Vitamin Deficiency		
• **Vit B3 deficiency (niacin)** Si/Sx- **Pellagra 3Ds:** Diarrhea Dermatitis Dementia	• **Vit B5 deficiency (pantothenate)** Si/Sx- dermatitis, enteritis (inflam intestines), **alopecia** (hair loss), adrenal insufficiency.	• **Vit B6 deficiency (pyridoxine)** Si/Sx- seborrheic dermatitis, **glossitis,** angular cheilitis, **peripheral neuropathy,** confusion, seizures, sideroblastic anemia.
17) Vitamin Deficiency		
• **Vit B12 deficiency** (cobalamin) Cx- **pernicious anemia** (most common) Si/Sx- macrocytic, megaloblastic anemia, **neurologic symps, glossitis.**	• **Folic acid deficiency** Assoc- **tea, toast, and canned food diet.** Si/Sx- macrocytic, megaloblastic anemia, **NO neurologic symps.** (most common vit def in the United States).	• **Vit C deficiency** (ascorbic acid) Si/Sx- **Scurvy; swollen gums,** bruising, anemia, poor wound healing.

EmergencyMed

18) Vitamin Deficiency		
• **Vit D deficiency** (↓bone mineralization) **Rickets** (child) Si/Sx- **craniotabes** (soft skull), **rachitis rosary** (costochondral joints knobs), **harrison groove** (groove along lower thorax), **thicken ends of long bones.** **Osteomalacia** (adults) Si/Sx- hypocalcemic, **TETANY.** Dx- ↓**Ca,** ↓**Ph,** ↑PTH.	• **Vit K deficiency** Dx- ↑**PT,** ↑**PTT,** with normal BT. All newborn babies should receive Vit K injection to prevent **hemorrhagic disease of newborn** (↑risk if born at home).	• **Zinc deficiency** Cx- **chronic TPN.** Si/Sx- alopecia, pustulous skin lesions around body orifices, impaired wound healing, **"abnormal TASTE"** (food does not taste normal).

19) Vitamin Deficiency		
• **Vit E deficiency** Increased **fragility** of RBCs. • **Biotin deficiency** Cx- ingest **RAW eggs.** Si/Sx- dermatitis, enteritis.	• **Magnesium deficiency** Si/Sx- weakness, muscle cramps, CNS hyperirritability, exacerbation of hypocalcemic tetany.	• **Selenium deficiency** Keshan disease (cardiomyopathy)

20) Postoperative FEVER 6 W		
• **WIND**: Atelectasis; **Resp alkalosis** from hyperventilating; ↑**pH,** ↓**Pco2,** ↓**PO2,** hypoxemia. Prevent; **incentive spirometry.** (postop day 1-2) • **WATER:** UTI (postop day 3-5)	• **WALKING**: DVT (postop day 4-6) • **WOUNDS**: abscess, infection (pain in wound, cloudy-gray discharge). Tx- urgent **surgical exploration.** (postop day 5-7)	• **WONDER drug**: drugs (postop day 7+) • **WOMB**: ob/gyn

EmergencyMed		
21) Types of SHOCK		
• **Cardiogenic shock** Cx- CHF, MI, MVA (myocardial contusion) ↓CO ↑**PCWP** ↑**PVR** • **Obstructive shock** Cx- PE, cardiac tamponade, tension pneumothorax ↓CO ↑**PCWP** ↑**PVR**	• **Septic shock** (distributive shock) Cx- bacteremia (esp gram neg) ↑**CO** ↓PCWP ↓PVR, **normal MVo2** (mixed venous O2 conc). • **Anaphylactic shock** (distributive shock) Cx- **bee stings,** food allergies, medications. Tx-IM epinephrine. ↑**CO** ↓PCWP ↓PVR • **Distributive Shock** Cx-sepsis, anaphylaxis, burns, CNS injury, drug reactions. ↑**CO** ↓PCWP ↓PVR	• **Hypovolemic shock** First sign- ↑pulse rate. Cx- ↓volume; burns, ↓blood, dehydration. Trauma- thorax, abdomen, pelvis, or femurs have potential to accumulate enough blood => to lead to **hypovolemic shock.** ↓CO ↓PCWP ↑**PVR**
22) Hyperthermia >104 (40C)		**23) Gynecomastia**
• **Malignant Hyperthermia** Cx- halothane, **succinylcholine.** Tx- **dantrolene.** **Clinical PEARL: Atracurium** Safe in pts with renal and liver disease. It is a neuromuscular blocking agent that is **metabolized in plasma** and hydrolyzed by serum esterases.	• **Neuroleptic Malignant Syndrome** Cx- antipsychotic (**haloperidol**). Si/Sx- hyperthermia, **muscle RIGIDITY,** autonomic instability, and AMS. Tx- **dantrolene** (muscle relaxant). Can also use **bromocriptine** (dopamine agonist), **amantadine** (antiviral with dopaminergic properties).	"Some Excellent Drugs Create Awesome Knockers." **S- Spironolactone** **E- Estrogens** **D- Digitalis** **C- Cimetidine** **A- Alcohol use** **K- Ketoconazole**

4 CHAPTER
ENDOCRINOLOGY

Endocrinology		
1) Diabetes Insipidus (DI)		
ADH dysfunction => failure to concentrate the urine. • **Central DI** Failure to secrete ADH. Cx- **Sheehan's/** ischemia, cerebral injury, infection. • **Nephrogenic DI** Kidneys failures to respond to ADH. Cx- **lithium,** renal dz, demeclocycline. Si/Sx- persistent thirst, polydipsia, polyuria, with **DILUTED urine.**	Si/Sx- pt may have dehydration with hypernatremia. Dx- Urine osmolality **<300mOsm/L.** **Water deprivation test**; pt continues to have high volume of **dilute urine** (this is the first test that should be done). **Desmopressin/ DDAVP stim test** (ADH analog): • **Central DI** ↓ urine output • **Nephrogenic DI** ↑ urine output (continues to be high)	Tx **Central DI**: intranasal **desmopressin** acetate (DDAVP). **Nephrogenic DI**: **restriction** of salt and water intake. If pt has **dehydration** fluid loss and ↑plasma osm give **IV infusion of normal saline** (IV crystalloid; 0.9% NaCl).

Endocrinology

2) SIADH

Syndrome of inappropriate antidiuretic hormone hypersecretion. Assoc: • **CNS disease**; head injury, tumor. • **Pulm disease**; sarcoid, pneumonia, **SCLC**. • **Drugs**; antipsychotics and antidepressants.	Si/Sx- edema, HTN, irritability, confusion, seizures, AMS from over stimulated ADH release=> **euvolemic hyponatremia**. Dx- ↓urine output, **↓serum osmolarity** (serum hyposmolarity), **↑urine osmolarity, urinary Na>20mEq/L**. Dx SIADH: • **↓Serum Osm** • **↑Urine Osm** • **↑Urine Na conc** Failure to correct with normal saline infusion.	**Tx- fluid restriction** (1st-line), **demeclocycline** (antagonizing ADH), **tolvaptan** (vasopressin agonist). **Clinical PEARL:** **Primary Polydipsia** (problem with excessive water ingestion) Dx- **hyponatremia** and maximally **dilute urine**. Confirm diagnosis by withholding water=> **↑urine osmolality**.

3) Adrenal Insufficiency

Primary Cx:	**Secondary** Cx:	Dx- "Salt wasting," hyponatremia, hyperkalemia. **Plasma ↓CORTISOL levels** (confirm, low <20 during high stress).
• **Addison's disease** (**adrenal** cortical destruction; ↑ACTH, **hyperpigmentation** of skin, non anion gap metabolic acidosis, ↑K, ↓Na). • **Autoimmune destruction**; type I DM, vitiligo, pernicious anemia, hypothyroidism, premature ovarian failure. • **Adrenal tuberculosis** (calcification on both adrenal glands).	• **Pituitary tumor** ↓ACTH production • **Glucocorticoids use** ↓ACTH production (Pts may have postoperative nausea, hypoglycemia, abd pain, hypotension). Si/Sx- weakness, fatigue, **hypotension,** anorexia, GI upset, **hyperpigmentation** (↑ACTH, Addison's). No hyperpigmentation think of pituitary tumor (↓ACTH) => ↓adrenal atrophy.	**Cosyntropin (ACTH) stimulation test-** after giving ACTH if **cortisol >20** this R/O adrenal insufficiency. Tx- **glucocorticoid w/ mineralocorticoids (fludrocorisone).** Pts on steroids ↑**dose** during major surgery, infxs, or trauma. **Tx Adrenal CRISIS** • **S- Salt** (0.9% saline) • **S- Steroids** (IV hydrocortisone) • **S- Support**

Endocrinology

4) Acromegaly (Gigantism in child)		
Benign **pituitary growth hormone (GH) adenoma.** Si/Sx- large **jaw, hands, feet, coarsening facial,** HTN, arthritis, carpal tunnel, bitemporal hemianopia, **diabetes** (glucose intolerance). Comp- CAD, cardiomyopathy, arrhythmias, LVH.	Dx- ↑ **IGF-1 level.** Confirm with **oral glucose suppression test**=> ↑ **GH remain high** (when glucose should suppress GH). **MRI** of pituitary shows sellar lesion. Tx- **Transsphenoidal surgical resection (1st-line), octreotide** (suppress GH), pegvisomant (blocks GH receptors).	**Clinical PEARL: Craniopharyngioma** Benign tumor, arising from Rathke's pouch. Si/Sx-HA, **bitemporal hemianopsia, hypo**pituitarism. Dx-CT or MRI shows **calcified** lesions **ABOVE sella turcica,** and **multiple cysts.** Tx- surgery and/or radiotherapy.
5) Hyper- prolactinemia		
Cx- **prolactinoma** (lactotroph adenoma), craniopharyngioma, cirrhosis. Si/Sx- amenorrhea, **galctorrhea, gynecomastia,** bitemporal hemianopia, **infertility,** hypogonadism, oligomenorrhea.	Dx- serum **PROLACTIN level >200** mg/mL. Overproduction of ↑ **prolactin** => androgen deficiency => ↓energy, ↓libido, ↓axillary, ↓pubic hair, and amenorrhea.	Tx-↑**dopamine agonist (1ˢᵗ line); cabergoline, bromocriptine.** Surgery considered for pregnancy or visual defects.

Endocrinology

6) Pheochromocytoma		
Tumor of **chromaffin** tissue of **adrenal medulla**=> **↑catecholamines**. Assoc- **MEN2,** Neurofibromatosis, Von Hippel-Lindau.	Si/Sx: **5P's**: • Palpitations • Perspiration • Pressure (BP) • Pain (headache) • Pallor Dx- CT or MRI may show **suprarenal mass,** plasma or 24hr urine **↑metanephrines. MIBG scan** can also be used.	Tx- **surgical resection, preOp use alpha-block** for BP, followed by **beta-blocker** for tachycardia. This is to avoid rapid ↑BP with beta blockers alone.
7) Hyper-aldosteronism		
↑↑Aldosterone from **zona glomerulosa** of the adrenal cortex. Cx- **adrenocortical hyperplasia** (70%), adrenal adenoma **(Conn's syndrome).** Si/Sx- **HTN, HA, polyuria,** muscle weakness, paresthesias, peripheral edema.	Dx- diastolic HTN, **NO edema. Mild hypernatremia,** hypokalemia, ↓H+. **↑Aldosterone/↓Renin ratio** (most specific for diagnosis), **↑bicarbonate** (metabolic alkalosis due to ↓H+). CT or MRI show **adrenal mass.**	Tx- **adrenalectomy** for adrenal tumor. For bilateral hyperplasia give **spironolactone** (aldosterone antagonist). **Clinical PEARL: Bartter/Gitelman** Syndrome Dx- **normal BP, normal serum Na, ↑Renin, ↑Aldosterone,** ↓K+, ↑bicarbonate, metabolic alkalosis, **↑urine Cl.**

Endocrinology

8) CAH

Congenital Adrenal Hyperplasia (AR) Cx- **21-hydroxylase** deficiency=> ↑ **17-OH progesterone** ↓ **cortisol** => ↑ACTH => ↑adrenal androgens. Si/Sx- **hypotension** **"salt wasting,"** severe cystic acne.	Si/Sx • Females- **ambiguous genitalia, virilization.** • Males- significant **growth acceleration,** macrogenitosomia. Dx-↑ **17-OH progesterone** and **androgens** in blood and urine.	Tx- **fluid** and **salt repletion,** administer **cortisol** => ↓ACTH and androgens. **Surgical** for ambiguous genitalia. • **21- hydroxylase def (AR)- HYPOtension** • 11-hydroxylase and 17-hydroxylase def **HYPERtension**

9) Type I Diabetes Mellitus	10) Types of Insulin	11) Type 2 Diabetes Mellitus
Autoimmune pancreatic **beta-cell destruction**=> insulin deficiency. Si/Sx- polyuria, polydipsia, polyphagia, **ketoacidosis.** Assoc- **HLA–DR3, HLA–DR4.** Dx- **fasting glucose >126, random >200** + symp, postprandial >200. Screen for microalbumin with urine **microalbumin/Cr ratio** (30-300 mg/24hr). Ophthalmologic screen for retinopathy (yrly). Tx- **insulin (goal blood glucose range; 80-120),** HbA1c <8.	• **Regular** duration 5–8hrs • **Humalog** (lispro) duration 6–8hrs • **NovoLog** (aspart) duration 3–5hrs • **Apidra** (glulisine) duration 1–2.5hrs • **NPH 18–28hrs** • **Levemir** (detemir) duration 20hrs • **Lantus (glargine)** duration 1–4hrs	"Insulin resistance" Assoc- **FH,** obesity. Si/Sx- polyuria, polydipsia, polyphagia, **CHARCOT joint** (neuropathic arthropathy), gastroparesis, **nonketotic hyperglycemia.** Dx- same DMI. Tx- **lifestyle modifications;** diet, weight loss, exercise. **Oral agents,** insulin, **statins** (LDL<100), **ACEIs; BP<130/80** (lowers nephropathy and retinopathy), **ASA** (antiplatelet).

Endocrinology

12) Diabetic Neuropathy	13) Neurogenic Arthropathy	14) Diabetic Retinopathy
Si/Sx- **"stocking glove"** sensory loss. Symmetric distal polyneuropathy and can have mononeuropathies. Pts can also get **foot ulcers** due to peripheral neuropathy. Dx-clinical Tx-tight glycemic control, **amitriptyline** (TCAs), **gabapentin** or pregabalin. Foot ulcers need debridement of necrotic tissue.	Also called, **"Charcot's joints."** Si/Sx- **PAIN** in **weight bearing** joints, **ulcers on SOLE of foot.** Dx- XR shows **osteophytes,** extrarticular bone fragments.	Sorbital (sugar alcohol) accumulating in lens. Si/Sx- blurred vision, trouble reading or driving. Dx- **funduscopic** exam shows **cotton wool spots, "FLAME" hemorrhages,** and dot-blot hemorrhages. Tx- argon laser **photocoagulation.**
15) Diabetic Retinopathy	**16) Gastroparesis**	**17) Dawn and Somogyi Effect**
Clinical PEARL: Vitreous Hemorrhage Si/Sx- sudden **loss of vision** and **new onset of "FLOATERS."** Assoc- **diabetic retinopathy.** Dx- immediate ophthalmologic consultation.	Delayed gastric emptying. Si/Sx- **early satiety,** chronic nausea, heartburn, abd pain, **bloating.** Dx- **manometry.** Tx- smaller meals, dopamine antagonist; **metoclopramide (1st-line),** domperidone. Can also use bethanechol or **erythromycin.**	• **Dawn Phenomenon** Si/Sx- morning hyperglycemia. Tx-↑**INSULIN closer to bedtime.** • **Somogyi Effect** Nocturnal **hypoglycemia** => **counter hormones** (epinephrine, norepinephrine, and glucagon release) => hyperglycemia in morning. Tx-↓**INSULIN closer to bedtime.**

Endocrinology

18) HONKS

Hyperosmolar Non-Ketotic Symdrome (HONKS) Assoc- recent URI, any physiologic stressor. Si/Sx- DM2 with **profound dehydration,** blurred vision, AMS, coma.	Dx ↑**GLUCOSE >600,** low/**no ketones, hyperosmolarity.** Tx- **normal saline.** Pt may require **8-10 liters** to reach euvolemic state.	Tx When serum **K<5.3mEq/L** replacement with IV **potassium chloride.**

19) Diabetic Ketoacidosis (DKA)

• **Diabetic ketoacidosis (DKA)-** hyperglycemia crisis in DMI. Assoc- infx, MI, trauma. Si/Sx- polyuria, abd pain, vomiting, **kussmaul breathing** (deep and labored breathing) and **"FRUITY" acetone breath,** AMS, metabolic acidosis.	Dx ↑**ANION GAP** (used to evaluate recovery). Hyperglycemia, **ketonemia,** osmotic diuresis, hyperkalemia (acidemia; H+ into cells and removing K+ from inside the cells).	Tx **IV normal saline** (IV crystalloid; 0.9% NaCl), **regular insulin.** Early **potassium supplementation,** possibly before giving insulin if already low. Insulin and IV fluids lead to rapid ↓serum potassium levels even if initially elevated.

20) DM2 Oral Agents

• **Sulfonylureas:** Glipizide, glyburide, and glimepiride. AE-**hypoglycemia,** weight gain. • **Meglitinides:** Repaglinide and nateglinide.	• **Metformin** (1st-line) inhibit gluconeogenesis. AE- **lactic acidosis** (rare), weight gain. • **Thiazolidinediones:** Glitazones. ↑Insulin sensitivity. AE-weight gain, edema, hepatotoxicity.	• **Alpha-glucosidase Inhibitor-**↓absorption. AE-flatulence • **DDP-4 inhibitor:** Sitagliptin. Inhibits degradation glucagon-like peptide-1.

Endocrinology

21) Metabolic Syndrome		
Comb of medical disorders that ↑risk of developing CVD and diabetes. Si/Sx- abd obesity, ↑BP, impaired glycemic control, dyslipidemia. Assoc-**NASH** (non-alcoholic steatohepatitis).	Dx- **3 out of 5:** • **Abd obesity** >40 inch • **Trig** >150mg/dL • **HDL** <40mg/dL • **BP** >130/85 mmHg • **Fasting glucose** >100mg/dL Tx- weight loss, **BP control, metformin, ↓cholesterol.**	**Clinical PEARL: Non-Alcoholic Steatohepatitis (NASH)** Dx- liver biopsy shows **steatosis.** Risk factors- obesity, DM, hyperlipidemia, corticosteroids.

22) Hyperthyroidism		
Cx- **Graves' disease,** toxic multinodular gotier, toxic adenoma, postviral thyroiditis. Si/Sx- palpitations, nervousness, fine tremor, ↓weight, ↑heat, ↑bowel, tachycardia or atrial-fib, **lid lag.** Graves' disease; **Exophthalmos** (periorbital lymphocytic infiltration) and **pretibial myxedema.** Comp- atrial fibrillation, rapid bone loss (↑osteo**clastic** activity in bone cells).	Dx- **↓TSH, ↑T4, ↑T3.** • **↑Uptake of RAIU** and **+ TSH receptor antibodies** (Grave's disease). • **↓Uptake of RAIU** (subacute thyroiditis). Tx- **radioactive 131I thyroid ablation.** Pts should be pretreated with **antithyroid** med to avoid exacerbations of thyrotoxic state.	Tx Radioiodine therapy AE: Hypothyroidism Antithyroid meds; **propylthiouracil** (PTU, safe in preg), **methimazole** (MMI). **Propranolol** for pts with acute symps and pts with a-fib. **Propylthiouracil** and **Methimazole** AE: **agranulocytosis,** so routine WBC count should be taken in pts taking antithyroid meds.

Endocrinology

23) Hypothyroidism

Cx- **Hashimoto's thyroiditis,** iatrogenic, iodine def, hypothyroid phase thyroiditis. Si/Sx **Cold intolerance, constipation,** dry/cold skin, hoarseness, **depression, memory changes,** bradycardia, **delayed relax of DTRs.** **Proximal muscle weakness** (hard time holding hand over head and trying to lower self into chair).	Si/Sx **Hyper-prolactinemia** as well (due to ↑**TRH** feedback to ↑TSH will also increase prolactin levels). In severe cases pts may become **paranoid** and have **hallucinations,** referred to as **"Myxedema Madness."** Risk- **thyroid lymphoma** in pts with Hashimoto's thyroiditis.	Dx-↑**TSH,** ↓T4, ↓T3. Elevation of **serum CK levels.** Hashimoto's dz has **anti-thyroid peroxidase (anti-TPO)** and **anti-thyroglobulin** antibodies. Tx- **levothyroxine.** If myxedema coma: IV levothyroxine, hydrocortisone. **Clinical PEARL: Sick Euthyroid Syndrome** Seen in pts with severe illness. Dx- **normal TSH, normal T4,** ↓**T3.**

24) Thyroiditis (Inflam Thyroid)   25) Papillary Thyroid Neoplasm

24) Thyroiditis (Inflam Thyroid)		25) Papillary Thyroid Neoplasm
Si/Sx- **subacute form** with **"TENDER"** thyroid. Dx-↓**uptake of RAIU.** Tx- **beta-blockers** for hyperthyroidism and **levothyroxine** for hypothyroidism.	**Subacute thyroiditis** is self-limited. Tx- **NSAIDs** (naproxen) **or corticosteroid.** **Clinical PEARL: NSAIDs** Inhib COX=> ↑leukotrienes, ↓prostacyclins, ↓prostaglandins, causes bronchoconstriction.	"**Most Po**pular thyroid neoplasm is **Papillary**" **P- Papillae** (branching) **P- Palpable** lymph nodes. **P- Pupil** nucei; Orphan Annie nuclei. **P- Psammoma** bodies with lesion (often). **P- Positive** prognosis

Endocrinology

26) Thyroid Neoplasms		27) Types of Thyroid Carcinoma
Si/Sx- asymp, +FH, **nodule, hoarseness,** anterior cervical lymph node may be **firm and fixed.** Assoc- **MEN2** with Medullary thyroid CA. Dx- **FNA, TFTs** (TSH to r/o hyperfunctioning gland), **U/S scan** (solid or cystic). **HOT nodule NEVER cancer=> no biopsy.**	Dx Genetic testing: **+RET proto-oncogene** mutation is diagnostic for **MENII** (medullary thyroid cancer). Tx Benign- **levothyroxine.** Malignant- **surgical resection** (1st line). **Clinical PEARL:** Most common benign thyroid nodule are **benign COLLOID nodules.**	• **Papillary** (75–80%) (most common) Slow growing, 90% survive 10yrs. • **Follicular** (20%) 90% survive 10yrs. Invasion of **tumor capsule and blood vessels,** early mets. Tx- **total thyroidectomy +** postoperative radioactive iodine (for **hematogenous** mets).

28) Types of Thyroid Carcinoma	29) MEN	
• **Medullary** (6%) Dx- **Calcitonin** producing **C-cells,** Check **calcitonin** levels (assoc **MEN2**). 80% survive 10yrs. • **Anaplastic** (<2%) Rapidly enlarges and metastasizes, only 10% >3yrs.	Multiple Endocrine Neoplasia (MEN) **MENI** (Wermer's) **"3P"** **P- Pancreas** (Zollinger-Ellison, VIPomas, insulinoma). **P- Pituitary** adenomas **P- Parathyroid**	**MEN2A** (Sipple's) **"2P"** **M- Medullary** thyroid cancer (↑calcitonin) **P-Pheochromocytoma** **P- Parathyroid** **MEN2B** **"1P"** **M- Medullary** thyroid cancer (↑calcitonin) **P-Pheochromocytoma** **M- Mucosal** neuromas **M- Marfanoid** habitus

Endocrinology

30) Osteoporosis (↓Bone Mass)		31) Paget's Disease
Bone mineral density (BMD) < 2.5 SDs from normal. Assoc- postmenopausal women, thin, caucasian. Risk factors: ↓estrogen, smoking, steroids, alcohol, caffeine. Si/Sx- asymp, hip, vertebral, and/or radius fractures. Comp- compression fractures.	Dx- DEXA; BMD <2.5 SDs from normal (gold standard). Screen all women >65yo. Tx • Ca and Vit D, weight-exercises. • Bisphosphonates (zoledronic acid, alendronate). • Raloxifene (agonist to bone, antagonist to breast and vaginal tissue, risk thromboembolism).	Osteitis Deformans; ↑rate bone turnover (osteoclastic bone resorption, bone remodeling)=> "MOSAIC" lamellar bone pattern. Most commonly locations are the femur, axial skeleton and skull. Assoc- viral infx, hyperparathyroidism.
32) Paget's Disease		
Si/Sx- HA, bone pain, joint pain, ↑hat size (skull deformities), "HEARING LOSS" (vestibulocochlear nerve compression) and femoral bowing. Comp- fractures, osteosarcoma. Dx- radionuclide bone scan (most sensitive test). Dx- Normal Ca, Ph, ↑Alkaline Phosphatase, urinary ↑Hydroxyproline.	Tx- there is no cure. Majority of pts are asymp and require no treatment. Pts that have symps can give: • Bisphosphonates (alendronate, risedronate, ibandronate, zoledronic acid) and calcitonin to slow bone resorption. • NSAIDs (naproxen AE: interstitial nephritis) and acetaminophen are used for arthritis.	Clinical PEARL: Drug-induced Interstitial Nephritis (papillary necrosis, interstitial nephritis) Si/Sx- painless hematuria. Cx- Drugs; • Cephalosporins • Penicillins • Sulfonamides • NSAIDs • Rifampin • Phenytoin • Allopurinol

Endocrinology

33) Hyperparathyroidism

Cx		Tx
• Primary- **adenoma**. • Secondary- **chronic kidney disease**. Si/Sx- asymp, HTN, nephrolithiasis, bone pain, fatigue, depression. **"Stones, bones, psychiatric overtones."** Risk- pseudogout, HTN. Dx- ↑**PTH**, ↑ **Ca**, ↓**Ph**. **Sestamibi scan**; highly sensitive to localize adenoma. Lithium and thiazides can exacerbate hyperparathyroidism.	• **STONES** (nephrolithiasis) • **BONES (bone pain,** nausea, vomiting, PUD, pancreatitis). • **PSYCHIATRIC Overtones** (fatigue, **depression,** anxiety, sleep disturbances). Comp- nausea, vomiting, bone disease, abd pain, AMS, coma.	**Parathyroidectomy** if one of the following: • <50yrs • Pt has symps • ↓Bone mass • Renal insufficient • ↑Ca or • Urine Ca >400 24hrs Tx- hypercalcemia=> give **FLUIDS, loop diuretics**, bisphosphonate, calcitonin. ↓Ph diet and use Ph binders, **Cinacalcet** (↓PTH, ↓Ca, ↓Ph).

34) Cushing's Syndrome

Cx	Si/Sx	Dx
• **Pituitary adenoma (Cushing's disease)**. • **Ectopic ACTH**; SCLC, carcinoid tumor. • **Adrenal** hyperplasia (secretion of **cortisol**). • **Iatrogenic** of **corticosteroids** (most common). Si/Sx- HTN, fatigue, **acne,** easy bruising, cataracts, androgen excess, **menstrual irregularities,** central **obesity, diabetes.**	Si/Sx- Pt may have classic **purple striae, hirsutism,** moon face, buffalo hump. Other symps are **depression,** infxs, osteoporosis, **proximal muscle weakness**. Dx Labs: ↑**CORTISOL**, ↓K+, ↑Na+, ↑Glu. **Dexamethasone Suppression Test** overnight: • If **LOW dose**=> ↓cortisol => normal. • If **HIGH dose**=> ↓cortisol => pituitary adenoma (Cushing's disease).	• **If Cortisol remains HIGH, abnormal** (ectopic ACTH, corticosteroids). Tx- **surgical resection** (pituitary adenoma), with hormone replacements. Can also use **ketoconazole, aminoglutethimide** (block adrenal steroidogenesis) may be useful.

5 CHAPTER
EPIDEMIOLOGY

Epidemiology

1) Prevalence vs Incidence	2) Sensitivity and Specificity	
• **Prevalence** (**cross-sectional study**) # of cases of disease in population at **one time**. • **Incidence** (**cohort study**) # **NEW** cases of disease in population **over time**. • **Prevalence** = (**incidence**) x (**time**)	• **Sensitivity** Probability pt **WITH disease** will have a + **test**. "**Screening Test**" Sensitivity= FN – 1 • **Specificity** (**SpIN rule IN**) Probability that pts **WITHOUT disease** will have **NEG test**. "**Confirm**" Specificity= FP- 1 ↑specificity=> ↑PPV ↑sensitivity=> ↑NPV	<table><tr><td></td><td>+ Dz</td><td>- Dz</td></tr><tr><td>+ Test</td><td>a TP</td><td>b FP</td></tr><tr><td>- Test</td><td>c FN</td><td>d TN</td></tr></table> Sensitivity = a/(a+c) Specificity = d/(b+d) PPV = a/(a+b) NPV = d/(c+d)
3) PPV and NPV		**4) Cohort Study** (Relative Risk)
• **Positive Predictive Value (PPV):** Pts with **positive test truly have disease.** ↑PPV with ↑prevalence, and ↓PPV with ↓prevalence (inverse is true with NPV).	• **Negative Predictive Value (NPV):** Pt with **NEG test** truly do **NOT have disease.** If pt has high probability of having disease=> ↓NPV. Low probability of having disease =>↑NPV.	**Cohort = longitudinal or incidence studies.** Best for determining **incidence**. **EXPOSED or UN-Exposed** group of people in which none have disease, but all could get disease. "**Prospective.**"

Epidemiology

5) Case-Control Studies (Odds Ratio)	6) Cross-Sectional Study	7) Other Studies
Two groups: disease (cases) vs non-disease (controls). " Back In Time" Measure possible RISK factors in both groups. Ex- smoking intake in lung cancer and w/o lung cancer. Matching is used in case-control studies to control confounding.	"SNAPSHOT study design" Exposure and outcome are measured simultaneously at a particular "point of time." Also known as a prevalence study.	• Two-Sample T Test Compare the means of TWO groups. • Chi-Square Test Categorical data and proportions. May use a 2x2 table to compare data. • ANOVA (analysis of variance) compare three or more means.

8) Other Studies	9) N-Null Hypothesis	10) Absolute Risk (AR)
• Meta-Analysis Pooling data from several studies for large statistical power. • Cross-Over Study One group with one tx for period of time and other group alternate tx. Two groups then switch tx for another period of time. • Factorial Design Study- randomized different interventions with two or more variables.	• N-Null Hypothesis N-NO relationship (no association) between exposure and the outcome ('p' value >0.05). • Null Hypothesis R-Rejected Means that there is a R-Relationship between exposure and outcome. If 'p' value is<0.05, the null hypothesis is rejected and there is a relationship.	• Absolute Risk (AR) Incidence of disease. • Absolute Risk Reduction (ARR) ARR= # of incidence with one tx minus # of incidence with other tx. • Number Needed to Treat (NNT) NNT= 1/ARR

Epidemiology

11) Relative Risk (RR)	12) Odds Ratio	13) Relative Risk vs Odds Ratio
How much more likely exposed to unexposed. **Relative Risk** = (disease **exposed**) **divided** (disease **UN-exposed**) Ex- RR = injuries involved knife **divided by** injuries with no knife. **Attributable Risk Percent (ARP)** **ARP**= (risk exposed **minus** risk unexposed) **divided** (risk exposed). **ARP=(RR-1)/RR**	Estimate relative risk in **Case-Control Studies** (retrospective study). **Odds Ratio**= (**disease** exposed) **divided** (**non-disease** exposed) ↓ **Disease incidence** (a rare disease) the more closely **odds ratio (OR)** approximates **relative risk (RR).**	<table><tr><td></td><td>**Dz**</td><td>**No Dz**</td></tr><tr><td>**Expo**</td><td>a</td><td>b</td></tr><tr><td>**No Expo**</td><td>c</td><td>d</td></tr></table> **RR =** **[a/(a+b)]/[c/(c+d)].** **RR**= (dz exposed) **divided** by (dz **un**exposed) **OR = ad/bc**

14) Randomized Control Trial	15) Types of Errors	
Prospective Study Subjects are **randomly** assigned to **treatment** or **control group.** **Matching and randomizing** (pts have similar baseline characteristics) are both used to minimize **bias and confounding**. **Double-blind** is used to prevents **observation bias.**	**TYPE I (alpha) Error** Say there is difference, but there is no difference. **"False positive"** (really neg) Ex. says he's rich, but he is really poor. **P- value: P<0.05** statistically significant. This means that there is <5% chance that the results were due to chance alone.	**TYPE II (beta) Error** Says there is no difference, but there is a difference. **"False negative"** (really +) Ex. he says he is not cheating, but he really is cheating. **POWER** Is the probability that a study will find a **significant difference** when one is TRULY there. **Power (beta)=** **1- Type II Error**

Epidemiology

16) Confidence Interval (CI)		17) Standard Deviation (SD)
Confidence interval expresses statistical significance **(P-value)**. **If CI is wide, power is low.** ↑ **Sample SIZE** will make confidence interval **tighter.** **Tighter CI** (↑ sample size) the more **precise** the results will be.	CI also includes the value corresponding to **relative risk of 1.0.** If **RR=1** there is **NO statistical significants** (zero difference with or without tx).	Normal (bell-shaped) distribution: **68%-** 1SD from mean **95%-** 2SD from mean **99.7%-**3SD from mean Mean= median= mode • **Median-** divide right and left data evenly. • **Mean-** add up all dataset and divide by # of datasets. **Outlier** sensitive. • **Mode-** most freq value of dataset.
18) Bias		
• **Measurement bias** Data-gathering methods (one group CT scan another by MRI). • **Selection bias** Pts are selected. Ex- loss to follow-up creates potential selection bias. **Selecting only sick pts is another ex.**	• **Susceptibility bias** Subgroup of **selection bias**. This bias does not take into account confounding variables. (can avoid with randomizing). • **Observer bias** Investigator's decision is adversely affected by knowledge of exposure status.	• **Confounding bias** There is a third variable. **Randomized** studies and **matching** can prevent confounding. • **Lead-time bias** Early detection of disease appears to prolong survival. Ex- new screening test.
19) Bias		
• **Recall bias** Past factors to recall Ex- cancer pt recalls more of the past episodes than non-cancerous pts. • **Length bias** Screening test detect slow progressive dz, but **misses rapid ones.**	• **Hawthorne effect** Tendency of study population to affect the outcome because they are aware they are being studied.	• **Effect modification** Effect of main exposure on **outcome is modified by another variable. NOT a bias.** It is not due to flaw in the design of the study. Ex- asbestos depends on smoking to get lung cancer.

6 CHAPTER
ETHICS AND LEGAL ISSUES

Ethics and Legal		
1) Ethics Principles	**2) Confidentiality**	**3) Unemancipated and Emancipated**
• **Respect for Autonomy** Respect pt's **right to choose.** • **B- Beneficence** Pt's **B- BEST** interest. • **Nonmaleficence** Do no HARM. • **Justice** Fairness to **equal pts**. • **Euthanasia** Administer lethal agent to pts.	**Protect pts privacy and confidentiality,** unless pt consents and **signs a legal document** allowing release of such information. **Clinical PEARL: Emergency setting** Treating pt without consent. Ex- Jehovah's Witness tx with blood transfusion regardless of spouse request (no blood refusal card) due to emergency setting.	Unemancipated **Minor:** Pt <18yo must have **consent from a parent** or legal **guardian.** Exceptions: **pregnancy, birth control, or STDs.** **Emancipated Minor:** Pt is <18yo, but can consent for there own care: • **Married** • **In the military** • **Lives separately** from parents and manages own finances.
4) Override Confidentiality	**5) Child Abuse**	
"WAIT a SEC" **W- Wounds** **A- Automobile** **I- Infectious** Disease **T- Tarasoff** **S- Suicide** **E- Elderly** abuse **C- Child** abuse	• **Documentation** of all signs of abuse. • Complete **skeletal survey**. • Notification to **child protective services**. • Pt should be **admitted** into hospital.	**Clinical PEARL: Mongolian spot** Si/Sx- **dark-purple skin**, present at birth. Dx- clinical, can **look like child abuse,** but is normal and disappears in several yrs.

Ethics and Legal

6) Informed Consent	7) Malpractice	8) Breaking Bad News
Pt should be **informed and understand** there procedure: **"BRAIN"** **B- Benefits** **R- Risks** **A- Alternatives** **I- Indications** **N- Nature**	**4 D's of Physician** • **Duty** to the pt • **Dereliction** of duty • **Damage** to the pt • **Direct** cause of damage to pt Conviction is made on **"Preponderance of evidence."**	**"SPIKES"** S- Set the stage P- Perception (pts knowledge of disease) I- Inform (events) K- Knowledge (allow pts to ask Q's) E- Emphathy S- Summary and strategy (review plan)

7 CHAPTER
GASTROINTESTINAL

GI		
1) Achalasia		
Impaired relaxation of the LES due to loss of inhibitory **ganglion cells in myenteric (Auerbach) plexus.** Si/Sx- dysphagia with **"liquids and solids,"** chest pain, regurgitation of undigested food.	**Dx- barium swallow** shows dilation with **"Bird's Beak."** **Manometry** shows ↑resting LES pressure. **Endoscopic evaluation** in pts >60yo with weight loss to r/o CA.	Tx- **nitrates**, CCBs, **Heller myotomy** surgery or can do balloon dilation. Comp- **esophageal rupture** from esophageal dilation procedure. May lead to mediastinitis.
2) Causes of Esophagitis		
• **Candida** Si/Sx- **ORAL THRUSH**; white plaques on mucosa that **"CAN SCRAPE OFF."** Dx- clinical, endoscopy. Tx- **fluconazole** PO.	• **CMV** Si/Sx- **superficial ulcerations,** retinitis, colitis. Dx- endoscopy Tx- **ganciclovir**	• **HSV** Si/Sx-**deep oral ulcers**. Dx- endoscopy, biopsy shows multinucleated giant cells. Tx- **acyclovir** • **Drugs** Potassium chloride, tetracyclines, aspirin, NSAIDs, bisphosphonates.
3) Zenker's Diverticulum		
Esophageal diverticulum due to **outpouching** of the cricopharyngeal muscle. Si/Sx- dysphagia, **halitosis** (bad breath), regurgitation of undigested food.	**Dx- barium swallow** shows outpouching (confirms diagnosis). In pts with dysphagia **barium esophagram** is usually performed before **endoscopy**.	Tx- cricopharyngeal **myotomy** (surgically cut muscle) of **cricopharyngeal muscle.**

GI

4) Diffuse Esophageal Spasm		5) BARRett's Esophagus
High amplitude **nonperistaltic** contractions=> **"Nutcracker esophagus."** Si/Sx- chest pain, **dysphagia** (difficulty swallowing), **odynophagia** (pain on swallowing) of **"HOT or COLD liquids,"** relieved by **nitroglycerin.**	Dx- **barium swallow** shows **"Corkscrew" esophageal.** **Manometry** shows **high-amplitude** contractions. Tx- symp relief with **nitrates, CCBs.** If severe esophageal **myotomy** surgery.	**BARRett's** • B- Become • A- Adenocarcinoma • R- Results from • R- Reflux **GERD=> BARRett's** esophagus=> adenoma.
6) GERD		
Transient LES relaxation due to incompetent LES. Assoc- caffeine, alcohol, chocolate, garlic, onions, mints and nicotine. Si/Sx- heartburn 30 mins after meal, **sour taste "WATER BRASH," worsens with reclining,** substernal chest pain, morning **hoarseness.**	Comp- **peptic esophageal stricture.** Dx- barium swallow, esophageal manometry. **24h esophgeal pH** (confirm diagnosis). **Esophagoscopy with biopsies** for pts that are unresponsive to tx. Tx- reduce meal size, antacids, H2 block (rani**tidine**, cime**tidine**), **PPIs** (ome**prazole**, lanso**prazole**).	Tx- Surgery for refractory disease with **Nissen fundoplication** (upper curve of stomach is wrapped around the esophagus). **Clinical PEARL: Infantile GERD** Si/Sx- freq vomiting in first few months of life with adequate weight gain. Tx- **thicken formula with rice cereal and upright positioning.** Resolution by 12mos.

GI

7) Esophageal CANCER

• Squamous cell cancer Cx- **alcohol, Smoking** • **Adenocarcinoma** Cx- **2nd Barrett's** (columnar metaplasia from **GERD**)	Si/Sx- dysphagia for **SOLIDS** (first)=> **liquids,** weight loss, odynophagia. **Firm, solitary lymph node** in cervical or submandibular.	Dx **Barium study** shows narrowing with irregular borders. **EGD** (esophago-gastro-duodenoscopy) and biopsy (confirm), **CT and endoscopic U/S scan** for staging.

8) Esophageal CANCER — 9) Gastritis

Dx	9) Gastritis	
Dx **PAN-ENDOSCOPY** (direct laryngoscopy, bronchoscopy, esophagoscopy) with **biopsies** of suspicious lesions. Do not perform open biopsy, it will interfere with surgical approach. Tx- surgical resection with chemotherapy and radiation. **Esophageal CA-** mets early due to esophagus **lacking serosa.**	**ACUTE Gastritis** Cx- **NSAIDs**, alcohol, H. Pylori, CNS Injury. **CHRONIC Gastritis** • **TYPE A** (10%) Autoantibodies to **parietal cells=> pernicious anemia** (lack intrinsic factor which is necessary to absorb B12). • **TYPE B (90%)** **H. pylori, NSAIDs.**	Si/Sx- asymp, nausea, vomiting, **epigastric pain, hematemesis**, unrelated to meal time or fatty foods. Dx- can detect **H. pylori** with "**UREASE Breath**" **Test** and stool antigen. Can also do endoscopy with biopsy. Tx- **H. pylor** use **triple therapy; omeprazole** (PPI), **clarithromycin,** and **amoxicillin.**

GI

10) Gastric Cancer		11) Hiatal Hernia
Adenocarcinomas (most common) Risk factors- H. pylori infx, pernicious anemia, high intake of N-nitroso (preserved, salted food). **TYPES:** • **Intestinal Type** Metaplasia of **gastric mucosal cells**. Assoc- high nitrites and salt diet, low veg diet, and H. pyloric infx. • **Diffuse Type Signet ring cells**, metastasizes to ovary, "**Krukenberg tumor.**"	Si/Sx- asymp, abd pain, loss of appetite, upper GI bleed. **Virchow's node** (enlarged **left supraclavicular** lymph node) Dx- **endoscopy with biopsy** in high risk individuals. CT scan is used to evaluate the extent of the disease. Tx-surgically remove tumor. Poor survival rate of <10% in 5 yrs.	**Herniation** of stomach into chest through diaphragmatic opening. **Types:** • **Sliding (95%)** Gastroesophageal junction. • **Paraesophageal (5%)** Fundus herniates into the mediastinum. Si/Sx- asymp, GERD. Dx- CXR, barium swallow or EGD (esophago-gastro-duodenoscopy). Tx- surgery with **gastropexy.**
12) Peptic Ulcer Disease (PUD)		
Cx- **H. pylori, NSAID,** corticosteroid, alcohol, tobacco. **Types:** • **Gastric-** Greater pain with meal. • **Duodenal-** Decreased pain with meal. Si/Sx- **burning epigastric pain,** hematemesis; "**COFFEE-ground**" emesis. Comp- **hemorrhage** (most common), **acute perforation, gastrocolic fistula** (gastric greater curvature with transverse colon).	Dx • **Upright AXR** to r/o perforation, which will shows "**FREE AIR**" **under diaphragm, emergent surgery** (exploratory laparotomy). • **NG lavage and rectal exam** to r/o active bleeding. • **Barium swallow** or **endoscopy** with biopsy (confirm). • **UREASE breath test** (H. pylori). • For recurrent or refractory order **serum gastrin** to screen for **Zollinger-Ellison** syndrome.	Tx • For mucosal protection give **antacids, sucralfate, misoprostol, and/or bismuth**. • Lower acid secretion with **H2 or PPI** (ome**prazole**, lanso**prazole**). • **H. pylori** + give **Triple therapy;** omeprazole, clarithromycin, amoxicillin. • For pts that require NSAID (for arthritis) give **misoprostol** as a substitute.

GI

13) PUD Complications	14) Zollinger-Ellison Syndrome	
HOPI **H- Hemorrhage** (most common risk factor, **posterior** into gastroduodenal artery)	**GASTRIN** producing tumor of duodenum and/or pancreas (non-beta cell islet tumor) => ↑**gastrin**.	Assoc- **MEN1** pancreas (gastrinoma) pituitary(prolactinoma) parathyroid tumor (hyperparathyroidism).
O- Obstruction **P- Perforation** (**anterior** ulcer) Emergent laparotomy! **I- Intractable** pain	Si/Sx- burning abd pain with **recurrent ulcers** in stomach and duodenum, that are **refractory to medical tx.** Pt may have nausea, vomiting, fatigue, and GI bleeding.	Dx- high-fasting serum gastrin, **serum GASTRIN >1000**. If fasting serum gastrin levels is non-diagnostic order **SECRETIN stim test** to show ↑**gastrin**. **Octreotide** scan can localize the tumor
Clinical PEARL: **MALT lymphoma** without metastasis Tx- **omeprazole, clarithromycin, and amoxicillin** (H. pylori triple therapy).	**Steatorrhea** may develop due to ↑stomach acid => inactivating pancreatic enzymes.	Tx- **high-dose PPI** (omeprazole, lansoprazole), surgical resection if possible.
15) LactOSE Intolerance	16) Small-Bowel Obstruction	
Unable to convert **lactose** => to glucose and galactose due to **lactASE deficiency**.	Cx- **Adhesions** (Adults) post abd surgery (60%), **hernias** (children).	Comp- **peritonitis**, surgical emergency.
Si/Sx- abd bloating, **flatulence** (flatus, fart, gas), cramping after **MILK ingestion.**	Si/Sx- **High-pitch tinkles** with **peristaltic rushes. Crescendo-decrescendo** pattern of abd pain that last for about 5-10mins at a time.	Dx- **Abd XR** shows **AIR-FLUID level** with **stepladder pattern** and **marked distention** of small-bowel loop (upright film).
Dx- "**HYDROGEN**" **breath test**=> ↑breath hydrogen following ingestion of **lactOSE** load.	There may be **vomiting** with proximal obstruction and **feculent** with distal obstructions.	Tx- partial obstruction; **NPO, NG suction, IV hydration.**
Tx- **avoid dairy products.** For pts that do not want to give up dairy products can give **lactase enzyme** replacements.		**Laparoscopy** or **laparotomy** for complete SBO.

GI

17) Ileus		18) Ischemic Colitis
Loss of peristalsis without obstruction. Risk factors: opioids, recent GI surgery, anticholinergics, hypothyroidism, hypokalemia slows GI. Si/Sx- nausea, vomiting, absence of bowel sounds or movement, abdominal distention.	Dx- Supine AXR shows distended loops of small and large bowel. Gastrografin study (radiocontrast agent) r/o obstruction. Tx- NPO, NG suction with parenteral feeds as necessary. Clinical PEARL: Pseudo-obstruction (Ogilvie syndrome) Si/Sx- abd pain, distention, nausea, dilated large bowel in post-operative period. Tx- IV neostigmine.	Lack of arterial blood supply to COLON. Assoc- atherosclerotic disease, coronary artery disease. Si/Sx- lower abd pain followed by bloody diarrhea. Pt have minimal abd findings on exam. Most common site is on the left side "water-shed" area, splenic flexure.
19) Ischemic Colitis	**20) Mesenteric Ischemia**	
Dx- colonoscopy or flexible sigmoidoscopy to assess colonic mucosa. Tx- bowel rest, IV fluids, broad-spectrum abxs. Surgery with resection if there is necrosis. Comp- ischemic colitis is a complication of AAA repair due to sacrifice of inferior mesenteric artery (IMA).	Ischemia of the SMALL bowel. Cx- arterial occlusion (SMA), thrombosis (atherosclerosis), embolism (atrial-fib). Si/Sx- severe abd pain out of proportion from exam with BLOODY stools. Pts also have weight loss, and food aversion. Dx- AXR and CT may reveal bowel edema, "Thumbprinting."	Dx- may see on labs: ↑LDH, ↑lactate, ↑amylase, and ↑CK. Mesenteric angiography (gold standard). Tx- laparotomy for acute arterial occlusive. Angioplasty and thrombectomy +/- stent for acute arterial thrombosis, or embolectomy for acute arterial embolism. Mortality rate >50%.

GI

21) Diverticular Disease		
Outpouching of mucosa and submucosa of the colon, **sigmoid** (most common). Si/Sx-asymp, **sudden "PAINLESS" lower GI BLEED.** • **Diverticulitis LLQ abd pain, fever,** nausea, vomiting, **+/-bleeding.** Comp-abscess, obstruction, fistula, **perforation** (may lead to peritonitis and shock).	Dx **CT scan** is the best test for diagnosing and for evaluating diverticulitis. It is also useful to r/o free air, obstruction, or ileus. Diverticula are not well seen on AXR. **Colonoscopy** should not be done in diverticulitis due to **risk of perforation.** R/O **angiodysplasia** (2nd most common cx of painless colonic bleed).	Tx- **bowel rest,** broad-spectrum antibiotics; **metronidazole, fluoroquinolone,** or **cephalosporin.** For **perforation** do **Hartmann's procedure** (resection of rectosigmoid colon). **Abscess-** CT guidance percutaneous abscess drainage. **Clinical PEARL: Pilonidal disease** Si/Sx- acute pain and swelling of **midline sacrococcygeal skin.** Assoc- ↑body hair.
22) Angiodysplasia	**23) Colorectal Cancer**	
2nd most common cause of lower GI bleed. Si/Sx- mild abd pain, **PAINLESS GI bleed.** Assoc- **aortic stenosis** (systolic ejection murmur at right 2nd intercostal space). Dx- **colonoscopy** or **angiography** (gold standard) shows slow-filling veins in colonic wall. Tx-**endoscopic ablation.**	Most colon cancers develop from polyps. The most premalignant are the **villous adenomas,** sessile adenomas, and >2.5cm. **Risk factors- HNPCC, FAP,** FH, IBD, polyps, low fiber diet. Assoc: • **Turcot's syndrome (brain tumors** with FAP or HNPCC). • **Gardner's syndrome** (colonic polyps and tumors throughout the body, **seed in body like a garden**).	Si/Sx- asymp (silent growth), vague abd pain, anemia. • **RIGHT side** Si/Sx- **ANEMIA** from chronic occult blood loss. • **LEFT side** Si/Sx- **change in BOWEL HABITS.** Dx- AXR or CT shows **"Apple-Core"** obstruction.

GI

24) Colorectal Cancer

Screening: DRE, +guaiac test, **colonoscopy >50yrs (every 10yrs).** If pt has 1st-degree relative begin screening 10yr before the age of relatives diagnoses. **Iron deficiency anemia in elderly pts with neg** DRE should still have **colonoscopy** to r/o CA. Dx- **CBC,** stool for occult blood, sigmoidoscopy or **colonoscopy** (determine left or right CA).	Dx **Air-contrast barium** to r/o additional lesions. Evaluate degree of invasion with **rectal U/S scan.** CXR, LFT, and **Abd CT scan** to r/o **mets.** Tx- **surgery resection;** • <10cm from anal verge => **remove rectum, anus and permanent colostomy.** • >10cm from anal verge => tx with **ananstomosis.**	Tx- **CEA monitoring** for recurrence. Chemo if +lymph. **FAP screening** (ACP gene) if 1st-degree relatives of FAP, start screening at 12yo. Once polyps identified, tx with **proctocolectomy.** Most common site of colon cancer **metastasis** is the **liver;** RUQ pain, mild ↑LFTs, hepatomegaly, small pleural effusion. Confirm with **Abd CT.**

25) Crohn's Disease

Site- **transmural inflam, discontinuous** spread, of any portion of **GI tract.** Assoc- **ashkenazi Jews** (both UC and CD). Si/Sx- **abd pain, watery diarrhea** (inflam type diarrhea), low-grade fever, abd tenderness.	Comp: Nephrolithiasis (**oxalate** stone formation), **perianal fissures** and/or **fistulas** (connection between bowel loops, or bladder).	**Clinical PEARL: Malabsorption** Calcium normally binds **oxalate** in gut and prevents absorption. If there is fat malabsorption, calcium binds fat and oxalate is absorbed=> leading to **oxalate stones.**

GI		
26) Crohn's Disease		**27) Ulcerative Colitis**
Dx- **AXR, CBC,** stool cultures, stool for ova and parasites, stool assay for C. difficile. **Upper GI** with small bowel follow-through. **Colonoscopy** shows; **cobblestoning** and **SKIPPED lesions,** creeping fat, **"NON-CASEATING"** **granulomas.** May also show **stellate ulcers** and/or strictures.	Dx **Biopsy** is definitive diagnosis that shows **TRANSMURAL** abnormalities with neutrophilic cryptitis. Tx- corticosteroids, **sulfasalazine,** and/or **mesalamine.** Pts may require surgical resection. **Infliximab** can be used if pt is not improving on other meds. **PPD screening** should be done before infliximab therapy.	Site- **mucosa, submucosa** of the large bowel with **continuous** spread in which the **rectum** is always involved. Assoc- **primary sclerosing cholangitis (PSC),** pyoderma gangrenosum, **erythema nodosum, uveitis, arthritis.**
28) Ulcerative Colitis		
Si/Sx- **abd pain, BLOODY diarrhea** (inflam type diarrhea), tenesmus, urgency, abd tenderness. Comp- **TOXIC megacolon.** Dx-**AXR** (confirm toxic megacolon with dilated colon >6cm). **CBC,** stool cultures, stool for ova and parasites, stool assay for C. difficile.	Dx **Colonoscopy** shows; continuous rectal involvement, **pseudopolyps, and** **"CRYPT abscessess."** **Biopsy** is definitive diagnosis and shows **superficial mucosal** ulcers with neutrophilic cryptitis. **Prevention:** Begin colonoscopy surveillance 8yrs after diagnosis. Once surveillance is started, **colonoscopy every 1-2yrs.**	Tx Corticosteroids (acute), **sulfasalazine, mesalamine enemas,** or azathioprine. **Oral 5-ASA** if cannot tolerate enemas. May require surgical resection, **total proctocolectomy is curative.** **Toxic megacolon** is a **medical emergency;** give IV fluids, NG decompression, IV steroids.

GI

29) Upper GI Bleeds		
Cx- **PUD,** esophageal varices, gastritis, **Mallory-Weiss tear** (ruptured submucosal arteries of distal esophagus and proximal stomach). Si/Sx- nausea, vomiting, **hematemesis** (vomiting blood), **MELENA (black stool),** and possible hematochezia (maroon stool).	Dx- NG tube and NG lavage, **endoscope.** Ongoing hemoptysis **intubate** and **emergent bronchoscopy** to visualize and stabilize bleeding.	Tx- first protect airway, IV fluids, and **PRBCs** if **Hb/Hct is <8g/L.** In pts has cardiac disease give PRBCs if <10g/L. Give **PPI** for PUD, **beta-blockers** for varices.
30) Lower GI Bleed		
Cx- **diverticulosis** (most common), hemorrhoids, IBD, Cancer. Si/Sx- abd pain, **HEMATOCHEZIA** (maroon stool), may have melena (black stool). Dx- **NG lavage** to r/o upper GI bleed. **Anoscopy** in office or in pts under 45yo with minimal bright red blood per rectum. Anoscopy is also very sensitive for diagnosing **hemorrhoids.**	Dx **Colonoscopy, arteriography or exploratory laparotomy** (if unstable). **Diagnositic studies** in relation to the **amount of bleeding:** • Bleeding **>2mL/min** do **angiogram.** • Bleeding <0.5mL/min order **colonoscopy.** • Bleeding between 0.5-2 mL/min, **technetium-99 labeled erythrocyte scintigraphy** (tagged RBC study).	Tx- underlying disease. **Endoscope, embolization,** or possibly surgery if pt has diverticular disease. **Ligament of Treiz;** the boundary between **upper and lower GI bleed** (between duodenum and the jejunum).

GI

31) Carcinoid Syndrome

Carcinoid tumors (Chromaffin cells) is from liver metastasis to the ileum and appendix => that produce **substance P** and **SEROTONIN.**

Locations:
Carcinoid tumors occur in bronchial tubes, small intestines, colon, and/or appendix.

Si/Sx- abd cramps, cutaneous
• **FLUSHING,**
• **DIARRHEA,**
• **WHEEZING,** and right valvular lesion of heart.

Comp- **Niacin def** (Vit B3): **3D's** diarrhea, dermatitis, dementia.

Dx- high **urine Serotonin** (5 hydroxy-tryptamine), **5-HIAA** (5-hydroxyindole acetic acid) are diagnostic.

Tx- **octreotide**, surgery if tumor is large.

32) DIRECT Inguinal Hernias

33) IN-DIRECT Inguinal Hernias

Defect **transversalis fascia** (through the floor of Hesselbach's triangle)

Hesselbach's TRIANGLE:
• **Inguinal ligament**
• **Rectus abdominus**
• **Inferior epigastric artery**

Si/Sx- abnormal **inguinal protrusion** from the abd contents going into the inguinal region.

Comp- **strangulation or incarceration.**

Dx- clinical
Tx- surgery to correct defect in **transversalis fascia.**

Congenital **patent processus vaginalis**; the abd contents go through **BOTH internal and external inguinal RINGS** into scrotum.

Si/Sx- abnormal **inguinal protrusion** from the abd contents going into the inguinal region.

Dx- clinical
Tx- surgery to reduce size of **internal inguinal ring,** allowing only spermatic cord through.

"MD don't LI"
• **MD**
M- Medial to inferior epigastric artery is a **D- Direct** inguinal hernia.

• **LI**
L- Lateral to inferior epigastric artery is a **I- Indirect** inguinal hernia.

Triangle of DOOM
• **Vas deferens** (medial)
• **Spermatic vessel** (lateral)
• **External iliac vessel** (inferior)

GI

34) BLOODY Diarrhea

• **Campylobacter jejuni** (most common) • **Salmonella** • **Shigella** • **Vibrio parahaemolyticus** Cx- seafood; shrimp, crab, raw oysters. • **E. coli O157:H7** (Entero**Invasive**) Risk- **HUS**, TTP. • **Cytomegalovirus**	**Clinical PEARL: Hemolytic Uremic Syndrome (HUS)** Si/Sx- recent diarrhea (E. coli) illness, with NEW onset of triad: • **Hemolytic anemia** • **Renal failure** • **Thrombocytopenia** ($\downarrow$platelets) Dx- peripheral blood smear shows schistocytes and giant platelets.	• **CMV** Si/Sx- SOB, abd pain, **bloody diarrhea,** GI ulcers, arthralgias, esophagitis. Assoc- post-BMT, HIV. Dx- CXR patchy infiltrates. **Colonoscopy** will show **multiple ulcers** and mucosal erosions. Tx- **ganciclovir.**

35) BLOODY Diarrhea

• **E. coli O157:H7** (Entero**invasive**) Cx- undercooked beef or **raw MEAT**. Si/Sx- abd pain, +/- **fever,** vomiting, **BLOODY diarrhea.** Comp- **HUS,** TTP. Dx- fecal RBCs, WBCs. Tx- supportive, **avoid antibiotics** => $\uparrow$risk of **HUS.**	• **Salmonella** Cx- **POULTRY or EGGS.** Si/Sx- HA, myalgia, abd pain, fever, weight loss, **bloody diarrhea,** RUQ pain, jaundice. Comp- **sepsis** in **sickle cell disease.** **Gallbladder cancer** with Salmonella typhi. Dx- fecal WBCs. Tx- oral quinolone, or **TMP-SMX.**	• **Shigella** Cx- contaminated food or water, person-to-person transmission, **"Extremely contagious."** Si/Sx- abd pain, **bloody diarrhea,** dehydration, seizures. Dx- fecal RBCs, WBCs Tx- **TMP-SMX.**

GI

36) BLOODY Diarrhea	37) NON-Bloody Diarrhea	
• Campylobacter (most common) Cx- contaminated food or water. Si/Sx- bloody diarrhea. Dx- fecal RBCs, WBCs Tx- Erythromycin Clinical PEARL: Celiac Disease Dx- D-xylose absorption is abnormal in both bacterial overgrowth and celiac disease. If pt cannot absorb D-xylose after abx tx then diagnosis is Celiac disease.	• Staph aureus • Clostridium difficile • E. histolytica • E. Coli (EnteroToxigenic) "Traveler's diarrhea" • Giardiasis (poor sanitary conditions) Tx-metronidazole • Legionella (pneumonia, abd pain, ↑ LFTs, hyponatremia). Dx- stool culture, stool for ova and parasites.	• Tropheryma whippelii (Whipple's) Si/Sx fever, diarrhea, lymphadenopathy, and arthritis. Dx- biopsy of small intestine; PAS-positive in lamina propria (diagnostic). • Tropical Sprue Si/Sx- hx of tropics, chronic diarrhea, borborygmi (rumbling of abd sounds) on exam. Dx- biopsy shows blunting of villi, inflam cells, eosinophils.
38) NON-Bloody Diarrhea		39) TRAVELER's Diarrhea
• Clostridium Difficile Cx- Clindamycin antibiotic treatment. Si/Sx- abd pain, fever, WATERY diarrhea. Comp: toxic megacolon; pseudomembranes. Dx-fecal RBCs, WBCs, sigmoidoscopy shows "Pseudomembranes." C. difficile TOXIN in stool (diagnostic). Tx- metronidazole, vancomycin.	• Entamoeba histolytica (protozoan) Cx- contaminated food or water. Si/Sx- abd pain, fever, diarrhea, with hx of TRAVEL (Mexico) to developing country. RUQ pain; "AMEBIC colitis." Dx- U/S scan of RUQ may show amebic liver abscess. Can also order serum antibody testing. Tx- metronidazole	Cx- EnteroToxigenic E. Coli (most common traveler's diarrhea) Si/Sx- NON-bloody diarrhea, abd cramps, malaise, watery diarrhea, that lacks mucous or fecal leukocytes. Avoid- salads, tap/ice water, unwashed fruits when traveling. Dx- stool culture, stool for ova and parasites.

GI

40) Cholelithiasis and Biliary Colic		
Cx **cholesterol** gallstones, **pigmented** gallstones (hemolysis, infection). **Risk factors "5F's:"** Female, Fat, Fertile, Forty, Flatulence. Si/Sx- **postprandial abd pain** with fatty meal (due to viscus distention of gallbladder). Pts may have nausea, vomiting, and right-sided shoulder or subscapular discomfort.	Dx- **U/S scan of RUQ** (best initial test). CT scan can miss many gallstones and is inferior to U/S scan. Tx- have pts **avoid fatty foods.** All symp pts that are stable should have **elective cholecystectomy.** **Triangle of CALOT:** common hepatic duct, cystic duct, and inferior border of liver; location of the **"cystic artery."**	Tx **Asymp** pt **do not** require any treatment. **ERCP** is used for common bile duct (CBD) stones. **Ursodeoxycholic acid** can be used for poor surgical candidates (high risk of relapse).
41) Choledocholithiasis		
Cx- **gallstone in common bile duct (CBD).** Si/Sx- asymp, jaundice, biliary colic, fever, pancreatitis.	Dx- ↑**AlkPh** and ↑**total bilirubin** (hallmark). **U/S scan of RUQ** (best initial test for evaluating gallbladder).	Tx- **ERCP**, elective **cholecystectomy.** Pts can have **post cholecystectomy pain** (functional pain or sphincter of oddi dysfunction).

GI

42) ACUTE Cholecystitis

Prolonged blockage of **CYSTIC DUCT** by **impacted stone**=> causing obstruction, distention, and **inflam.** Si/Sx- nausea, vomiting, **RUQ pain, FEVER,** + **Murphy's.** Dx- U/S, **HIDA Scan** (**non-visualize** of the gallbladder on HIDA is a **positive test**).	Tx- broad-spectrum **IV antibiotics** and **IV fluids,** and early **cholecystectomy** (within **24-48hrs** if possible). **Clinical PEARL: Gallbladder Cancer** Dx- CT scan shows **calcified rim** in gallbladder wall, **"Porcelain gallbladder."**	**Clinical PEARL: Emphysematous Cholecystitis** (a form of acute cholecystitis) Infx of gallbladder wall with **GAS-forming bacteria.** Dx- U/S shows **AIR-fluid levels in gallbladder,** but no gallstones.

43) Acalculous Cholecystitis

Cholecystokinin (CCK) stasis results in **bile "SLUDGE."** Cx- **CRITICALLY Ill,** TPN, extensive burns. Si/Sx- **critically Ill patient** with biliary colic, and RUQ abd pain.	Dx- **RUQ U/S scan** (best initial test) shows **no stone, bile SLUDGE,** with pericholecystic fluid. **CT scan and HIDA scan** (more sensitive for diagnosis).	Tx- supportive. Critically ill pts should be started on **abxs** followed by **percutaneous cholecystostomy.**

GI

44) ASCENDING Cholangitis

Acute bacterial INFECTION secondary to **gallstones** obstruction in **CBD** (common bile duct).

Si/Sx- cystic duct stone => obstructive jaundice (**Mirizzi** syndrome)

Charcot's TRIAD:
• **RUQ pain**
• **Jaundice**
• **FEVER/chills**

Reynolds PENTAD:
• RUQ pain
• Jaundice
• Fever +
• **Septic shock**
• **AMS**

Dx
Labs: ↑↑↑**AlkPh,**
↑Amylase, ↑Lipase,
↑LDH, leukocytosis,
↑bilirubin. **U/S** or CT scan can be done.
ERCP for both Dx and Tx (biliary drainage).

Tx- **broad-spectrum abxs,** possibly ICU adm. If pt does not improve, emergent **bile duct decompression via ERCP** (therapeutic and diagnostic).

Alternatives are **percutaneous transhepatic cholangiography (PTC)** or open surgery.

45) Hepatocellular Carcinoma

Cx- **cirrhosis** and chronic **hepatitis** (HCV) are the most common in the United States. In developing countries **aflatoxins** (aspergillus) and **HBV**.

Si/Sx- RUQ pain, abd distention, **jaundice,** easy bruisability and coagulopathy.

Dx- serum ↑**AFP** (serum tumor marker, first step in evaluation for carcinoma), followed by **U/S scan or CT scan.**

Tx- underlying disease, liver transplant.

46) Hepatitis

Inflam of liver => cell injury and necrosis of the liver.

Cx
• **Viral**
(HAV, HBV, HCV).

• **Drug-induced**
(ETOH, acetaminophen, methyldopa, INH).

• **Autoimmune hepatitis**

• **Hereditary**
(Wilson's disease, hemochromatosis, alpha-antitrypsin def).

Si/Sx- **jaundice,** nausea, vomiting, **RUQ tenderness,** fatigue, **scleral icterus, hepatosplenomegaly.**

Dx
• **Hepatocellular** injury
↑AST, ↑ALT

• **Cholestasis**
↑AlkPh, ↑bilirubin

• **Post-Operative cholestasis** (blood loss)
↑AlkPh, ↑bilirubin

• **Hyperbilirubinemia**
↑Bilirubin

Dx
↑**AST, ↑ALT,**
↑**AlkPh, ↑bilirubin, hypoalbuminemia**
(↓plasma oncotic pressure), ↑**PT,**
↑clotting factors.

Hepatitis serology to diagnose viral hepatitis.

AST/ALT ratio >2
"you're to**AST**ed"=> alcoholic hepatitis.

Alcoholic hepatitis
Can be **reversible** with cessation of alcohol intake.

GI

47) Hepatitis

Dx **Autoimmune**; order **ANA,** **anti-smooth muscle** (autoimmune hepatitis) **antimitochondrial** **antibodies** (primary biliary cirrhosis). **Hereditary**; order **iron studies** (hemochromatosis), ↓**ceruloplasmin** (wilson's disease). **Clinical PEARL:** **Intrahepatic** **Cholestasis of** **Pregnancy** (ICP) Si/Sx- **jaundice,** **pruritus** hand and feet. Dx- ↑**bile acids,** ↑AST, ↑ALT, ↑GGT.	Tx- etiology, **steroids** for severe cases, add **azathioprine** for autoimmune hepatitis. **Liver transplantation** for end stage liver failure. Screen pts that have had blood transfusion in the past for: HCV (<1992), HBV (<1986). Tx HBV with **IFN-alpha,** **lamivudine, or** **adefovir.** HCV with **interferon and** **ribavirin (combo).** Asymp HCV pts with normal LFTs **do not** require tx.	Tx Chronic HCV should recieve **vaccination** **against Hepatitis A** **and B** (also safe to give in pregnancy). Newborns of **HBV** **mothers** should be given **Hep B immune** **globulin (HBIG)** and **HBV vaccine.** **Clinical PEARL:** **Hepatic Adenoma** Si/Sx- young women with RUQ pain on **oral** **contraceptives (OCP).** Dx- U/S scan of RUQ. Biopsy cells with **glycogen and lipids.** Risk- hemorrhage (highly vascular), malignancy.

48) Hepatitis Serologic Markers

• **IgM HAVAb** IgM antibody HAV **ACTIVE** Hepatitis A. • **HBsAg- Surface** of HBV, **carrier STATE.** • **HBsAb** - provides **IMMUNITY** to HBV. • **HBcAg-** antigen assoc with **CORE** of HBV.	• **HBcAb- WINDOW** **PERIOD,** IgM HBcAb **recent disease.** **Screening** for acute HBV: **HBsAg and HBcAb** (won't miss window period when HBsAg disappeares and HBsAb has not appeared yet).	• **HBEAg** transmite **BEware!** High rate of **fulminant** **hepatitis** (↑PT, ↑LFT) in **pregnancy,** esp in 3rd trimester. • **HBeAb-** low transmission **Ag- Antigen** (foreign to the body) **Ab- Antibody** (body army, destroy invaders)

GI

49) PSC		
Primary Sclerosing Cholangitis (PSC); autoimmune inflam, fibrosis, and strictures of **EXTRAhepatic** and **INTRAhepatic bile ducts.** Assoc- young **MEN** with **ulcerative colitis.** P-ANCA (perinuclear antineutrophil cytoplasmic antibodies).	Si/Sx- fatigue, jaundice, pruritus. Comp: **Cholangiocarcioma** (screen pts with colonoscopy). Dx-↑AlkPh, ↑bilirubin, MRCP/**ERCP** show **multiple bile-duct strictures.**	Dx- liver biopsy shows periductal sclerosis, **"ONION skinning."** Tx- **ursodeoxycholic acid**, stenting for bile strictures, severe pts liver transplantation.
50) Primary Biliary Cirrhosis (PBC)		
Autoimmune destruction of **INTRAhepatic bile ducts.** Assoc- middle-aged **WOMEN, xanthelasma** (cholesterol-filled yellow plaques) on eyelids. Si/Sx- pruritus, jaundice, fat vit **KADE** malabsorption.	Dx-↑AlkPh, ↑bilirubin, ↑cholesterol, **anti-mitochondrial antibody** (diagnostic). Liver biopsy shows **ductopenia** (vanishing bile duct syndrome). Tx- **ursodeoxycholic acid**, cholestyramine (pruritus), severe cases will need liver transplantation.	**Clinical PEARL: Choledochal Cyst** Si/Sx- RUQ abd pain, jaundice, recurrent pancreatitis. Dx- U/S shows **cystic extra hepatic mass** and gall bladder **separated** from the mass. May see dilatation of **intra and/or extra** hepatic biliary ducts. Risk- cholangio-carcinoma.

GI

51) Cirrhosis

Hepatocellular injury=> **fibrosis and nodular** regeneration. Cx- chronic hepatitis, PBC, PSC, Budd-Chiari syndrome (hepatic vein thrombosis). Si/Sx- jaundice, **ascites, varices,** spontaneous bacterial **peritonitis, hepatic encephalopathy** (asterixis, AMS).	Dx-↑ **bilirubin,** ↓ **albumin,** ↑ **PT/PTT.** U/S scan for liver size and evaluate ascites, **SAAG>1.1.** **CT scan** may show large, intrahepatic multifocal tumor. **Liver biopsy** show **bridging fibrosis and nodular** regeneration. Also obtain serologies, autoimmune studies.	Dx Screen all cirrhosis pts for **esophageal varices** with **endoscopy.** Prophylaxis with **beta-blockers.** Tx- **ascites** with salt and water restriction, diuretics (spironolactone, loop diuretic), possibly paracentesis. Consider **TIPS placement** in refractory pleural effusion.

52) Serum-Ascites Albumin Gradient

SAAG= **serum** albumin minus **ascites** albumin. **SAGG<1.1 PROTEIN leak** (↑capillary permeability, **exudative**): Cx- nephrotic syndrome, TB, malignancy.	**SAGG>1.1 PORTAL HTN** (↑capillary hydrostatic pressure, **transudative**): • **PRE-Sinusoidal** Cx- portal vein thrombosis, **splenic vein thrombosis,** or schistosomiasis.	• **Sinusoidal** Cx-**cirrhosis,** metastases. • **POST-Sinusoidal** Cx- constrictive pericarditis, **right heart failure,** Budd-Chiari syndrome (**hepatic vein thrombosis**).

GI

53) Effects of Liver Failure		54) Effects Portal HTN
• Jaundice • Gynecomastia • Spider nevi (telangiectasia; central red-spot radiate outward) • Scleral icterus (yellow eyes) • Fetor hepaticus (breath corpse) • Hypothalamic pituitary dysfunction (hypothyroidism)	• Anemia • Bleeding (↑PT) • Testicular atrophy • Edema • Loss sexual hair • Asterixis (flap tremor) Clinical PEARL: Hyperestrogenism; gynecomastia, spider angiomas, testicular atrophy, ↓body hair, palmar erythema.	• Ascites • Hemorrhoids • Peptic ulcers • Melena • Splenomegaly • Esophageal varices • Hematemesis (vomiting blood) • Caput medusae
55) Cirrhosis Complications		
• Ascites Tx- ↓Na diet, diuretics; **furosemide and spironolactone.** Paracentesis to r/o infx, or cancer and obtain SAAG.	• Esophageal varices Tx- **beta-blockers (1st-line),** octreotide. If severe **band ligation** or portocaval shunt, possibly liver transplantation for advanced disease.	• Spontaneous Bacterial Peritonitis Si/Sx- abd pain, fever, AMS. Dx- **paracentesis; >250 PMNs or >500 WBCs** in ascitic fluid. Tx- **IV antibiotics** (3rd cephalosporin).
56) Cirrhosis Complications		**57) Wilson's Disease**
• Hepatic Encephalopathy Si/Sx- confusion, AMS, coma. Dx- ↑↑AMMONIA. Tx- **lactulose** (nonabsorbable disaccharide syrup, ammonia trapped in GI). Can also use abxs **neomycin or rifaximin.** Pts should be put on a **low protein diet.**	• Hepatorenal Syndrome Si/Sx- **cirrhosis** with **NEW onset of renal failure** that does not respond to volume resuscitation. Dx- of exclusion. Tx- octreotide, **liver transplantation** (1st-line).	"ABCD" A- Asterixis (flapping tremors) B- Basal ganglia deterioration. C-↓Ceruloplasmin, ↑Copper, Choreiform (involuntary movement) Cirrhosis, Carcinoma. D- Dementia

GI

58) Wilson's Disease (AR)		
Hepatolenticular degeneration disease=> ↑COPPER, ↓ceruloplasmin (copper carry protein). Si/Sx- jaundice, **tremors,** anxiety, mania, depression, asterixis, **choreiform** movements, brown-green cornea.	Dx- serum ↑**copper,** ↓**ceruloplasmin,** ↑**urinary COPPER.** **Kayser-Feischer ring (green-brown cornea,** copper in descemet's membrane, diagnostic).	Tx- **penicillamine** (copper chelator), zinc (fecal excretion), diet copper restriction (avoid shellfish, liver, legumes).

59) Hemochromatosis		
Hyperabsorption of ↑**IRON** with **hemosiderin** => accumulate in liver, pancreas, heart, kidney, testes, pituitary, and adrenals. Cx- **HFE gene (AR),** alcoholics, alpha-thalassemia. Si/Sx-abd pain, **testicular atrophy,** arthropathy of MCP jts.	Si/Sx- **BRONZE diabetes skin pigment** (pancreatic fibrosis) hepatomegaly, **cirrhosis, CHF.** Comp: **Yersinia, Vibrio,** and **Listeria** monocytogenes infxs **(iron-loving bacteria). Hepatocellular carcinoma,** cardiac conduction block.	Dx-↑**serum IRON,** ↑**Ferritin** (stores), ↓transferrin (transport**), glucose intolerance.** **Liver biopsy** shows **hemosiderin** deposits. **HFE gene** mutation screening. Tx- wkly phlebotomy, with possibly **deferoxamine** (chelate iron).

GI

60) Pancreatitis

Risk factors: **GALLSTONES,** **ALCOHOLISM** (two most common) hyperparathyroidism, hypercholesterolemia (eruptive xanthomas), thiazide diuretics, cystic fibrosis. Si/Sx- epigastric pain, nausea, vomiting, abd pain that **RADIATES** **to the BACK.** **Steatorrhea** (pale, foul-smelling stools), possibly hypotension (capillary leak, vasodilation).	Si/Sx • **Grey Turner's sign** (flank discoloration). • **Cullen's sign** (periumbilical discoloration). Comp- **pseudocyst,** **fistula** formation. Dx- Labs: ↑**AMYLASE,** ↑**lipase,** ↓**Ca** (labs for **acute** pancreatitis). **U/S scan of RUQ** if suspecting gallstones, or first attack of acute pancreatitis to r/o gallstones.	Dx **CT scan** (best initial diagnostic test for **chronic** pancreatitis) may show **sentinel** **loop, colon cut-off** **sign,** abscess, or pseudocyst. ↑**ELASTASE** in stool (**chronic** diagnosis). **Secretin stimulation** **test** for pts with chronic pancreatitis to r/o Zollinger-Ellison syndrome (gastrinoma). Tx- **bowel rest,** NG suction, analgesia.

61) Ranson's Criteria

Ranson's criteria **on admission.** **GA LAW:** **G- Glucose** >200 **A- Age** >55 yrs **L- LDH** >350 **A- AST** >250 **W- WBC** >16,000	Ranson's Criteria **AFTER 48 hrs** **C HOBBS:** **C- Ca2+** < 8.0 **H-** ↓**Hematocrit** >10% **O- PaO2** <60 **B- Base excess** >4 **B-** ↑**BUN** >5 **S- Sequestered** **fluid**>6L	**Ranson's Criteria** **Mortality Risk** 20% 3–4 signs, 40% 5–6 signs, 100% >7 signs. Comp- **pancreatitis** **abscess** (10-14days), **pseudocyst** (>6wks).

GI

62) Pancreatic Cancer

Adenocarcinomas of the head of the pancreas.

Risk factors:
SMOKING, FH, DM, obesity, high-fat diet, chronic pancreatitis.

Si/Sx- asymp, abd pain **radiating to the back, weight loss,** fatigue, **obstructive jaundice.**

Si/Sx
• **Courvoisier's sign** (nontender gallbladder)

• **Trousseau's sign** (migratory thrombophlebitis).

Clinical PEARL: Mirgratory Thrombophlebitits All pts with mirgratory thrombophlebitis should have a work up for cancer with **CT scan of the abdomen.**

Dx
U/S scan may also show dilated, thin-walled gallbladder, no stones (**obstructive jaundice**).

Labs: ↑↑**AlkPh,** ↑**conjugated** bilirubin, ↑**CA-19-9**.

Abd CT scan (best initial test, very sensitive and specific for diagnosis) shows pancreatic mass and metastases to liver.

63) Pancreatic Cancer

No screening in asymptomatic pts.

Tx
Whipple procedure (pancreatico-duodenectomy). Chemotherapy with 5-FU and gemcitabine.

Comp:
If obstruction of the common bile duct (CBD) occurs; **ERCP placement of a common bile duct STENT** to relieve obstruction.

Clinical PEARL: VIPoma (rare tumor) Si/Sx- **facial flushing,** abd pain, weight loss, watery bloody **diarrhea, leg cramps**. Dx- **hypokalemia,** ↑**VIP (vasoactive intestinal peptide)** in blood (diagnositic). Abd CT shows mass in head of pancreas.

8 CHAPTER
HEMATOLOGY

Hematology

1) Megaloblastic Anemia MCV>100

Cx • **Folate def**; alcoholism, malabsorption, drugs; phenytoin, methotrexate, trimethoprim. • **Vit B12 def** (cobalamin, cofactor for purine synthesis); **pernicious anemia** (most common), malabsorption, diphyllobothrium latum (tapeworm). Si/Sx- **fatigue, pallor,** HA, diarrhea, and possibly **numbness, tingling of hand/feet** (neurologic symps are ONLY vit B12 def).	Dx-↑**MCV >100, hypersegmented neutrophils.** **Schilling test** Ingestion of radiolabeled **Vit B12** with and w/out intrinsic factor. In dietary def, give Vit B12 => leads to absorption in the gut and excreted by kidneys in normal amount. Dx **Vit B12 def:** • ↑**MMA** (Methylmalonic acid) • ↑**Homocysteine** **Folate def:** • **Normal MMA** • ↑**Homocysteine** Tx-underlying cause.	**Metabolism of Homocysteine:** **Vit B6, folate,** and **Vit B12** are all involved in homocysteine metabolism. So, if one vitamin is deficient there will be a increase in homocysteine level. **Clinical PEARL: Diamond-Blackfan Anemia** Si/Sx- cleft lip, short stature, webbed neck, shielded chest (like Turner's syndrome), **triphalangeal thumbs** (five long fingers). Dx- **macrocytic anemia** that is pure RBC.

Hematology

2) Microcytic Anemia MCV <80		
Cx- **TICS**: **T- Thalassemia** **I- Iron def** **C- Chronic disease** **S- Sideroblastic anemia** (assoc with myelodysplastic syndrome) Si/Sx- fatigue, pallor, weakness. **Clinical PEARL:** **Myelodysplastic Syndrome (MDS)** Dx- MCV>100, **ovalo-macrocyte RBC**, and neutrophils with ↓**segmentation.** BM biopsy (confirms diagnosis).	Dx • **Iron def:** ↓**IRON**, ↓**FERRITIN** ↑**TIBC**, ↑**transferrin** (but transferrin saturation in low), ↑**RDW (>20%)** (normal RDW in thalassemia). • **Chronic disease:** ↓iron, ↓ferritin, ↓**TIBC, normal transferrin**	Dx • **Thalassemia:** **NORMAL iron studies**, with normal TIBC, ferritin, and **normal RDW.** **Hemoglobin electrophoresis** (confirm diagnosis in beta-thalassemia, but is normal in alpha-thalassemia) • **Sideroblastic anemia:** sideroblasts on blood smear. Tx- underlying cause.
3) Iron Deficiency Anemia		
Cx- NSAIDs, **chronic blood loss** (should r/o GI bleed or colorectal cancer), low intake, malnutrition, hookworm. Si/Sx- asymp, fatigue, weakness, **glossitis, angular cheilitis, koilonychia** (spoon nails), **PICA** (craving to eat odd things like paper, ice, clay, or dirt).	Dx- microcytic anemia **MCV<80,** blood smear shows **hypochromic and microcytic RBCs.** • ↓**IRON** • ↓**Reticulocyte count** • ↓**FERRITIN** (confirm diagnosis, ↓iron stores) • ↑**TIBC** • ↑**Transferrin** • ↑**RDW (>20%)** (normal RDW in thalassemia)	Tx- **oral iron sulfate** or oral **ferrous salts** replace iron 4–6 mos. **Iron sulfate AE:** constipation, nausea, diarrhea, abd pain. **Clinical PEARL:** **Angiofibroma** (↑blood vessels) Si/Sx- frequent epistaxis (nosebleeds), **nasal MASS, bony erosion** in back of the nose.

Hematology

4) Direct and Indirect Coombs		5) Hemolytic Anemia
• IN-DIRECT Coombs "Antibodies in serum **not directly** on RBC." Ex- ABO, Rh D. Used to detect **antibody-antigen reactions**. Used to detect **antibodies in PLASMA/serum** prior to blood transfusion.	• DIRECT Coombs "Antibodies **DIRECTLY** on RBC surface" Ex- SLE, penicillin allergy, mononucleosis. Used to detect if **antibodies** on the **RBC SURFACE antigens.**	↑Destruction of circulating blood cells. Si/Sx- **fatigue, pallor,** tachypnea, tachycardia, jaundice. Cx: • **Sickle Cell disease** Beta-globin mutation. • **Mechanical hemolysis anemia** Mechanical valve. • **Microangiopathic hemolytic anemia**: TTP, HUS, DIC.
6) Hemolytic Anemia		
Cx • **G6PD def (XR)** ↑Oxidative stress; sulfa drugs, primaquine, dapsone, nitrofurantoin, chloroquine, quinidine, or fava beans. Dx- peripheral smear shows **BITE cells and HEINZ bodies.** (G6PD level may be normal during hemolytic episode). • **Paroxysmal Nocturnal Hemoglobinuria** (PNH) cells sensitivity to **complement.** Assoc- **portal vein thrombosis** (Budd-Chiari syndrome)	Cx • **Autoimmune destruction** 2nd EBV, CLL, RA, mycoplasmal, meds. Dx- **Neg Family Hx,** + **Coombs' test.** • **Hereditary spherocytosis (AD)** Abn RBC membrane. Dx- +**Family Hx, Neg Coombs' test.** Positive osmotic fragility test. Si/Sx- **fatigue, pallor,** tachypnea, tachycardia, jaundice.	Dx- clinical, **Coombs test** detect autoimmune hemolysis. Labs: ↓**HAPTOGLOBIN,** ↑indirect bilirubin, urine dark with hemoglobinuria, ↑**urobilinogen** in urine, and/or fecal. ↑**reticulocyte >2.5.** Tx- **corticosteroids (1st-line), iron supplements** for urine loss. Daily **folic acid** (sustain erythropoiesis from ↑RBC turnover). **Splenectomy** if severe.

Hematology

7) Splenectomy		
Post-splenectomy risk of infxs of **encapsulated infx**: S. pneumoniae, N. meningitidis and H. influenzae (impaired phagocytosis).	Dx- **Howell-Jolly bodies** on peripheral blood smear (blue inclusions in RBC typically removed by spleen).	Tx- wks before splenectomy give **anti-pneumococcal, haemophilus, and meningococcal** vaccines. Followed by **daily oral penicillin** prophylaxis for 3-5yrs.

8) Aplastic Anemia		
Failure all three cell lines; ↓RBC, ↓WBC and ↓platelet production due to **destruction BM cells.** Cx Hereditary, fanconi's anemia, **autoimmune, viral** (HIV, parvovirus B19), **toxins, radiation**.	Si/Sx- anemia, pallor, **weakness, petechiae,** bruising, bleeding, **infections.** Dx- **BM biopsy** shows **hypocellularity** and space occupied by **fat.** Labs- **pancytopenia;** ↓RBC, ↓WBC, ↓platelets. Tx- blood transfusion and stem-cell transplantation.	**Clinical PEARL: Fanconi's anemia** Si/Sx- café au lait spots, short stature, **radial/thumb hypoplasia,** strabismus, low-set ears, **aplastic anemia.** Dx- genetic analysis shows **chrom breaks.** Tx- BMT

Hematology

9) Sickle Cell Disease		
Beta chain mutation, Glutamine replaced by **Valine**. (AR) Assoc-young African American (AA) male. Si/Sx- asymp, anemia (hemolytic anemia), **DACTYLITIS** (hand-foot swelling). Pts may have jaundice, **cholelithiasis (black pigment** gallstones; due to excessive hemoglobin breakdown), delayed growth.	Si/Sx **Hyposthenuria** (RBC sickling in vasa rectae of inner medulla). Dx Blood smear shows **sickle cells, TARGET cells, reticulocytosis** (attempt to compensate for chronic hemolysis). **Hemoglobin electrophoresis** identifies HgbS, HgbSC the two most common forms (gold standard). CXR may show **H-SHAPED vertebrae** (bone infarctions).	Dx **Howell-Jolly bodies** (nuclear remnants of RBCs) might be seen on peripheral smear if pt has functional **asplenia or splenectomy**. **Clinical PEARL: Sickle Cell Trait** (HbS) Si/Sx-the most common finding is **painless hematuria.** HbS also gives some protection against **malaria.**
10) Sickle Cell Disease		
Tx **Hydroxyurea** (↑Hgb F) which will help ↓painful episodes. **Folic acid** to help in erythropoiesis and **prevent aplastic crisis.** Cholelithiasis treat with **cholecystectomy**. **Vaso-occlusion crisis (Osteonecrosis)** Give IV fluids, O2, and pain management.	Tx **Exchange transfusion** in stroke ↓percentage of sickle cells and prevent secondary infarct from occuring. Prevent pneumococcal sepsis with: **pneumococcal vaccination plus penicillin** prophylaxis. Comp: • **Osteomyelitis** • **Pneumococcal sepsis** • **Avascular necrosis** of the **HIP**.	Comp: • **Aplastic Crisis** Dx- acute **severe anemia,** ↓reticulocytes. • **Vaso-occlusive crisis (Osteonecrosis)** Triggered by infx, dehydration, cold temp. Si/Sx- diffuse musculoskeletal pain. • **Splenic infarction** • **Parvovirus B19** infxs • **Bacteremia** Cx- strep pneumoniae (most common).

Hematology

11) Beta Thalassemia		
Mutation in **one or both beta-hemoglobin.** Assoc- **mediterranean** descent. • **Beta-Major** (pt has zero out of two beta chains) Si/Sx- microcytic anemia at first year of life.	• **Beta-Minor** (pt has only one out of two beta chains) Si/Sx- **asymp** Dx- **Normal iron studies, NORMAL RDW** and MCHC. **TARGET cells** on blood smear. **Electrophoresis** shows ↑**HbF** (major), ↑**hemoglobin A2** (minor). DNA studies.	Tx • **Beta-Major** Tx- is **transfusion** dependent. Can also give **deferoxamine** (iron chelators) to prevent iron overload. • **Beta-Minor** Tx- NONE, **Reassurance.**

12) Alpha Thalassemia		
Mutation of one or more of the **four genes** for **alpha-hemoglobin.** • **Hydrops Fetalis** (none of the four alpha) Pt does not survive. • **Hemoglobin-H** (has one of four alpha) Si/Sx- **severe anemia** Dx-severe hypochromic, microcytic anemia.	• **Alpha Trait** (has two of four alpha) Si/Sx- **asymp**, mild fatigability. Dx-↓**MCV**, target cells. Tx- **reassurance**. • **Silent carrier** (three of four alpha) Si/Sx- none.	Dx- Normal RDW, normal iron studies. **TARGET cells** on blood smear. **Normal Electrophoresis.** DNA studies. Tx- Hemoglobin-H treat anemia. **Alpha trait** give **reassurance**.

Hematology

13) Polycythemias		
Erythrocytosis (↑RBC production, or ↓plasma volume) Cx- • **Polycythemia vera** • **Delayed clamping of umbilical cord** • **Cancer** • **Steroid** drug abuse • **Hypoxemia;** lung disease, obstructive sleep apnea, smoking, high altitudes.	Si/Sx Blurred vision, bruising, bleeding, **flushing, pruritus esp after hot shower,** fatigue, dizziness, facial plethora, hepatosplenomegaly. **Newborns** may have respiratory distress, poor feeding, and neurologic manifestations.	Dx- clinically, **↑Hematocrit >65%.** **Polycythemia vera** Dx **↑Hematocrit >65%,** **↑RBCs, ↑**platelets, and ↓**erythropoietin** (also absence of erythropoetin in urine). Tx- underlying cause, **ASA** (to reduce hyperviscosity state). **Phlebotomy** (with a target hematocrit of <45%), **hydroxyurea** (↑fetal hemoglobin).

14) Hemolytic Transfusion	15) NON-Hemolytic Febrile Reaction	16) ALLERGIC Reaction
Antibodies against donor erythrocytes. Cx- mismatched blood, **ABO mismatch.** Si/Sx- symps start **HOURS DURING transfusion;** of flush, burning at IV site, **fever**, chills, nausea, tachycardia, tachypnea, hypotension, **hemolysis, shock, DIC.** Tx- life-threatening, **stop transfusion, IV fluids, ↑**urine output (diuretics and pressors).	**Cytokine** form in **storage** of the blood. Si/Sx- malaise, **FEVER, chills, rigors** within **1–6hrs AFTER transfusion.** Prevention: Leukocyte depletion techniques, like **CELL WASHING** can lower febrile, nonhemolytic transfusion reaction. Tx- clinical, control fever with acetaminophen, and r/o infxs.	IgA against donor proteins. Si/Sx- **urticaria** (rash), anaphylactic reaction; starts **seconds to minutes DURING** transfusion **wheezing, (bronchospasm), hypotension,** but **no fever**. Tx- **antihistamine.** If reaction severe or anaphylactic reaction **stop transfusion** and give **epinephrine**, IV fluids, vasopressors. **Prevent transfusion reactions-** pretreat with acetaminophen and diphenhydramine.

Hematology

17) Porphyria		18) AML
Abn heme production=> **↑ porphyrins**. Si/Sx- **colicky abd pain, "Pink URINE,"** **skin erythema**, blisters, photodermatitis, neuropsychiatric, and seizures. Ex-college student consumes **alcohol and barbiturates** at party, and then has acute episode of: "**Abd pain and brown urine**" the next day.	Dx- clinincal, **↑porphyrins** in serum, urine, and stool. Tx **Avoid triggers**; alcohol, OCPs, barbiturates. Give glucose for mild case, IV hematin (hydroxide of heme) for severe attacks.	**Acute Myelogenous Leukemia (AML)**; immature blood cells **"BLASTS,"** overwhelm bone marrow to produce normal cells. Si/Sx- **RAPID** progression of **fatigue, malaise, and infxs**. Dx- **↑ blasts** (immature blood cells) peripheral blood, **AUER Rods**, myeloperoxidase positive, BM biopsy shows **>20% blast** cells (definitive diagnosis).
19) AML	**20) ALL**	
• **Good prognosis:** If pts have marker AML M3 responds to **all-trans-retinoic acid (ATRA)**. • **Poor prognosis:** If pt is >60yo, or have markers; CD34+, MDR1+, FAB M7. Tx- **chemotherapy, allopurinol** (prevent hyperuricemia), and **BMT.** If M3 acute promyelocytic leukemia give **all-trans-retinoid acid (ATRA).**	**Acute Lymphocytic Leukemia (ALL)** Si/Sx- anemia, anorexia, irritability, lethargy, fatigue, malaise, and infxs. Pts may have pallor, petechiae, hepato-splenomegaly, lymphadenopathy. Dx **↑ Blasts** (immature blood cells) peripheral blood, **lack** auer rods, **Neg** myeloperoxidase, BM biopsy >20% **LYMPHOBLASTS** (definitive diagnosis).	Dx- cytoplasmic aggregates of **periodic acid Schiff (PAS) positive** material. Immunostaining shows positive **terminal deoxynucleotidyl-transferase (TdT)**. TdT expressed only by pre-B lymphoblasts and pre-T lymphoblasts. **Poor prognosis:** Age <1yr, >10yrs, ↑WBC >50,000. Tx- **chemotherapy, allopurinol** (prevent hyperuricemia), and **BMT.**

Hematology

21) CLL

Chronic Lymphocytic Leukemia (CLL) malignant **lymphocytes** that accumulate in BM and in peripheral blood. Si/Sx- chronic fatigue, malaise, splenomegaly, **lymphadenopathy** and infxs.	Dx- clinical, peripheral smear shows **"SMUDGE cells."** Dx- **FLOW CYTOMETRY** show lymphocyte clonality (confirms diagnosis). **Thrombocytopenia** is a indication of poor prognosis.	Tx- **HOLD treatment** until pt has **symps.** **Rituximab** (monoclonal antibody against CD20 antigen on B lymphocytes) used to treat **pts that are symptomatic.** Give chemotherapy for pt to have a longer life, only palliative.

22) CML

Chronic Myelogenous Leukemia (CML) clonal expansion of myeloid progenitor cells from **BCR-ABL translocation, Philadelphia t(9,22).** Si/Sx- chronic anemia, splenomegaly with LUQ pain, weight loss anorexia, fever and chills.	**Phases:** • **Chronic** Dx- ↓ **Leukocyte Alkaline Phosphatase,** with no tx 3–5yrs. Tx- **Imatinib** (Gleevec) inhibitor of **BCR-ABL tyrosine kinase.** • **Accelerated BLAST crisis** Dx-↓ **LAP,** ↑basophils, thrombocytopenia. Live 3–6mo. Tx- **dasatinib + BMT.**	Labs: ↑↑WBC >100,000, ↑LDH, ↑uric acid, Vit B12, ↓ **Leukocyte Alkaline Phosphatase (↓ LAP).** Dx Cytogenetic analysis shows **Philadelphia chromosome.** **Clinical PEARL: Leukemoid Reaction** Si/Sx- infxs and inflam Dx- ↑ **Leukocyte Alkaline Phosphatase (↑ LAP).**

Hematology

23) Hairly Cell Leukemia		24) Hodgkin's Disease
Maligant disorder of well-differentiated B lymphocytes. Assoc- **older males** Si/Sx- weakness, fatigue, anemia, bruising, petechia, **infxs** (mycobacterium avium intracellulare, **MAC**), splenomegaly.	Dx- **TRAP stain** (tartrate-resistant acid phosphatase) shows **"HAIRY" cells** on electron microscopy, and **flow cytometry**. Tx: **CLADRIBINE** (1st-line for hairy cell leukemia).	**B-cell malignancy** of unclear etiology. Assoc- **EBV** Si/Sx- **cervical adenopathy, B symps** (temp>38.5C, night sweats, weight loss), **mediastinal mass,** hepatosplenomegaly. **Pel-Ebstein Fevers** (1–2wk ↑**fever** alter 1–2wk afebrile).
25) Hodgkin's Disease		
TYPES: • **Nodular sclerosing** (most common) large tumor nodules with scattered **lacunar Reed Sternberg (RS) cells,** pts 30's. • **Mixed-cellularity** (subtype) • **Lymphocyte-depleted** (rare) pts are older. Dx- **excisional** lymph node biopsy shows **Reed-Sternberg cells, "OWL's Eye"** (fine needle biopsy is usually nondiagnostic).	Dx- **chest CT** scan may show **mediastinal lymphadenopathy.** **Clinical PEARL: Anterior Mediastinal Mass "4 T's"** • **Thymoma** • **Teratoma** (and other germ cell tumors; seminoma ↑Beta-HCG, nonseminomatous ↑Beta-HCG, ↑AFP) • **Thyroid neoplasm** • **Terrible lymphoma**	**Staging** is based on the number of nodes, presence of B symp, and if cross diaphragm. Tx- stage dependent, involve chemo and/or radiation. **Stage I, II** 90% 5yr survival**.** **Stage III** 84% survival. **Stage IV** 65% survival. Tx- chemotherapy and radiation. **Radiation** is directed toward involved lymph node. Chemotherapy; **ABVD, MOPP.**

Hematology

26) Hodgkin's Disease	27) Non-Hodgkin's Lymphoma (NHL)	
Chemotherapy; • **ABVD** **A- Adriamycin** **B- Bleomycin** **V- Vinblastine** **D- Dacrbazine** • **MOPP** **M- Mechlorethamine** **O- Oncovin** **P- Procarbazine** **P- Prednisone**	Progressive clonal expansion of B cells, T cells and NK cells from **translocation t(14,18).** Most are **B-cell origin (85%).** Assoc- H. pylori and MALT gastric lymphoma.	Si/Sx- painless peripheral adenopathy, fatigue, weakness, **B symp** (temp >38.5, night sweats, weight loss), splenomegaly, hepatomegaly. Dx- **excisional lymph node biopsy** (diagnosis). Disease staging is based on #nodes and if it crosses the diaphragm.

28) Non-Hodgkin's Lymphoma Tx	29) Eosinophilia	30) Neutropenia
Tx- based on histopathologic. Radiation and chemo. **CHOP:** **C- Cyclophosphamide** **H- Hydroxy- daunorubicin** **O- Oncovin** **P- Prednisone**	**Cx- allergies, asthma, parasites,** collagen vascular disease, neoplasm. Si/Sx- anemia, fever. Pt may have had recent **travel hx,** change in medication, or diet. Comp- **eosinophilic fasciitis** (orange peel skin). Dx- absolute ↑**eosinophil** count (normal <350), CSF for eosinophilia. Tx- **corticosteroids.**	Absolute Neutrophil Count (**ANC**) **<1500.** Assoc- staph aureus, E. coli, klebsiella, pseudomonas, proteus, sepsis. Si/Sx- ↑**infxs,** sinusitis, gingivitis, stomatitis, perirectal infx, splenomegaly. Dx- CBC with **absolute neutrophil count (ANC) <1,500.**

Hematology

31) Neutropenia	32) Amyloidosis	
Tx **Broad-spectrum antibiotics. G-CSF** can shorten the duration of neutropenia. **Cefepime or ceftazidime** should be started in **febrile** neutropenic pts. If severe give **IVIG** and **allogeneic BM** transplant.	**Extracellular** deposit of protein fibrils. Assoc- psoriasis, IBD, RA, chronic infxs, IV drug abuse. Si/Sx- symp of cardiomyopathy, hepatomegaly, nephrotic syndrome, peripheral neuropathy.	**Alzheimer's disease** type is limited to just the brain. Dx- biopsy; **Congo-red staining, apple-green birefringence** under polarized light. Tx- chemo, possibly transplantation.
33) Types of Amyloidosis		
• **AL-Amyloid** Deposits of **Amyloid LIGHT-chain.** Assoc- multiple myeloma and Waldenstrom's.	• **AA-Amyloid** Deposits **Amyloid A protein.** Assoc- rheumatoid arthritis, infxs, neoplasms.	• **Dialysis-Amyloid** Deposits **BETA- 2 microglobulin** in pts on long-term **dialysis.** • **Senile-Amyloid** Systemic deposit **transthyretin.**

Hematology

34) Multiple Myeloma

Excessive **monoclonal immunoglobulins** (kappa/lambda **light chains**). Si/Sx- **anemia, bone pain,** back pain, **lytic bone lesions,** infxs, **renal abn** (bence jones proteins). **Hypercalcemia; constipation,** anorexia, weakness, AMS.	**CRABS** C-↑ **Calcium** R- **Renal disease** A- **Anemia** B- **Bone lytic lesions** S- **Spike monoclonal protein (↑IgG)** **Clinical PEARL: Waldenstrom macroglobulinemia Dx- ↑IgM,** does not have a ↑Ca, and does not have lytic bone lesions (which are seen in multiple myeloma).	Dx- ↑ESR, ↑BUN/Cr, ↑ **monoclonal proteins** serum/urine. **Rouleaux formation** on blood smear. U/A shows **casts** with paraproteins; **bence jones proteins** (damage renal tubules). **Triad:** • **>10% plasma cells** in the BM. • **M protein (↑IgG)** • ↑ **lytic bone lesions** Tx- chemotherapy. Pts with **MDR gene** makes myeloma cells resistant to drug txs.

Hematology

35) Waldenstrom's Macroglobulinemia

Malignant monoclonal gammopathy; ↑**IgM** => hyperviscosity, ↑coagulation. (↑IgG is in multiple myeloma)

Assoc- amyloidosis, cryoglobulinemia, cold agglutinin disease, hyperviscosity syndrome.

MGUS (monoclonal gammopathy of undetermined significance) is precursor for disease (just like it is for **multiple myeloma**).

Si/Sx- ↓weight, lethargy, **raynaud's phenomenon**, blurry vision, AMS, peripheral neuropathy.

Symps due to **hyperviscosity** from ↑**IgM LARGE molecule** (IgG is SMALL molecule in multiple myeloma and does not cause hyperviscosity, AMS).

There are no lytic bone lesions and no↑**Ca** (which are in multiple myeloma).

Dx- ↑ESR, ↑uric acid, ↑LDH, ↑AlkPh.

BM biopsy and aspirate shows **Dutcher bodies** (**PAS+ IgM** deposits around nucleus in plasma cells).

Electrophoresis shows **M-Monoclonal SPIKE** (↑**IgM).**

Pt with **MGUS** should have **bone XR** to r/o multiple myeloma.

Tx- **plasmapheresis** (remove excess immunoglobulins), chemotherapy for lymphoma.

36) Heparin

↑**PTT** (Partial Thromboplastin Time), activates antithrombin III affect **intrinsic pathway** and ↓fibrinogen.

Enoxaprin (LMWH) inhibit Xa, does not have to be monitored, 1–2x a daily.

Tx- **Protamine sulfate** antidote.

Clinical PEARL: Heparin Induced Thrombocytopenia Antibodies against heparin-platelet **factor-4 complex.** Si/Sx- **arterial**/venous **thrombosis** in pt receiving heparin therapy.

Hematology

37) Warfarin

↑ **PT** (Prothrombin Time), inhibit Vit K and affect **extrinsic pathway.** Warfarin- **inhibits** synthesis of **Vit K** dependent factors **II, VII, IX, and X** (prothrombin), **protein C,** and **protein S**.	**Goal INR 2.0-3.0 (2.5–3.5** in pts with **mechanical valves).** Heparin-to-warfarin conversion to avoid transient **paradoxical hypercoagulability.** Tx- **fresh frozen plasma (FFP)** rapid reversal of anticoagulation of warfarin. **Vit K** takes **8-12 hrs** to be effective.	Comp- **skin necrosis** secondary to thrombus formation. ↑Risk of skin necrosis in pts with **protein C def.** Warfarin protect against embolic events, but also inhibits anticoagulants, protein C and S. **Warfarin** interacts with **many DRUGS,** remember this when initiating new drug therapies. **Carefully follow INR.**

38) Hemophilia (XR)

Deficiency of clot **factor VIII and IX**. Si/Sx- hemorrhage into **tissues and joints**. Disease is almost always **MALE,** due to **XR.** Dx- ↑**PTT,** normal PT. Also normal thrombin time, fibrinogen, and BT. If ↑**PTT** order a **mixing study.**	Dx **MIXING study:** • If PTT corrects this r/o factor deficiency. • If PTT remain elevated => abnormal. Next obtain **factor assays** for VIII or IX. **Hemophilia A (VIII) (90%),** hemophila B (IX) (9%).	Tx- mild treat **desmopression (DDAVP).** Replace factor if pt does not improve with **desmopression.**

Hematology

39) Von Willebrand's (AD)		40) Factor V Leiden
Deficiency of **vWF with ↓VIII,** which is carried by vWF (most common inherited bleeding disorder). Si/Sx- easy **bruising, mucosal bleeding,** worse with ↑ASA, ↑bleeding risk. "A **platelet** type of bleeding with a **NORMAL platelet count"** = von Willebrand's disease.	Dx- +FH, **NORMAL platelets and PT.** ↑**aPTT,** ↑**BT** as result of VIII def. **Ristocetin cofactor assay** measure **vWF** to agglutinate platelets (confirm diagnosis). Tx- **desmopressin (DDAVP),** menorrhagia treat **OCPs,** and avoid ASA. If severe give **IVIG.**	↑**Protein C,** ↑**APC** (activated protein C) due to resistant to inactivity by **protein C or APC** which leads to a **hypercoagulable state.** Si/Sx- **recurrent** DVT, PE, **arterial** thrombosis, MI, and stroke. Tx- **heparin** for DVT or PE followed by **3–6mo warfarin.** 6–12mo for second event, lifelong warfarin if it is the third event.
41) DIC		**42) Platelet vs Factor deficiencies**
Disseminated intravascular coagulation (DIC) from ↑deposition of **fibrin** (overwelming the system) => leads to **thrombosis and hemorrhage.** This depletion of **clotting factors and platelets** gives way to ↑bleeding. Si/Sx- bleed out of **venipuncture** sites with **petechiae,** bruising, mucosal bleeding, and thrombophlebitis.	Assoc- neoplasms, acute promyelocytic leukemia, obstetric complications, drug reactions. Dx -↑**PT,** ↑**PTT,** ↑**TT** (thrombin time), ↑**FDPs** (fibrin degeneration products), ↑**D-dimer,** ↓**platelets,** ↓**clotting factors.** Tx- underlying illness. Transfuse platelets if <20,000.	"P and C " • **Platelet deficiency** P- **Petechiae** suggest P- **Platelet** deficiency • **Factor deficiency** bleeding into body C- **Cavities** or joints suggest => C- **Clotting factor** def 3 cx for **MHA** (microangiopathic hemolytic anemia): **HUS, TTP, DIC**

Hematology

43) ITP

Idiopathic Thrombocytopenic Purpura (ITP) **IgG antibodies** against pts **platelets.** Assoc- lymphoma, leukemia, SLE, HIV, and HCV. **Clinical PEARL: Porphyria Cutanea Tarda** Uroporphyrinogen decarboxylase def (for heme synthesis) Assoc-**HCV** Si/Sx-painless blisters, hyperpigmentation.	Ex- **healthy adult** following a **viral illness** with no other medical problems. A **child** 2–6yrs old, following a **viral illness.** Si/Sx- following viral infx, epistaxis, menorrhagia, oral bleeding, **petechiae, purpura,** bleeding mucocutaneous, no splenomegaly. Dx- Normal coagulation studies. **Low platelets** on peripheral smear. BM ↑ **megakaryocytes** in marrow.	Tx- watchful management. Give high-dose oral **prednisone** (initial tx) until normal platelet count. **IVIG** in bleeding emergencies, and **splenectomy** (definitive therapy). **Platelet transfusion is of no benefit** (unless below 30,000 to 50,000 or bleeding symps). Other emerging therapies for ITP is anti-D (Rh) and rituximab.

Hematology

44) TTP		45) HUS, HELLP, DIC
Thrombotic Thrombocytopenic Purpura (TTP) Assoc- **HUS,** HELLP syndrome. Si/Sx- 5 symp: • **↓Renal function** • **Hemolytic anemia** • **Thrombocytopenia** • **AMS** (delirium, seizure, stroke) • **FEVER**	Dx- Labs: coagulation factors are NORMAL. **Low platelets, ↑creatinine (↑BUN/Cr).** Peripheral blood smear will show **schistocytes.** Tx- **Plasmapheresis (plasma exchange)** 1st-line. Platelet transfusion is **contraindicated.**	• **HUS** Cx- **E. Coli** (0157:H7) Si/Sx- **triad:** - **↓Renal function** - **Hemolytic anemia** - **Thrombocytopenia** (HUS > TTP) • **HELLP syndrome** Pregnant women assoc with **preeclampsia.** H- Hemolysis, EL- Elevated Liver, LP-Low Platelets. • **DIC**- distinguished from TTP by prolonged **PT, PTT.**
46) Bernard-Soulier Syndrome (AR)		
↓Dysfunctional platelets=> disorder with **thrombocytopenia and LARGE platelets.** Si/Sx- **easy bruising, nosebleeds,** mucosal bleeding, bleeding.	Assoc- with surgical procedures, and menorrhagia. Dx- **↓**dysfunctional platelets, peripheral smear shows **LARGE platelets.**	Dx- diagnostic; • **Do NOT** aggregate to **Ristocetin.** • Aggregation to **adenosine diphosphate (ADP), epinephrine,** and **collagen.**
47) Glanzmann Thrombasthenia		
Platelet glycoprotein IIb/IIIa complex deficiency => defective platelet aggregation. (AR) Si/Sx- **easy bruising, mucosa bleeding,** nosebleeds, GI bleeding, menorrhagia.	Dx Normal PT, PTT, and normal platelet count. • **Aggregate to RISTOCETIN.**	Dx • **Do NOT** aggregate to adenosine diphosphate (ADP), epinephrine, and collagen. Tx- pts who are bleeding require **platelet transfusion.**

9 CHAPTER
INFECTIOUS DISEASE

Infectious

1) Gram-Positive Cocci	2) MRSA	3) Gram-Positive and Gram Neg
Oxacillin, cloxacillin, dicloxacillin, nafcillin "Methicillin sensitive drugs" "Antistaphylococcal penicillins." Tx- **staph, strep**	**Vancomycin** (most common), **linezolid,** daptomycin, ceftaroline, tigecycline. "Methicillin-resistant staphylococcus aureus" (MRSA). Tx- **MRSA,** also use instead of penicillins in life threatening **penicillin allergies**.	Penicillin G, penicillin VK, ampicillin, amoxicillin. Tx- **strep** pyogenes, strep viridans, strep pneumonia, **Neissera.** Ampicillin or amoxicillin. Tx- enterococci, **Listeria.** **Ampicillin** can also treat **E. coli** infxs.
4) Cephalosporins		
Tx- **staph, strep,** some **gram-negative organisms**. • **1st- Generation:** Cefazolin, cephalexin cefadroxil. Tx- staph, strep, **E. coli, Moraxella.**	• **2nd- Generation:** Cefoxitin, cefprozil, cefotetan, cefuroxime, loracarbef. Tx- staph, strep, E. coli, Moraxella, **Haemophilus, Klebsiella, Proteus, Providencia, Citrobacter, Morganella.** 2nd-generations **does not** cover **Pseudomonas.**	• **3rd- Generation:** Ceftazidime, ceftriaxone, cefotaxime • **4th- Generation:** Cefepime Tx- **broad-spectrum antibiotic** covering both gram positive and gram negative. Only cefepime and ceftazidime cover **Pseudomonas.**

Infectious

5) Penicillin Allergic		6) Gram-Negative Bacilli
Si/Sx- **RASH** Tx- **cephalosporins** instead of penicillins. Si/Sx-**Anaphylaxis** Tx- **macrolide** (azithro**mycin**, clarithro**mycin**) or **fluoroquinolones** (levo**floxacin**, gemi**floxacin**, moxi**floxacin**).	Si/Sx **LIFE-Threatening** penicillin allergies. Tx- **vancomycin,** linezolid, daptomycin, or tigecycline.	**Penicillins**; piperacillin, mezlocillin, ticarcillin. Tx- gram-negative bacilli; **Pseudomonas,** and Enterobacteriaceae (**E. coli, Klebsiella, Serratia, Morganella, Proteus, Enterobacter, Citrobacter**).

7) Gram-Negative Bacilli	8) Aminoglycosides	
Penicillins; piperacillin, mezlocillin, ticarcillin. Tx- **gram-negative + coverage for staph** need to add a beta-lactamase inhibitor: • **piperacillin/** tazobactam, • **ticarcillin/** clavulanate, • **amoxicillin/** clavulanate, • **ampicillin/** sulbactam.	**Gentamicin, tobramycin, amikacin.** Tx- "exclusively" **gram-negative coverage** such as **enterobacteriaceae;** E. coli, Klebsiella, Enterobacter, Haemophilius, Serratia, Moraxella, Morganella, Citrobacter.	Tx For **gram positive** coverage must be **comb** with a penicillin.

9) Macrolides and Fluoroquinolones		
Macrolides; azithro**mycin**, clarithro**mycin**, erythro**mycin**. Fluoroquinolones; Levo**floxacin**, gemi**floxacin**, moxi**floxacin**.	**Alternatives** to penicillins and cephalosporins for gram positive infxs. Tx- **staph** (not in serious staph infxs), **strep** (except ciprofloxacin does not cover strep).	Tx **Fluoroquinolones** also cover gram negative **Enterobacteriaceae;** E. coli, Klebsiella, Enterobacter, Haemophilius, Serratia, Moraxella, Morganella, Citrobacter.

Infectious

10) Quinolones		11) Carbapenems
Levo**fl**oxacin, cipro**fl**oxacin, gemi**fl**oxacin, moxi**fl**oxacin, o**fl**oxacin. Tx **Enterobacteriaceae;** E. coli, Klebsiella, Enterobacter, Haemophilius, Serratia, Moraxella, Morganella, Citrobacter.	Tx First line treatment for **pneumonia** because they cover **Legionella, Mycoplasma, Chlamydia.** Only **ciprofloxacin** covers **Pseudomonas** out of the quinolones (but ciprofloxacin does not cover strep).	Imi**penem**, mero**penem**, erta**penem**, dori**penem**. Tx **Enterobacteriaceae;** E. coli, Klebsiella, Enterobacter, Haemophilius, Serratia, Moraxella, Morganella, Citrobacter. Also cover **Pseudomonas** (except ertapenem). Also have "excellent" **staph** and **ANAEROBIC coverage.**
12) Anaerobes		
Metronidazole, clindamycin. Tx **Metronidazole** Covers **anaerobic,** gram negative bacteria in **bowel;** Bacteroides fragilis. **Metronidazole** 1st-line against **Clostridium difficile.**	Tx **Clindamycin** covers **anaerobic** infxs **ABOVE the diaphragm.** Other agents that will cover **anaerobic infxs;** carbapenems and beta-lactam/beta-lactamase comb.	Beta-lactam/ beta-lactamase comb: • **Piperacillin/ tazobactam** • **Ticarcillin/ clavulanate** • **Ampicillin/ sulbactam** • **Amoxicillin/ clavulanate**

Infectious

13) Gram Stain	14) Sinusitis	
• **Strep** gram + **diplococci** • **Staph** gram + **cocci clusters** • **Listeria, Bacillus** gram + **rod** • **Neisseria** gram **neg cocci** • **Pseudomonas,** **Haemophilus,** **Legionella** gram **neg rods** • **Klebsiella** gram **neg bacilli**	Inflam paranasal sinus. • **ACUTE <1mos** Most common **VIRAL** **upper resp infx**. Pt can get 2nd acute **bacterial** **sinusitis** after viral URI. • **CHRONIC >3mos** • **Diabetics** consider **mucormycosis** (rhizopus) Si/Sx- fever, **nasal** **congestion,** facial pain, HA. Always consider **occult sinusitis** in febrile ICU pts.	**Bacterial sinusitis:** **Strep pneumoniae** (most common), H. influenzae, Moraxella catarrhalis. Dx- **clinical,** CT is not required for acute sinusitis. For chronic sinusitis **CT scan** (test of choice), and **bacterial culture** (gold standard). Tx- **viral sinusitis** is self-limiting. Can give decongestants and antihistamines. **Acute bacterial** **sinusitis** (<7day) use **Amoxicillin** +/- clavulanate for 10days.

Infectious

15) Sinusitis	16) Acute Pharyngitis	
Tx For chronic bacterial (4–12mo) give **corticosteroids, decongestants,** and **antihistamines.** **Mucormycosis** tx: **amphotericin B + incision and drainage.**	Cx- **VIRAL** (most common, 90%), **strep phyaryngitis** (**GAS**/strep pyogenes). Si/Sx- **sore throat,** fever, pharyngeal erythema, **tonsillar exudate.** Dx- clinical, **rapid GAS antigen testing** (>90%), throat culture. **Antistreptolysin-O (ASO)** titer is high in strep phyaryngitis. Comp: Poststrepococcal **glomerulonephritis, rheumatic fever,** peritonsillar abscess.	Tx **VIRAL infx** is **self-limiting** and no treatment is needed. **Penicillin** for 10days for strep phyaryngitis. Amoxicillin, cephalosporins, and azithromycin are alternatives. Can give **aspirin for arthralgias** (risk of **Reye syndrome** in viral infxs leading to fulminant hepatic failure). Important to tx strep phyaryngitis in children to prevent **Rheumatic FEVER**.
17) Influenza		
Cx- **orthomyxovirus** transmitted by droplets. **Types**: A, B, and C. **Influenza A** (H5N1, H1N1). Si/Sx- weakness, fever, chills, **myalgias, cough, coryza.** Comp- post-influenza infx with **staph aureus pneumonia.** Pts can also get **multiple nodular infiltrates** in lungs (small abscesses).	• **Antigenic DRIFT** Small changes from **point mutations.** Pts can be infected multiple times. • **Antigenic SHIFT** Major change in **subtype=> pandemic**. Dx- clinical, nasopharyngeal swab, viral culture or **direct immunofluorescence assay (DFA) tests** (definitive diagnosis).	Tx- bed rest and simple analgesics (acetaminophen). El**tamivir**, osel**tamivir**, or zan**amivir** is most effective when **used within 2 DAYS of onset.** Rimantadine and amantadine are other options, but only cover Influenza A.

Infectious

18) Pneumonia

Cx
• **Child** (6wk–18yr)
RSV, chlamydia,
mycoplasma, strep
pneumoniae.

• **Adults** (18–40yr)
Strep pneumoniae,
mycoplasma (young
healthy adults, "**walking**
pneumonia," with
+cold agglutinins),
chlamydia.

• **Adults** (40–65yr)
Strep pneumoniae,
H. influenzae,
anaerobes, viruses.

• **Elderly** (>65yr)
Strep pneumoniae,
H. influenzae, viruses,
anaerobes.

• **Community**
Acquired
Strep pneumoniae,
H. influenzae,
moraxella catarrhalis.

Tx
Outpt: macrolide
(azithromycin or
clarithromycin),
alternatives
doxycycline,
levofloxacin.

Inpt: fluoroquinolone
(cover gram neg,
gram+, atypical).

Prevent: **pneumovax**
vaccination (strep
pneumonia).

Special Groups:

• **Atypical-** chlamydia,
mycoplasma, legionella

• **Aspiration-**anaerobes
(also **bacteroides,**
fusobacterium)

• **Alcoholics-** klebsiella
(Friedlander's,
currant jelly-sputum)

• **HIV-** pneumocystic
jiroveci (PCP)

• **Nosocomial**(hospital)
staph, anaerobes,
gram neg rods (GNRs).

• **Neonate-** Group B
Strep (**GBS**) "**Baby,**"
E. coli.

• **Postviral-** staph

19) Pneumonia

Si/Sx- fever, cough,
yellow-green sputum,
dyspnea, night sweats.
↓breath sounds, rales,
wheezing.

Atypical: dry cough,
myalgias, sore throat.

Dx- **CXR,** sputum
gram stain and culture.
Also order blood
cultures, ABG and
nasopharyngeal
aspirate.

Atypical Dx:

• **Chlamydia-** culture,
serologic testing, **PCR.**

• **Legionella- urine**
legionella antigen test.

• **Mycoplasma**
cold agglutinin and
mycoplasma antigen.

Infectious

20) Pneumonia Tx

Community-Acquired	Community-Acquired + Hospitalization	HOSPITAL Acquired
Tx- **Outpt:** • **Macrolides** (azithromycin or clarithromycin) • **Fluoroquinolone** (levofloxacin, moxifloxacin, gatifloxacin) • Alternative **doxycycline** (AE: **phototoxicity**).	Tx- **Inpt:** • **Fluoroquinolone;** levofloxacin or moxifloxacin (1st-line for inpt CAP). • **Cephalosporin** (ceftriaxone, cefotaxime) or beta-lactam inhibitor plus a **macrolide** (often azithromycin) or doxycycline.	Tx **Cephalosporin** (ceftriaxone, cefotaxime) or carbapenem. **Critically Ill** Add **vancomycin** or **linezolid** for **MRSA.** **Aspiration pneumonia** (anaerobic) Assoc- seizures, drug overdose, alcoholism, CVA, intubation. Tx- **Clindamycin**

21) Legionella Pneumonia   22) Mycoplasma Pneumoniae

21) Legionella Pneumonia		22) Mycoplasma Pneumoniae
Intracellular gram negative rod. Spread by **cooling towers** and **water supplies.** Assoc- cruise ships, hotel water supplies. Si/Sx- cough, pneumonia, **abd pain, ↑LFT, hyponatremia.**	Dx- **urine antigen testing** or culture on charcoal agar. ↑**LFT** (↑**AST,** ↑**ALT**), **hyponatremia.** Sputum stain shows many neutrophils, but no organisms (intracellular). Tx- macrolides; **azithromycin** or newer generation fluoroquinolones; **levofloxacin.**	Si/Sx- **YOUNG adult, non-productive cough,** low grade fever, HA, sore throat, **erythema multiforme** (commonly shows up on hands and feet). Dx- **No cell wall,** does not stain with gram stain. Tx- **erythromycin,** doxycycline, or quinolones.

Infectious

23) Tuberculosis (TB)

Cx- **mycobacterium tuberculosis**.

Si/Sx- >3wk of symps of fatigue, **fever, night sweats, hemoptysis,** weight loss. Latent TB infx may be asymp.

Comp- **adrenal insufficiency** from milliary TB infx.

Dx- **CXR** may show **cavity infiltrate** in upper lobe, culture sputum (gold standard, takes wks).

Dx
Pts should be put in **respiratory isolation** to prevent spread while r/o disease.

Sputum **acid-fast stain**; three AFB stain and culture are advised to r/o TB. If **AFB neg** with high suspicion, **bronchoscopy with bronchoalveolar lavage.**

Test for **latent TB** with **PPD**, followed by CXR if positive.

PPD
• **>5mm**- HIV, close TB contact. If a child is in close contact and PPD <5mm, tx and re-test in several wks.

• **>10mm**- homeless, health care.

• **>15mm**- everyone else.

BCG vaccination
May give false+ test.

24) Tuberculosis Tx

25) TB Drugs Adverse Effects

Tx- **"RIPE"**
R- Rifampin
I- Isoniazid (INH)
P- Pyrazinamide
E- Ethambutol

• **Active TB**
2mos of **RIPE: rifampin, INH, pyrazinamide, ethambutol,** followed by 4 mos of **INH.** Add **Vit B6 (pyridoxine)** to prevent peripheral neuritis.

Tx
• **Latent TB**
(+PPD with no symps)
INH for 9mos or INH 6mos then rifampin 4mos. Add **Vit B6 (pyridoxine).**

Clinical PEARL: Contraindications for Breastfeeding
• Tuberculosis
• HIV/AIDS
• Active DRUG abuse (are contraindication to breastfeeding).

• **Rifampin**
AE- turn body fluids **red-orange** (benign red urine).

• **Ethambutol**
AE- optic neuritis (↓color vision, ↓visual acuity).

• **INH**
AE- peripheral neuritis and **hepatitis (↑LFTs).** Add **pyridoxine** (Vit B6) to avoid peripheral neuritis.

Infectious

26) Leprosy

Chronic granulomatous disease=> affects **peripheral nerves and skin.** Cx- **Mycobacterium leprae.**	Si/Sx- **insensate** (lacking sensation), hypopigmented patch of skin, **muscle atrophy.** Crippling deformities affecting face, eyebrows, ears, wrists, knees, and buttocks.	Dx- **SKIN biopsy** shows **acid-fast bacilli** (diagnostic). Tx- multidrug therapy (MDT) combining all three; **clofazimine, rifampicin, dapsone.**

27) Meningitis

Cx • **Newborn (0–6mo) GBS,** E. coli/GNRs, listeria, echovirus. • **Child (6mo–6yr) Strep pneumoniae,** neisseria/ meningococcal, H. influenzae (↓cases due to vaccine), **enteroviruses.** • **6–60yrs Strep pneumoniae,** HSV, neisseria, enteroviruses.	• **>60yrs Strep pneumoniae,** listeria, neisseria, GNRs. • **HIV Cryptococcus,** CMV, HSV, VZV, TB, **toxoplasmosis, JC virus.** • **Immigrant** H. influenzae, due to lack of vaccination.	**Risks factors:** Sinusitis, sick contacts, recent ear infection, immunodeficiency. Si/Sx- **HA, fever, neck stiffness,** photophobia, nausea, vomiting. **+Kernig's sign** and **+Brudzinski's sign.** **Clinical PEARL: Meningococcal** (neisseria) meningitis has **petechiae RASH** and/or skin lesions. Tx- highly contagious, pt need **hospital isolation** and started on IV abxs.

Infectious

28) Meningitis

Dx- blood cultures, **LP CSF gram stain and culture**. If there is **papilledema** (↑ICP) do not do a LP. If there is ↑ICP start **abxs and order CT** or MRI. Viral **PCRs** (HSV). Crytococcal antigen in HIV pts.	Tx- **ceftriaxone and vancomycin after LP**. Important: if LP cannot be done and CT is ordered, then start **abxs before CT.** Add **ampicillin** for pts that are **>60yo,** have chronic illness, or in immunocompromised individuals.	**Clinical PEARL: Menigococcemia** Risk of **Waterhouse Friderichsen syndrome** (adrenal hemorrhage). Si/Sx- vasomotor collapse, with **PETECHIAE RASH** in pt that has menigitis.

29) Meningitis	30) Encephalitis	
Tx Close contact with pts that have **meningococcal meningitis** give prophylaxis **rifampin**, ciprofloxacin, or ceftriaxone. **Tx for different ages:** • **<1mos**- ampicillin + cefotaxime or gentamicin. • **1mos-adulthood vancomycin IV +** **ceftriaxone** or cefotaxime. • **>60 yo or chronic illness**- ampicillin + **vancomycin +** **ceftriaxone** or cefotaxime.	Cx- **HSV (herpes simplex virus),** most common), arboviruses, CMV, toxoplasmosis. Si/Sx- HA, fever, neck stiffness, **AMS, CONFUSION, seizures,** photophobia, nausea, vomiting. Dx CSF shows; normal glucose level, ↑ **LYMPH**, ↑ **protein**, ↑↑ **RBCs** (hemorrhagic destruction of frontotemporal lobes). **PCR for HSV**, VZV, CMV, EBV, and enterovirus. **MRI** with contrast for lesion in **temporal lobe** (bizarre behavior) seen in **HSV.**	Tx • **HSV Encephalitis** IV **acyclovir** (start without waiting for PCR testing). • **CMV** Encephalitis **IV ganciclovir +/-** **foscarnet**. • **Doxycycline** for Rocky Mountain Spotted Fever, Lyme disease, or **ehrlichiosis** (tick bite, leukopenia, thrombocytopenia, ↑aminotransferases). Doxycycline AE: **Phototoxicity**, pts may have sudden-onset of redness and **rash after going in sun** with use.

Infectious

31) Bacterial Meningitis	32) Viral Meningitis	33) SAH
• ↑WBC >1000 PMNs • ↓glucose • ↑protein • CLOUDY	• ↑WBC Lymphs • normal glucose • normal/↑protein • CLEAR	• ↑↑RBC, ↑WBC • normal glucose • normal/↑protein • YELLOW/RED

34) Brain Abscess		
Infection of the brain parenchyma, with "ring-enhancing" lesion. Cx- strep, staph, anaerobes, often multiple organisms. Si/Sx- triad: HA, fever, and focal neurologic deficit. Seizures, ↑ICP and can lead to CNIII and CNVI deficits.	Types of Spread: • Direct spread- otitis media, mastoiditis, or dental infection. • Hematogenous spread- multiple abscesses at gray-white junction. • Direct inoculation head trauma, or neurosurgergical. Dx- ↑ESR, ↑CRP. CT scan shows ring-enhancing lesion. CSF analysis is not needed.	Tx- broad-spectrum IV abxs and surgical drainage. If <2cm may only need abxs alone. 3rd-generation cephalosporin, metronidazole and vancomycin IV for 6–8wks following by 2–3wks PO. In severe cases use dexamethasone (↓cerebral edema), and/or IV mannitol (↓ICP).

Infectious

35) HIV

Acquired Immune Deficiency Syndrome (AIDS). • **CD4+ count- degree** of immunosuppression. • **Viral load- rate** of progression, **RNA PCR** (viral load).	Assoc- **multiple sex partners**, unprotected sex, men having sex with men, IV drug abuse. Si/Sx- **asymp, flu-like illness;** nausea, vomiting, fever, pharyngitis, maculopapular rash, ↓weight, HA, lymphadenopathy, **"mononucleosis-like."**	Dx-**ELISA test** (↑sens, ↓spec) for **screening. Rapid HIV test** now available. **Western blot** (↓sens, ↑spec) **confirmatory.** **CCR5 mutation** gives resistance to HIV infx.

36) HIV

Tx- initial **3 meds:** 2 **NRTI** + 1 **NNRTI** or 1 **protease inhibitor.** **Protease inhibitor** AE: crystal induced nepropathy.	**Avoid efavirenz** in pregnancy. **Efavirenz** AE: **teratogenic,** insomnia, **bizarre dreams.** Tx- pts that are pregnant give **zidovudine (AZT)** intrapartum and also to infants postpartum for 6wk.	HIV pts should **NOT breastfeed** and it is an absolute contraindication. **Needle stick** from HIV pt: draw blood for HIV serology and start **three drug antiretroviral** prophylaxis.

37) Infx Risks of Low CD4+ Counts

• **CD4 >500** HSV, HZV, TB, Kaposi's sarcoma (HHV-8), vaginal candidiasis, hairy leukoplakia.	• **CD4 <200** PCP, toxoplasmosis, **cryptococcosis,** cryptosporidiosis, pneumonia, **PML (JC virus).**	• **CD4 <50** **MAC, CMV retinitis** (**painless, fluffy,** yellow-white patches and hemorrhages), histoplasmosis, CNS lymphoma.

Infectious

38) Prophylaxis for HIV

Vaccines:
MMR, pneumococcal vaccine in pts with CD4>200.

Annual **influenza** in all HIV pts.

• **Pneumocystis (PCP)**
CD4+<200
Tx- **TMP-SMX** (1st-line) or dapsone +/- pyrimethamine. Steroids ↓mortality in severe PCP infxs (PaO2<70).

• **Toxoplasma**
CD4+ <100
Tx- **TMP-SMX**

• **MAC**- CD4+<50-100 Tx- wkly azithro**mycin** or daily clarithro**mycin**.	• **HSV** Tx- acy**clovir**, famci**clovir**, or valacy**clovir**.
• **Candida**- esophagitis Tx- flucon**azole**, or **nystatin**.	• **Strep pneumonia** Tx- **pneumovax** (every 5yrs when CD4 <200).
• **TB**- PPD >5mm. Tx- **INH 9mos**, or rifampin +/- pyrazinamide 2mos. (Add **Vit B6/ pyridoxine** with INH)	• **Influenza** Tx- vaccine yrly.

39) PML (JC virus)

Progressive Multifocal Leukoencephalopathy (PML); **demyelination** disease of **white matter.**

Cx- **JC virus** (named after first pts to be discovered with disease).

Assoc- **HIV with CD4<200,** or pt that is immunosuppressed.

Si/Sx- hemiparesis, ataxia, aphasia, ↓cognition, visual field deficits.

Dx- CT or MRI shows **patchy, focal**, and **non-enhancing** lesions of the **white matter.**
Tx- underlying disease.

Clinical PEARL: Cryptosporidium parvum
Si/Sx- chronic diarrhea in HIV pts with **CD4<200.**
Dx-acid-fast stain shows **oocysts in stool.**

Infectious

40) Aspergillus (fungal)	41) Nocardiosis	42) Candidiasis
Si/Sx- cough, SOB. Dx **CXR shows cavitary lesion that "MOVES" with change in position.** **CT scan** shows pulmonary nodules with **"HALO sign"** or lesions with an air crescent. **KOH shows 45% angle branching septate hyphae.** Tx- **voriconazole (1st-line)**, amphotericin (AE nephrotoxicity).	Cx- Nocardia asteroides (found in **soil** worldwide). Assoc- **HIV,** lymphoma, pts that have had transplanted organs. Si/Sx- subacute pneumonia, CNS, and/or **cutaneous** manifestations. Dx- gram stain shows aerobic, **gram positive, "PARTIALLY ACID-FAST," BRANCHING Rods.** Tx- **TMP-SMX (1st-line).**	Cx- esophagitis, thrush. Si/Sx- soft white plaques **CAN rub off** (oral hairy leukoplakia **cannot** rub off). Dx- clinical, KOH show **pseudohyphae,** budding yeast. Tx- flucona**zole,** clotrima**zole,** or **nystatin.**
43) Blastomycosis (fungal)	44) Bacillary angiomatosis	45) Other Opportunists Infxs
Si/Sx- cough, SOB, flu-like, **bone lesions, SKIN ulcers;** initially papulopustular => become **crusted, heaped up and warty,** with a violaceous hue. Assoc- OHIO Dx- **Broad-based budding** yeast. Tx-**itraconazole,** amphotericin B.	Cx- **Bartonella** henselae, **Bartonella** quintana (gram neg bacillus) Si/Sx- **"BRIGHT RED,"** firm friable, exophytic nodules. Pt may have fever, ↓weight, malaise, abd pain, **skin lesions and viscera.** Assoc-**AIDS,** chemo pts, organ transplant recipients. Dx- tissue biopsy, **"risk of hemorrhage."** Tx- oral **erythromycin** (1st-line).	• **Cryptococcus** Cx- meningitis Dx- CSF cultures **encapsulated yeast.** Tx- IV **amphotericin + flucytosine.** • **Mucor** Cx-sinusitis Dx- irregular broad **non-septate** hyphae, **WIDE-angle** branching. Tx: **amphotericin B + incision and drainage.**

Infectious

46) Cryptococcal Meningitis (fungal)	47) Coccidioidomycosis	
Risk factors: **AIDS pts** (CD4 <200), exposure to **pigeon droppings.**	**"San Joaquin Valley Fever"**	Dx- **bronchoalveolar lavage** with fungal culture of sputum. If severe and serology indeterminate do **bronchoscopy with fine-needle biopsy.**
Si/Sx- HA, fever, neck stiffness, nausea, vomiting.	Pulm **fungal** infxs found in southwest U.S. (Arizona, California).	
Dx- **LP CSF** ↓glucose, ↑**protein,** ↑leukocyte, ↑↑open pressure, **ENCAPSULATED** yeast.	Cx- coccidioides immitis.	If **titers are >1:16** most likely disseminated infx.
India-ink stain, fungal culture, +**CSF cryptococcal antigen test.**	Si/Sx- recent travel hx, HA, fever, dyspnea, **dry cough, night sweats,** flulike illness, and/or pleuritic chest pain.	**CXR** may be normal, or may show hilar adenopathy, cavity, or nodules.
Tx- **IV amphotericin B** + **flucytosine** x 2wks. Lifelong fluconazole (or until CD4 >200 for 6mos).	Pt may have **erythema multiforme** (common on hands and feet) erythema nodosum, arthralgias, soft tissue infxs, or bone lesions.	Tx- PO fluconazole or itraconazole for mild infx. For severe infx use **IV amphotericin.**

Infectious

48) Histoplasmosis (fungal)		49) CMV
Dimorphic fungus found as mold in soil. Risk factors: **Spelunking, bird or BAT droppings. Ohio, Mississippi rivers,** and Central America. Assoc- **AIDS** pts (CD4<50). Si/Sx- asymp or flu-like; fever, dyspnea, cough. Disseminated **palatal ulcers, hepato-splenomegaly, lymphadenopathy.** Dx- **CXR** shows **nodular densities** that are diffused. Disseminated infxs may have pancytopenia.	Dx- order **urine** or serum **polysaccharide antigen test.** Yeast form shows **SILVER stain** on lymph node biopsy or broncho-alveolar lavage. Pt may have pancytopenia, ↑LFTs, ↑ferritin. Tx- supportive for mild pulm infx. **Itraconazole (1st-line)** For severe infxs **amphotericin B** for 3–10days followed by **itraconazole** for 12wks. If there are cavitary lesions give **itraconazole >1yr.**	**Cytomegalovirus (CMV)** Risk factors: Immunocompromised pts, unprotected sex, **breast milk**, daycare facilities, blood transfusions. Si/Sx- **retinitis, GI symps, bloody diarrhea,** pneumonitis (fever, cough, sputum). **Encephalitis** in HIV when CD4+ <50. Dx- culture, **serum PCR.** CT or MRI of head may show periventricular calcifications. Tx- ganciclovir or **foscarnet.**

Infectious

50) MAC		51) Toxoplasmosis
Mycobacter Avium Complex (MAC) Assoc- COPD, TB, or CF, **AIDS (CD4<50),** healthy nonsmokers (Lady Windermere syndrome). Si/Sx- SOB, weakness, anemia, fever, ↓weight, lymphadenopathy, hepatosplenomegaly.	Dx- blood cultures, ↑**AlkPh,** ↑**LDH.** Biopsy shows **foamy macrophages** with **acid-fast bacilli.** Tx- **ethambutol** and clarithromycin +/- **rifabutin** and **HAART** for >12mo and until CD4>100 for 6mo. Prevention: Weekly **azithromycin** if CD4<50.	Risk- **CAT litter, RAW undercooked meat.** "Don't change kitty litter while pregnant." Assoc: AIDS, pregnancy, immunosuppressed. Si/Sx- asymp, **encephalitis in AIDS** have fever, HA, **AMS,** seizures.
52) Toxoplasmosis	53) Pneumoncystic Jiroveci (PCP)	
Dx- **serology, PCR.** CT scan show **multiple HYPODENSE, ring-enhancing** lesions. MRI may show lesions in **basal ganglia.** Tx- PO **sulfadiazine-pyrimethamine,** and leukovorin for 4-8wks. If pt does not improve R/O CNS lymphoma. Prophylaxis: **TMP-SMX** or **pyrimethamine + dapsone** for pts with CD4+ <100 and +Toxo IgG.	Risk factor: **AIDS,** impaired immunity. Si/Sx- fever, nonproductive cough, dyspnea on exertion, impaired O_2. Dx-**ABG, CXR** shows **bilateral, diffused infiltrates** with ground-glass appearance.	**Bronchoalveolar lavage (BAL);** cystology from **bronchoscopy** with **silver stain** and **immunofluorescence** (diagnosis). Tx- high dose **TMP-SMX** for 21days. If pt has sulfa allergy use **clindamycin and primaquine.** Pts with severe hypoxemia (PaO_2<70) give **prednisone.**

Infectious

54) Neurocysticercosis

Cx- **Taenia solium** (pork **tapeworm/** parasitic).	Si/Sx- **immigrant** (Mexico) with a NEW-onset of **seizure.**	Dx- positive enzyme linked immunotransfer blot assay in CSF.
Assoc- **eating pork** or vegetables irrigated with **contaminated water,** or in area where **"PIGS" are raised.**	Dx- **CT scan** of head may show **multiple, small** (usually <1cm), **"FLUID-filled cysts"** in brain parenchyma.	Tx- **albendazole** (use bendazole for bending tapeworm infxs), glucocorticoids, surgery if cysts are located.

55) Syphilis

Cx- Treponema pallidum (spirochete). • **Primary** Si/Sx- **"CHANCRE,"** a **painLESS ulcer.** (appears 10–90 days after infx). • **Secondary Early latent <1yr,** no symp, **+serology.** **Late latent >1yr,** no symp, +/- serology.	• **Secondary** Si/Sx- low grade fever, lymphadenopathy, maculopapular **RASH** on face, trunk, extremities, **soles and palms.** **Condylomata lata** (verrucous lesions) 4–8wks after **chancre** disappears.	• **Tertiary** (1-20yrs) Si/Sx- granulomatous **GUMMAS** (soft, noncancerous growth), aortic root aneurysms. **Neurosyphilis;** meningitis, **Argyll Robertson pupil** (accommodate but don't react), **tabes dorsalis** (post column degeneration).

56) Syphilis

Dx • **VDRL/RPR** for screening **(rapid and cheap).** Pts that have AIDS with **+RPR** r/o neurosyphilis. • **FTA-ABS** (confirms diagnosis).	• **Dark-Field microscopy** identifies spirochetes (in primary and secondary syphilis).	**False+ VDRL:** • **V-** Viruses • **D-** Drugs • **R-** Rheumatic fever • **R-** Rheumatoid (RA) • **L-** Leprosy • **L-** SLE

121

Infectious

57) Syphilis Tx

Tx **Benzathine Penicillin IM x 1day** (primary and secondary syphilis). For penicillin-allergic pts give **azithromycin** (single dose). Can also use **tetracycline,** or **doxycycline** for 14 days.	• **Pregnant** and tertiary syphilis must be **desenitized for penicillin.** • **Latent- benzathine penicillin** 1x weekly x 3weeks. • **Neurosyphilis** penicillin **IV.**	• **Jarisch-Herxheimer Reaction** may follow tx which is a acute flulike illness, HA, myalgias in **first 24hrs** of therapy.

58) Chlamydia

Most common bacterial **STD** infx. Cx- Chlamydia trachomatis. Risk factors: unprotected sex, multiple sex partners. Assoc- **coexist with gonorrhoeae** infxs.	Si/Sx- asymp, **adnexal tenderness,** painless, papule, ulcer, **lymphogranuloma venereum** (infx of the lymphatics), or anal pruritus. Pts can also have mucopurulent **urethritis, cervicitis,** or **PID.**	**Clinical PEARL: Chlamydial Urethritis** (most common urethritis) Assoc- ↑sex partners. Si/Sx- **mucopurulent urethral discharge,** dysuria, urinary frequency. Dx- U/A shows absent bacteriuria, ↑WBCs.

59) Chlamydia

Dx- clinical, **culture** (gold standard), **gram stain** may show **PMNs,** but no bacteria because infx is **intracellular.** **Screen-** all sexually active pts that are under <24 yo.	Tx Azithromycin x1day or doxycycline BID x7days. In pregnant pts use **erythromycin.** Treat pts at the same time for **N. gonorrhea** with **ceftriaxone** or cefepime. **Sexual partners** should also be treated for **both chlamydia and gonorrhea.**	Comp: • **PID** • **Ectopic pregnancy** • **Reiter's syndrome** Si/Sx- conjunctivitis, urethritis, arthritis. **"Cannot see, pee, or climb a tree."** • **Fitz-Hugh-Curtis syndrome** Si/Sx- perihepatic inflam and fibrosis.

Infectious

60) Gonorrhea

Cx- **N. gonorrhoeae** (gram neg intracellular diplococcus) Si/Sx- **greenish-yellow discharge**, adnexal pain, dysuria, purulent urethral discharge (in men). Dx- **gram stain** and **culture** (gold standard).	**Clinical PEARL: Disseminated Gonorrhea** Si/Sx- fever, chills, triad: • **Migratory polyarthralgias** • **Tenosynovitis** • **RASH**/ skin lesions (vesiculopustular).	Dx- **nucleic acid amplification test** of vaginal tissue or urine. Tx- **ceftriaxone** IM or cefepime PO x 1dose. Pts with septic arthritis give ceftriaxone (1st-line). Also treat coinfection **chlamydia** with **azithromycin** x1day or **doxycycline** BID x7days.

61) Urinary Tract Infections (UTI)

Ascending urinary tract infection. Cx- **E. Coli** (most common, 80%), enterobacter, serratia, saprophyticus (sex), klebsiella, **proteus,** pseudomonas. **Proteus-** produce urease, which makes **urine alkaline ↑pH.** Risk- care facilities.	**Risk factors:** ↑ **sexual intercourse** (most common), previous UTIs, pyelonephritis, pregnancy, catheters, vesicoureteral reflux (VUR), DM, BPH.	Si/Sx- urgency, dysuria, frequency, **suprapubic pain,** foul-smelling urine. Child may present with **bed-wetting.** Comp- **acute pyelonephritis**.

Infectious

62) Urinary Tract Infections (UTI)		
Dx- clinical, **U/A** check for ↑ **leukocyte esterase** (WBCs), ↑ **nitrites** (bacteria). ↑ **urine pH** (**proteus**), and **hematuria** (possibly cystitis). **Urine culture** is the gold standard. Also r/o bacteremia.	Tx • **Uncomplicated UTI**: PO **TMP-SMX**, or fluoroquinolone x3day, **nitrofurantoin** x7days. • **Complicated UTI:** same tx but **7–14 days.**	Tx • Pregnant pts give 7 day course of **amoxicillin, nitrofurantoin** or **cephalosporin**. • In pregnancy avoid fluoroquinolones, tetracyclines, and TMP-SMX.
63) Pyelonephritis		
Si/Sx- dysuria, urgency, frequency, UTI. **"FLANK pain," fever, chills,** nausea, vomit. Dx **U/A and culture,** look for **WBC CASTS.** **Blood cultures** to r/o urosepsis. **U/S scan** to r/o obstruction. **CT scan** is test of choice (imaging is not needed to diagnose).	Tx- blood cultures first followed by abxs. ↑ **PO fluids** and **fluoroquinolones** (1st-line). **Cephalosporins, carbapenem**, or beta-lactam/lactamase inhibitors (2nd-line). If pt is **pregnant** or has other underlying illness **admit and give IV abxs.** If pt does not respond to abxs after **48-72hrs** order **renal U/S** to r/o obstruction or abscess.	**Clinical PEARL: Interstitial Cystitis** Si/Sx- urinary urgency, frequency, pelvic pain, relieved by voiding. Dx- **CYSTOSCOPY** shows submucosal petechiae or ulcers. Tx- **TMP/SMX** or **nitrofurantoin** (**1st-line**), fluoroquinolone (for complicated cystitis)

Infectious

64) Sepsis

Systemic Inflammatory Response Syndrome (**SIRS**). Si/Sx- **abrupt fever, chills,** tachycardia, tachypnea, and AMS. **Neonatal sepsis** Si/Sx- ill-appearing, jaundice, hypothermia, lethargy, poor feeding.	• **Septic shock WARM** skin, hypotension. • **Cardio shock COLD** skin. • **Gram Positive shock** (staph, strep) 2nd to fluid loss by **EXOtoxins.**	• **Gram NEG shock** (E. coli, klebsiella, proteus, and pseudomonas) 2nd to vasodilation by **ENDOtoxins (lipopolysaccharide).** • **Neonates shock GBS, E. coli**, listeria.

65) Sepsis

• **Severe sepsis** Sepsis with hypotension and **organ dysfunction.** Dx- **culture ALL;** blood, sputum, CSF, wound, and urine. Labs may show ↑bands, leukocytosis, thrombocytopenia, ↑LFTs, ↑BUN/Cr (all signs of ↓tissue perfusion).	Tx- Maintain BP and perfusion to end organs; **IV fluids, pressors, empiric abxs.** Remove infected lines and possibly foley catheter.	Dx- **2+** of following: • **Temp** >101.3, < 95F • **Pulse** >90/min • **Resp** >20/min • **WBC** >12,000, <4000 or >10% bands.

Infectious

66) Malaria (protozoal)		
Bite from female **anopheles mosquito** that carries the protozoa. Cx- **Plasmodium**; vivax, ovale, malariae, and Falciparum (most Fatal). Comp- hemolytic anemia, pulm edema, coma. ATN **"blackwater fever"** (dark urine).	Si/Sx- recent hx of travel, nausea, vomiting, HA, malaise and myalgia are commonly seen. **Periodic attacks of CHILLS and FEVER** (>41C). Pt are asymp between attacks for 2-3 days. Pt get **anemia and splenomegaly** within four days of onset of infection. Dx- **Giemsa- and Wright** for strain and degree of parasitemia.	Tx- **chloroquine** (standard treatment) or atovaquone/proguanil. ↑**Resistance use mefloquine** or doxycycline (Sub-Saharan Africa, India, Pakistan, and Bangladesh). **P. vivax, P. ovale dormant in liver.** Chloroquine resistant use **primaquine.** Sever infection use **IV quinidine.** Newer combo **proguanil/ atovaquone.**
67) Pinworm (parasite)		
Cx- **Enterobius vermicularis** (most common helminthic infection in the U.S.) Female migrate at night from cecum or appendix => to **rectum** onto perianal skin to deposit eggs.	Si/Sx- nocturnal **perianal pruritus.** Pt may also have abd pain, nausea, vomiting, or **vulvovaginitis.**	Dx **"SCOTCH TAPE"** test which demonstrates the presence of **pinworms.** Tx- Al**bendazole** or me**bendazole** **(1st-line), pyrantel pamoate** is alternative.

Infectious

68) Trichinellosis (parasite)		69) Hydatid Cysts (parasite)
Cx- trichinella (roundworm) Assoc- eating **undercooked PORK.** Si/Sx- abd pain, nausea, vomiting, diarrhea, **"SPLINTER"** hemorrhages, **retinal hemorrhages.** **"Trichinellosis is tricky"** because it can look like endocarditis, with no valvular lesions.	Si/Sx periorbital edema, and chemosis, muscle pain, weakness. Triad: • **Periorbital edema** • **Myositis** • **Eosinophilia** Dx- ↑Eosinophilia.	Cx- **Echinococcus granulosus** (tapeworm) Assoc-contact with **DOGS, sheep breeder.** Si/Sx- **asymp,** RUQ pain. Dx- U/S or CT shows **"EGGSHELL" Ca** of **hydatid cysts** (fluid-filled cyst) in liver. Tx- surgical resection under the coverage of **albendazole.**

70) Sporotrichosis (fungal)	71) Animal or Human Bites	72) Actinomycosis
Cx- Sporothrix schenckii (found in bark of trees, shrubs, garden plants) Assoc- **GARDENERS** (thorn prick). Si/Sx- initial lesion is a **reddish nodule** that becomes **ulcerated.** Dx-clinical Tx- **itraconazole (1st-line), fluconazole.** Severe infxs use IV amphotericin B with flucytosine (sporotrichosis meningitis).	Cx- **polymicrobial** (gram+, gram neg, and anaerobes) Assoc- **"fight bite,"** clenched fist injury into someones mouth is also a bite wound of the hand. **Dog or cat bites.** Tx- **Amoxicillin-Clavulanate (1st-line)** prophylaxis/treatment. **Clinical PEARL: Cat-Scratch Disease** Si/Sx- scratches, **not bite.** Cx-Bartonella henselae. Tx- **Azithromycin.**	Cx **Actinomyces israelii** (anaerobic, gram+, **branching bacteria**). Si/Sx- **cervical-facial,** thoracic, or abd are common infected areas. Non-tender, indurated mass that **DRAINS yellow fluid.** Dx- fluid contains **SULFUR granules** (yellow). Tx-**high-dose penicillin** for 6-12wks.

Infectious

73) FEVER of Unknown Origin		74) Neutropenic Fever
Cx- **infxs and cancer** (>60%). • **Infectious** Osteomyelitis, endocarditis, TB, dengue fever (watch for hemorrhagic shock), abscess, catheter. HIV; MAC, CMV, lymphoma. • **Autoimmune** SLE, cryoglobulinemia, PAN's, sarcoidosis, Still's disease (inflam arthritis).	• **Neoplastic** Hepatic, renal cell CA, lymphomas, leukemias. • **Other Cx** Drug fever, PE, alcoholic hepatitis, factitious fever. Dx-CBC, blood/sputum gram stain and culture, U/A. CT chest and abd. Tx- **stop unnecessary meds**. Treat underlying disease.	**Common in cancer** pts that are undergoing chemotherapy. Dx- CBC with differential, BUN/Cr, **culture sputum, blood, urine, stool, wound.** Avoid rectal exam, due to risk of bleeding. Tx- empiric abxs; **cefepime.** If fever persists >72hrs after abxs, start antifungal tx.
75) RASH and FEVER	**76) Mononucleosis "KISSING dz"**	
"Tiny **GERMS**" T- **Typhoid** Fever G- **Gonococcemia** E- **Endocarditis** R- **Rocky** Mountain Spotted Fever M- **Meningococcemia** S- **Sepsis** (bacterial) **Clinical PEARL: Unilateral Cervical Lymphadenitis** Cx- staphylococcus aureus (most common), GAS (group A strep). Si/Sx- tender, warm, erythematous, enlarged lymph node.	Cx- **EBV** Si/Sx- triad; • **Fever** • **Pharyngitis** • **Posterior cervical lymphadenopathy** Pts may also have bilateral upper eyelid edema, tonsillitis, and **tonsillar exudates.** **2-3wks** after initial onset pts can get **autoimmune hemolytic anemia** and thrombocytopenia. Comp- **SPLENIC rupture,** airway obstruction, CNS infxs.	Risk- **maculopapular RASH with ampicillin**. Dx- **Heterophilic antibody (Monospot) test.** EBV-specific antibodies can be ordered. If **NEG** monospot and EBV antibody, **"think CMV."** Assoc- **IgM cold agglutinin antibodies** (Coombs'-test positive). Tx- supportive. Advise pt to **avoid CONTACT SPORTS** to prevent splenic rupture until pt has a normal physical exam.

USMLE FINAL REVIEW STEP 2&3

Infectious

77) Lyme Disease

Cx- **Ixodes** tick-borne disease caused by spirochete **Borrelia burgdorferi.** Si/Sx- hx of **camping, HIKING** in woods, **fever, rash,** with or without recall of tick bite (most pts do not remember tick bite). **Clinical PEARL:** If pt has **tick bite** and **SPLENECTOMY,** think **"Babesiosis"** (parasite Babesia), **NOT** lymes disease.	Si/Sx **Erythema migrans; "BULL's EYE" rash.** If disease disseminates pts may get **"BELL's PALSY" (CNVII),** meningitis, polyarthropathies. Late in disease pts may have **waxing and waning monoarthritis** or oligoarthritis and/or **encephalitis.**	Dx- **erythema migrans** (bull's eye rash) **ELISA** (screen), **western blot** (confirm). **tissue culture PCR.** Tx **DOXYCYCLINE.** **Children <9mos** or if pt is **pregnant** give **amoxicillin.** If severe with arthritis or CNS finding give **ceftriaxone.** The best way to remove tick is with **tweezers.**

78) Rocky Mountain Spotted Fever / 79) Anthrax

78) Rocky Mountain Spotted Fever	79) Anthrax	
Cx- **rickettsia rickettsii** carried by **dog tick**=> small vessel vasculitis. Si/Sx- fever, HA, and **petechial rash** starts on WRISTS and ANKLES => **spread central**. Dx- clinical, indirect immunofluorescence (confirms diagnosis). Tx- **doxycycline** or chloramphenicol. Begin tx while awaiting for labs, disease is rapidly fatal.	Cx- **bacillus anthracis** (spore-forming gram+) Assoc- **farmers, veterinarians,** contact with animal wool. Si/Sx: • **Inhalation** Si/Sx- fever, dyspnea, hypoxia, hypotension (due to **hemorrhagic mediastinitis**). • **Cutaneous** Si/Sx-pruritic papule=> **"Black ESCHAR"** in 7–10 days.	• **GI infx** Si/Sx- GI upset from **poorly cooked,** contaminated meat. Dx- occupation, CXR may show **wide mediastinum.** Aerobic culture and gram stain of **ulcer exudate.** Tx- **ciprofloxacin** or doxycycline. Prophylaxis for postexposure-**ciprofloxacin.**

Infectious

80) Infective Endocarditis		
Cx • **ACUTE** Staph aureus (normal valve). • **Subacute** Viridans group strep (preexist valvular disease). Locations: • **Mitral valve** (most common, LEFT sided murmur, mitral regurgitation, murmur ↑ expiration). • **Tricuspid valve** (IV drug abuse, murmur ↑ inspiration).	Risk factors: **Rheumatic fever,** congenital infx, IV drug abuse, prosthetic valve, AIDS, organ transplant. Assoc: • **GI malignancy (strep bovis)** • **UTI, pyelonephritis (Enterococci)** • **URI (GAS/viridans strep; S. mutans)** • **Skin infx** (staph)	Si/Sx- fatigue, fever, weight loss, **migratory polyarthritis, sydenham chorea,** subcutaneous nodules, erythema marginatum, **NEW heart murmur.** **Clinical PEARL: Right sided heart lesions** (IV drug abuse) can give **septic emboli,** resulting in multiple cavitations and nodules in lungs.

81) Infective Endocarditis		
Si/Sx • **Janeway lesions (painless,** peripheral hemorrhages) • **Roth's spots** (retinal hemorrhages) • **Splinter hemorrhages** (subungual petechiae) • **Osler's nodes (painful,** tender nodules finger and toe pads)	Dx- **duke criteria,** CBC, blood cultures, ↑ESR. Rising titers of **anti-DNase B, antistreptolysin O, antihyaluronidase.** **Clinical PEARL: Septic emboli to spleen** from endocarditis. Si/Sx- fever, chills, LUQ pain, and **splenic fluid collection.**	Tx- Start antibiotics **after blood cultures** have been done with IV **vancomycin** or **nafcillin + gentamicin.** Prophylaxis- with **penicillin** to prevent further attacks.

Infectious

82) Duke Criteria (Endocarditis)		83) Endocarditis
MAJOR Criteria:	**MINOR Criteria:**	**JR. has NO FAME**
• **2+ cultures** • **Bacteremia** • **1+culture coxiella** burnetii • **Carditis** • **Polyarthritis** • **Chorea** • **RASH** (erythema marginatum) • **Subcutaneous** nodules	• **Predisposing RISK** • **Fever** • **Vascular- janeway** lesions, septic emboli, infarct, aneurysm. • **Immunologic-** osler's nodes, roth's spots, glomerulonephritis. • **↑PR interval**	**J-** Janeway lesions **R-** Roth's spots **N- Nail bed** (splinter) **O- Osler's** nodes **F- Fever** **A- Anemia** **M- Murmur** **E- Emboli**
84) Orbital Celluitis		
Infx of **paranasal sinuses** that can lead to blindness. Cx- strep, staph (MRSA), H influenzae. In **diabetics**; **mucormycosis** (**rhizopus** species).	Si/Sx- acute **fever, ocular pain, proptosis, ↓EOM.** Pt may have hx of **sinusitis or ocular trauma.** **Mucor (rhizopus)** are often assoc with **cavernous sinus thrombosis.** Dx- **clinical,** CT not needed for diagnosis, but used to r/o oral abscess.	Tx- **IV abxs** and **ophthalmologic** consult. For diabetic give **amphotericin B and surgical debridement** if mucor/rhizopus. **Clinical PEARL:** Every case **leukocoria "WHITE REFLEX in EYE"** is **Retinoblastoma,** until proven otherwise. Prompt referral to ophthalmologist.
85) Dacryocystitis		
Infection of **lacrimal sac=> blocking tear duct.** Cx- staph, strep. Si/Sx- painful, swelling over **inner aspect of the eye.**	Si/Sx- pt may have tenderness, edema redness, over medial canthus, **excessive TEARING** and mucoid material secretions. Dx- clinical Tx-massage, clensing eyelid 3x daily.	**Clinical PEARL: Adenoid Cystic CA** Salivary glands tumor of oral cavity. Dx- **CT mass in** lacrimal gland.

Infectious

86) Infectious Conjunctivitis		87) Bacterial Conjunctivitis
Inflammation of the **conjunctiva.** Cx- bacterial, viral, allergic, chemical, or fungal. Dx- clinical Tx- abx drops or abx ointment. R/O **corneal abrasion**; inspection of eye, with topical anesthetic (**tetracaine**), with fundoscopy and **fluorescein slip-lamp exam.**	**Clinical PEARL: Herpes Simplex Keratitis** Most common corneal blindness in U.S. Si/Sx- pain, redness, photophobia, blurred visioin, and tearing. Dx- **corneal "VESICLES"** and **dendritic ulcers.** Tx- antiviral therapy (oral or topical).	Cx- **staph, strep,** pseudomonas, haemophilus. Si/Sx- **unilateral, MUCOPURULENT discharge,** sensation of foreign body in eye. Dx- **clinical,** gram stain and culture if severe. Tx- abx drops or abx ointment; **sulfa ophthalmic** drops. **Erythromycin** ointment (best for children) or quinolones (2nd-line).
88) Chlamydia Conjuctivitis		
Cx- **C. trachoma.** Most common **neonatal** conjunctivitis. Si/Sx- **keratitis,** possibly corneal scarring. In newborns develops **>5 DAYS after birth** with **purulent discharge.**	Dx- **Giemsa stain,** chlamydial cultures. Follicular conjunctivitis and neovascularization formation in **cornea.**	Tx- **oral azithromycin, erythromycin,** or tetracycline. Oral treatment is given to lower the risk of **chlamydial pneumonia.**

Infectious

89) N. Gonorrhea Conjunctivitis	90) Viral Conjunctivitis	91) Allergic Conjunctivitis
Cx- N. Gonorrhea	Cx- adenovirus	Cx- allergies, seasonal.
Si/Sx- copious amount of **purulent drainage** in **NEWBORN** that is **TWO to FIVE days old.**	Si/Sx- hx URI, **bilateral, "WATERY"** **discharge,** preauricular lymphadenopathy, sandy feeling.	Si/Sx- **bilateral, RED eyes,** pruritus, burning, with **watery discharge**. Assoc- **asthma**.
Dx- gram stain shows gram neg, intracellular. Culture should be performed on **Thayer-Martin media.** Tx- **emergency** due to possible blindness, give **PO ciprofloxacin, ofloxacin,** or IM ceftriaxone.	Dx- clinical Tx- **self-limiting** (viral conjunctivitis is **contagious**)	Dx- clinical, eye exam may show **chemosis**, large **cobblestone**-appearing **papillae** on upper tarsal conjunctiva. Tx- topical **anti-histamines, ketotifen** (mast cell stabilizer).

92) Allergic Rhinitis		
Si/Sx- itchy, watery eyes, **CLEAR NASAL discharge,** during spring and fall seasons. Pts may have swollen inferior turbinates, and/or boggy nasal mucosa. Assoc- **allergic conjunctivitis**.	Dx- clinical, **nasal smear has EOSINOPHILS** (characteristic). If severe order CT scan of sinuses. Tx- intranasal **glucocorticoids,** oral **antihistamine** (loratadine), or **phenylephrine** spray (nasal vasoconstrictor).	Tx Pt that fail to respond, give short course of **10-day oral glucocorticoids.** **Clinical PEARL: Pseudo-Allergic Reaction** Cx- **ASPIRIN** Si/Sx- breathing difficulty, **wheezing,** persistent **nasal blockage.** Tx- d/c aspirin.

Infectious

93) Otitis Externa "Swim Ear"		
Inflammation of **EXTERNAL auditory canal**. Cx- **Pseudomonas** (most common), enterobacteriaceae. Si/Sx- **purulent discharge, pruritus,** PAIN with movement of **tragus/pinna** (with otitis media no pain of tragus/pinna).	Dx- clinical. Tx Abxs and steroid eardrops. **Pseudomonas** infxs **ciprofloxacin** (1st-line). Can also use **cefepime**, or **piperacillin-tazobactam**.	**Clinical PEARL Malignant Otitis Externa** Assoc- **DIABETIC** Cx- **Pseudomonas** Si/Sx- granulation tissue in ear canal, ear pain and drainage. Dx- CT or MRI (confirm diagnosis) Tx- **ciprofloxacin** (1st-line).
94) Osteomyelitis		
Bone infx secondary to: Cx- **staph aureus** (most common). • **IV drugs** (staph, pseudomonas) • **Sickle cell** (**Salmonella,** staph) • **Hip replace** (staph epidermidis) • **Foot wound** (**pseudomonas**) • **Diabetic** (polymicrobial, pseudomonas, staph, strep, anaerobes)	• **Direct spread** soft tissue infx (**80%** cases). • **Hematogenous** Seeding (20%) **IV drugs (vertebral bodies).** Si/Sx- +/- fever, chills, **localized bone pain** and tenderness. Dx-↑WBC, ↑**CRP,** ↑**ESR>100,** +/- blood cultures, **bone aspiration** with gram stain and culture (definitive dx). **XR** may show **"PERIOSTEAL" Elevation.** MRI (test of choice).	Tx **Surgical debridement** followed by **IV abxs** for 4–6wk; **clindamycin +** ciprofloxacin, ampicillin/sulbactam, or oxacillin/nafcillin. Pseudomonas infx give **cefepime** or **piperacillin-tazobactam**. Comp: **Marjolin's ulcer** (squamous-cell CA).

Infectious

95) Type of Vaccinations		
• LIVE- MMR, polio (sabin), yellow fever, influenza (nasal spray). • KILLED- cholera, influenza, HAV, polio (SalK), rabies, influenza (injection). • Subunit- HBV, pertussis, strep pneumoniae, HPV, meningococcus. • Toxoid- diphtheria, tetanus. • Conjugate- Hib, strep pneumoniae	• Td- tetanus diphtheria toxoid • TIG- tetanus immune globulin Tetanus Prophylaxis • Unimmunized or Last Td >10yrs: - Minor wound (TOXOID only) - Major wound (TOXOID, Globulin) • Last Td <10yrs: - Minor wounds (no toxoid) - Major wounds (TOXOID, if latest booster given >5yrs ago).	• DTaP- diphtheria, tetanus, pertussis • Hib- H influenzae B • PCV- pneumococcal (induces a T-cell independent B-cell response) • IPV- inactive poliovirus • MMR- measles, mumps, rubella. • HepA- hepatitis A • MCV-meningococcal Clinical PEARL: Tularemia Cx- Francisella tularensis. Si/Sx- rabbit bite, fever, ulcer, necrosis. Tx-streptomycin.

Infectious

96) Vaccination Birth–6 yrs	97) Vaccination 7–18 yrs	98) Vaccination 19–65 yrs
• **Hep B** Birth,1–2mos, 6–18mos	• **Hep B** • **IPV** • **MMR and** • **Varicella** 7–18yr (catch-up imm)	• **Hep B**- 3 doses • **HPV**-3 doses (females)
2, 4, 6 mos • **Rotavirus**- 2, 4, 6 mos • **DTaP**-2, 4, 6 mos • **Hib**- 2, 4, 6 mos • **PCV**- 2, 4, 6 mos • **IPV**-2, 4, 6 mos	• **HPV** • **DTaP** 11–12yr, 13–18yr (series)	• **DTaP**-1x dose, every 10yrs • **Hib**- 1 dose annually • **Influenza**- yrly
• **Hib** 2, 4, 6, 12–15mos	• **PCV** • **HepA** 7–18yr (if high risk)	• **PCV**-1 dose • **MMR**- 1 dose • **MCV**- 1 dose • **Zoster**- >60yr 1 dose
• **Influenza** 6mos, then **yrly**	• **Influenza**- yrly	• **Varicella**- 2 doses • **HepA**- 2 doses
• **MMR and** • **Varicella** 12–15 mos, 4–6yr (not before 1yo)	• **MCV** 7–10yr, 11–12yr, 13–18yr	
• **HepA** 12–23mos (2x's), 2–6yr		
• **MCV**- 2-6yr		
99) Vaccinations		
• **HepB**- pepatitis B • **DTaP**- diphtheria, tetanus, pertussis	• **PCV**- pneumococcal (induces a T-cell independent B-cell response) • **IPV**- inactive poliovirus	• **Hib**- H influenzae B • **MMR**- measles, mumps, rubella. • **HepA**- hepatitis A • **MCV**-meningococcal

10 CHAPTER
MUSCULOSKELETAL

Musculoskeletal		
1) Fractures		
• **BOXER's fracture**	• **COLLE's fracture**	• **ULNER fracture**
Fracture of the fifth metacarpal of the hand, from **"PUNCHING"** **a wall.** Tx- closed reduction, abxs; **amoxicillin-clavulanate.**	Fracture of distal **radius** from **"FALL on outstretched hand."** Tx- closed reduction with long-arm cast.	**Ulnar** shaft from **SELF-DEFENSE** against **blunt object.** Tx- open reduction and internal fixation.
2) Fractures		
• **HIP fracture** Cx- osteoporosis, displaced femoral neck. Comp- **avascular necrosis (AVN), DVT.** Tx- **arthroplasty** (hip replace). In elderly pts assess preoperative risk prior to surgical correction.	• **STRESS (hairline) fracture** Risk factors: athletes; dancers, runners, military recruits. Locations- 2nd **metatarsal** of foot, anterior **tibia** of leg. Dx- clinical, XR may look normal. Tx- **rest, analgesia,** hard-soled shoe.	• **FEMORAL fracture** Cx- direct trauma, motor vehicle accident (MVA). Comp- **"FAT emboli"** (fever, SOB, AMS, petechial rash). In **children** perform **skeletal survey** (70% are inflicted).

Musculoskeletal

3) Fractures

• **RIB fracture** Assoc- MVA Si/Sx- chest pain, hypoventilation. Dx- CXR Tx- **ensure appropriate analgesia** with NSAIDS or opiates to reduce the risk of atelectasis and pneumonia.	Comp:**"FLAIL Chest"** Si/Sx- chest retract on inspiration, bulge on expiration, the opposite of what it should do. Dx- positive pressure mechanical ventilation cx flail chest to **move normally**.	• **BURST fracture of vertebra** (anterior cord syndrome) Si/Sx- **loss of motor** function below level of lesion with **loss of pain and temp** on both sides. With intact proprioception. Dx- **CT scan of spine** shows burst fracture.

4) Fractures

• **HUMERUS fracture** **Radial nerve** fracture of midshaft of the humerus. Si/Sx- **WRIST drop,** loss of abduction of the thumb. Tx- splint and/or sling.	• **SCAPHOID fracture** Si/Sx- assume fracture if tender in **"SNUFF BOX."** Dx- **normal XR,** can take up to 10 days to show abn on XR. Tx- **thumb spica cast** and repeat XR in 2wks.	• **PENILE fracture** Risk- intercourse with female on top. Tx- surgical emergency retrograde urethrogram followed by surgical exploration of penis. **Clinical PEARL Amputation injury** Tx- wrap in saline moistened gauze, sealed in plastic bag, placed on ice.

Musculoskeletal

5) Fractures		
• **Osteogenesis Imperfecta (AD)** Mutation in **type 1** collagen. Si/Sx- **BLUE sclera, HEARING loss**, joint laxity, short stature, scoliosis, **reccurent fractures.**	• **De Quervain Tenosynovitis** New mothers who hold their new infants with **thumb outstretched (abducted/extended).** Si/Sx- pain on lateral side of wrist from holding baby.	• **Morton Neuroma** (enlarged nerve in third inerspace of foot) Si/Sx- **pain** between **third and fourth toes.** • **Clubfoot** (talipes equinovarus) Si/Sx- at birth of infant. Tx- stretching, manipulation, and **reassurance.**
6) MCL	**7) ACL**	**8) PCL**
Medial Collateral Ligament (MCL) Most common injured ligament of knee. Cx- **abduction** of knee. Si/Sx- **swollen joint.** Dx- **MRI** (best test). Tx- bracing, early ambulation. Surgery is rarely required.	**Anterior Cruciate Ligament (ACL)** Cx-**hyperextension**, or impact to extended knee. Dx- **+ANTERIOR Draw Test**. Tx- graft	**Posterior Cruciate Ligament (PCL)** Cx- **hyperextension.** Dx- **+POSTERIOR Draw Test**. Tx- none, unless severe.
9) Meniscal Tear (Knee Injuries)		
Si/Sx **Twisting injury** to the knee when the foot is planted. Pain is not severe enough to stop activities.	Si/Sx Pt may feel a **"POPPING"** sensation at time of injury. **Clicking** or **locking** may be found on exam. Pt may also have **pain with squatting.**	Dx- **+McMurray test** (pop or click with flex or extension of the jt). Tx- none.

Musculoskeletal

10) Rotator Cuff Tears	11) Compartment Syndrome	
Tendons of muscles: • **Supraspinatus** (most common injured) • **Infraspinatus** • **Teres minor** • **Subscapularis** Cx- FALL on outstretched hands. Si/Sx severe **shoulder pain,** edema following traumatic event. Unable to **abduct arm past 90 degress.** Dx- "+**DROP ARM**" **Sign**; arm drops rapidly when near the **90 degree position.**	↑**Pressure** that compromises nerve, muscle, and soft tissue => soft tissue swelling. Risk factor: burn, crush injuries. Si/Sx- **6P's** P- **Pain** P- **Pallor** P- **Paresthesias** P- **Paralysis** P- **Pulselessness** P- **Poikilothermia**	Comp- **Volkmann's contracture** (dead muscle has been replaced with fibrous tissue). Dx- measure compartment pressure (normal >**30mmHg**). Tx- **emergent FASCIOTOMY.**
12) Shoulder Dislocation		**13) Hip Dislocation**
• **ANTERIOR dislocation** (most common) Si/Sx- arm will be **abduction** and **external rotation.** Pts has arm held close to body and forearm **rotated OUTWARD as if preparing to "SHAKE hands."** Comp- **AXILLARY** artery and nerve injury.	• **Posterior dislocation** (rare) Assoc- **SEIZURES (tonic-clonic).** Si/Sx- arm will be **adducted** and **internal rotation.** Dx- clinical Tx- sling.	• **POSTERIOR dislocation** (most common) Risk- **sciatic nerve** injury and avascular necrosis (AVN). • **Anterior dislocation** Risk- possibly injure **obturator nerve.** Dx-clinical Tx- **closed reduction** and CT scan, followed by abduction bracing.

Musculoskeletal

14) Tendinitis	15) Bursitis	16) Carpal Tunnel Syndrome
Inflam commonly to the supraspinatus, wrists, patellar, and achilles **tendons.**	**Inflam of BURSA** from repetitive use, infx, trauma, or systemic inflam.	Inflam of the wrist leading to **median nerve** entrapment at the wrist.
Risk facotr: **Fluroquinolones** ↑risk of **tendon rupture** and tendinitis.	Si/Sx- localized tenderness, edema, ↓ROM, and erythema.	Si/Sx- aching, paresthesia, and numbness over **thenar area** of hand that is **worse at night.**
Si/Sx- **pain at tendon insertion** that is worse with **repetitive movement and stress.**	Dx- clinical, **normal XR.** Needle aspiration if septic bursitis is suspected.	Dx- clinical; • **Phalen's maneuver** (wrist flex) • **Tinel's sign** (tap wrist)
Dx- clinical, radiographics. Tx- **rest, NSAIDs, ICE 24–48hrs,** splint, strength exercises. NEVER inject achilles tendon.	Tx- **NSAIDs, rest, ice,** possibly intrabursal **corticosteroid injections.** Abxs for septic bursitis for 7–10 days.	Tx- **NSAIDs, wrist splinting.** Possibly corticosteroid injection of carpal canal. If severe surgery.

17) Herniated Disk	18) Spinal Stenosis	
Most common- **L4-L5, L5-S1.**	Narrowing of spinal canal secondary to **degenerative joint disease.**	Dx- XR shows **disk space narrow.** CT or **MRI** will show spinal stenosis.
Si/Sx- lower back pain, **sciatica,** ↑PAIN with **passive straight LEG RAISE, cauda equina syndrome** (↓anal sphincter tone).	Si/Sx- neck or back pain that **radiates to buttocks and legs.**	Tx- **NSAIDs, corticosteroid injections.** If severe surgical with **laminectomy.**
Dx- ESR, radiograph, **MRI** for cauda equina syndrome.	Leg cramping is **worse walking, standing, and at REST** (pseudo-claudication).	**Clinical PEARL:** In **children** with back pain think cancer or
Tx- **NSAIDs,** physical therapy, local heat for 4wks, **80% resolve.**	Pain **improves** with **LEANING forward.**	**Spondylolisthesis** (palpable **"step-off"** at lumbosacral area).

Musculoskeletal

19) Regional Pain Syndrome		20) Gout Acute Monoarticular
Pain and loss of function after trauma at trauma site (reflex sympathetic dystrophy). Assoc- DM Si/Sx- diffuse pain and loss of function with ↓skin temp and ↓hair growth.	Dx- clinical Tx- NSAIDs, corticosteroids, TCAs, pregabalin, gabapentin. Sympathetic chemical block may also relieve symps.	Disorder of urate metabolism=> leads to acute monoarticular arthritis. Cx- monosodium urate crystals. Assoc- diet; red wine, alcohol, ↑red meat. Myeloproliferative disease (polycythemia vera).
21) Gout Acute Monoarticular		
Si/Sx- sudden joint pain that awakes pt from sleep. Podagra (first MTP joint of big toe) with TOPHI (urate crystal deposit) that may have a chalky white appearance. Dx- serum ↑uric acid, but could be normal (NOT diagnostic).	Dx Joint fluid aspirate shows; NEEDLE shaped NEG birefringent crystals. Gout crystals appear yeLLow when paraLLel.	Tx- lifestyle modifications (1st-line); alcohol cessation, weight loss, ↓red wine, ↓red meat. Acute: NSAIDs (indomethacin), Colchicine (acute) in gout flare. Chronic: Allopurinol (overproducers), Probenecid (undersecretors).

Musculoskeletal

22) Pseudogout

Calcium Pyrophosphate Dihydrate Crystal (CPPD) disease. Dx- joint fluid aspirate shows **"RHOMBOID"** shaped, **POSITIVE birefringence crystals**. (**Gout- NEEDLE** shaped, **NEG** birefringence crystal)	Comp: **chondrocalcinosis** (calcification of articular cartilage) Tx- **colchicine** (acute).	**Clinical PEARL:** **Lesch-Nyhan** Cx- **def HPRT**; Hypoxanthine-guanine PhosphoRibosyl Transferase (HPRT). Si/Sx- child with **GOUTY arthritis, self-mutilation**, MR, dystonia, spasticity.

23) Osteosarcoma

Malignant bone tumor found in **metaphyseal of distal femur, proximal tibia,** and proximal humerus. Si/Sx- **bone pain** in affected area that is **worse at night.**	Dx- XR may shows **Codman's triangle** (periosteal new bone formation), or **SUNBURST pattern.** **Clinical PEARL:** **Ewing's sarcoma** Dx- XR shows **onion skinning.**	Tx- surgical and chemotherapy. **Clinical PEARL:** **Osteochondroma** most common **BENIGN** bone tumor.

24) Osteoarthritis (OA)

Degenerative joint disease; NON-inflam chronic arthritis of synovial joints with **deterioration of articular cartilage.** Risk factors: **joint trauma,** obesity, +FH.	Si/Sx- **morning stiffness <30min,** bony enlargement, tenderness, that **lacks warmth of joint**. Asymmetric pain in **knee, hip, spine and/or fingers,** often monarticular.	Si/Sx- ↓ROM, bony crepitus, pain that is **WORSE over course of the day,** may **IMPROVES with REST.** Also, involving the **Heberden nodes (DIP), Bouchard nodes (PIP),** and sparing MCP.

Musculoskeletal

25) Osteoarthritis (OA)		
Si/Sx **SPINAL osteoarthritis (pseudoclaudication)** lower extremity pain that occurs with walking and **does NOT improve with standing or rest.** Pain is **worse when pt walks DOWNHILL.**	Dx **XR shows joint space narrowing with osteophyte** formation, subchondral sclerosis. Synovial fluid shows **straw-color fluid** and WBCs <2000cells/uL.	Tx- **NSAIDs (1st-line),** ↓weight (if BMI>30), and possibly corticosteroid injections. If severe joint replacement.
26) Polymyalgia Rheumatica (PMR)		
PAIN, tenderness, and stiffness in large joints. Risk factors: female, >50yrs. Assoc- **anemia, giant cell arteritis.**	Si/Sx- fever, malaise, **tenderness with PAIN and stiffness** in neck, **SHOULDER and PELVIC girdle** muscles.	Si/Sx-morning stiffness **lasts >1hr.** Pt also have **difficulty getting out of CHAIR.** Dx- clinical,↑ESR. Normal CPK. Tx- **prednisone (low-dose, 10-20mg)**
27) Rheumatoid Arthritis (RA)		
Symmetric inflam arthritis with **synovial** hypertrophy and **PANNUS formation=>** that leads to **erosion** adjacent cartilage, tendons, and bone. Si/Sx- pts have **morning stiffness >1hr** in small joints; wrists, MCP, PIP, knees, elbows for **>6wks.** **Anemia of chronic disease** with NSAID treatment.	Si/Sx **Boutonniere deformities, ulnar deviation, SWAN neck deformities.** Comp: • **Osteopenia,** osteoporosis. • **Septic arthritis** Si/Sx- fever and monoarticular joint pain in preexisting joint disease. Dx- arthrocentesis. Tx- IV antibiotics.	Comp: • **Baker cysts** Si/Sx- **popliteal fossa** with inflamed synovium. • **Atlantoaxial subluxation** (atlas C1, axis C2). Dx- XR of **cervical spine** before intubation, anesthesia. **Clinical PEARL: Cervical spine injuries** should have orotracheal intubation to establish the airway.

Musculoskeletal

28) Rheumatoid Arthritis (RA)		
Assoc- Sjogren's (keratoconjunctivitis), Felty's syndrome, Caplan syndrome. **Felty's syndrome:** • **RA** • **Splenomegaly** • **Neutropenia** **Caplan syndrome:** • RA, pneumoconiosis.	Dx- ↑ANA, ↑ESR, **↑Rheumatoid factor (RF)** IgM abs against Fc IgG. As well as **Anti-Cyclic Citrullinated Peptide (anti-CCP).**	Dx **Synovial fluid** shows turbid fluid, ↑WBC 3,000-50,000. XR- may show soft-tissue swelling, **space narrowing and erosions.**

29) Rheumatoid Arthritis (RA)		
Tx- **NSAIDs,** DMARD (disease modifying antirheumatic drugs), **methotrexate** (antimetabolite agent), **hydroxychloroquine,** sulfasalazine.	**Methotrexate** AE: stomatitis (oral ulcers), anemia, **hepatitis,** pneumonitis. **Hydroxychloroquine** AE: retinopathy.	Tx 2nd Line: **TNF** inhibitors, rituximab, leflunomide. **Screen** for latent TB with **PPD** before starting treatment with **TNF inhibitors.**

30) Juvenile Idiopathic Arthritis		
Monoarthritis and polyarthritis with bony destruction in **<16yr, for >6wk.** Si/Sx- **arthritis with nodules, fatigue, fever,** erythematous **rash.** Pts can also have pericarditis. **↑Risk- Iridocyclitis** (anterior uveitis).	Si/Sx Pt can have **arthritis** with **daily SPIKING fever and SALMON colored rash.** Dx- clinical, +ANA, ↑ESR, +/-RF. Eye exam to r/o **iridocyclitis** (anterior uveitis).	Pts with **+ANA** (antinuclear antibodies) have an excellent prognosis. Tx- **NSAIDs,** corticosteroids, or methotrexate (2nd line). Most resolved by puberty (95%).

Musculoskeletal

31) Common Antibodies

• **Anti-dsDNA, Anti-Smith** (SLE)	• **C-ANCA** (Wegener's)	• **Anti-Jo-1** (Polymyositis, Dermatomyositis)
• **Anti-CCP** (RA)	• **P-ANCA** (Microscopic polyangiitis)	• **Anti-Mitochondrial** (Primary biliary cirrhosis)
• **Anti-Centromere** (CREST syndrome)	• **U1RNP antibody** (Mixed connective tissue disease)	• **Anti-Scl-70** (Scleroderma)
• **Anti-TSH** (Graves Disease)	• **Anti-Histone** (Drug SLE)	

32) Ankylosing Spondylitis

Apophyseal joint arthritis; chronic inflam of **SPINE and PELVIS** causing **sacroilitis =>** **fusion** of affected joints.	Dx- ↑**ESR,** ↑**CRP,** **neg RF,** neg ANA, **HLA-B27** (95%).	Other **Seronegative spondyloarthropathy** that should be r/o:
Assoc- **HLA-B27, IBD** (both assoc +P-ANCA).	Radiograph may show **fusion of the sacroiliac joint** and **"BAMBOO spine"** (diagnostic).	• **Reiter's syndrome** Si/Sx- arthritis, uveitis, and urethritis after **infx.** **"Cannot pee, see or climb a tree."**
Si/Sx- fatigue, **shoulder, hip, and lower back** pain with stiffness, **worse in the morning. IMPROVES with ACTIVITY, worse with inactivity.**	Schober test + (↓spine flexion). Tx- NSAIDs **(indomethacin)**, physical therapy, **exercise improves.**	• **Psoriatic arthritis** Si/Sx- psoriatic skin changes, arthritis including the **DIP** joints, and **dactylitis**; **"SAUSAGE"** digits.
Comp- **anterior uveitis, heart block,** vertebral fractures.	In severe cases use TNF inhibitor or sulfasalazine.	**Clinical PEARL: Enthesitis** Si/Sx- inflam and pain where tendon and ligaments attach. Sites: iliac crests, tibial tuberosities, heels.

Musculoskeletal

33) Sjogren Syndrome		
Chronic autoimmune disease; lymphocytic infiltration of exocrine glands. Assoc- RA, SLE, PBC (primary biliary cirrhosis). Risk- lymphoma	Si/Sx- **ITCHY, "DRY" eyes, sandy feeling,** xerostomia (dry mouth), **dental caries,** parotid enlargement. Dx- **Schirmer's test** (↓TEAR production). **Rose Bengal stain** (stain damaged corneal cells and conjunctival) may show corneal ulcerations.	Dx- +ANA, **anti-Ro (SSA) and anti-La (SSB).** Tx- no cure, **artificial tears.** Pilocarpine, cevimeline (↑acteylcholine) which can help to ↑**tears and** ↑**saliva.**

34) Dermatomyositis		35) Polymyositis
Systemic connective tissue disease. Si/Sx- symmetric **PROXIMAL muscle PAIN and weakness** with **RASH:** • **Gottron's papules** (rash over **hand** bony prominences). • **Heliotrope RASH** (periorbital rash). • **Shawl sign** (rash over shoulder, chest, and back). Assoc- **malignancies** (most commonly **ovarian cancer**).	Dx-↑**CK, Anti-Jo-1** antibodies, **muscle biopsy** shows inflam muscle in various stages of disease. Tx- high-dose **corticosteroids** (taper after 4-6wk). **Methotrexate** and/or **azathioprine** can be used instead of steroids. **Methotrexate** AE: anemia, stomatitis (mouth ulcers), alopecia (hair loss), hepatitis, pneumonitis. Tx- **folic acid** (improves symptoms).	Si/Sx- symmetric, **PROXIMAL muscle WEAKNESS.** Problems breathing and swallowing are seen late in the disease. Dx-↑**CPK, Anti-Jo-1** antibodies, **muscle biopsy** shows inflam muscle in various stages of disease. Tx- **corticosteroids. Methotrexate** and/or **azathioprine** can be used instead of steroids.

Musculoskeletal

36) Fibromyalgia		37) Scleroderma
Chronic "PAIN" disorder. Assoc- women **30-50yo**, IBD, depression, **sleep disorders.** Si/Sx- soft tissue tenderness, **muscle "PAIN" and axial skeletal PAIN.** With no joint pain, no muscle weakness, and no inflam. **PAIN is worse with exercise.**	Dx- **>11 multiple, diffuse tender (PAIN) points** over all four body quadrants (diagnosis). Tx- antidepressants **(SSRI/TCA combo),** muscle relaxants, **physical therapy.** Pregabalin, gabapentin, are also used.	Systemic sclerosis inflammation=> **tissue fibrosis,** ↑deposit type I, II collagen. Si/Sx- **CREST** C- Calcinosis R- Raynaud's E- Esophageal S- Sclerodactyly T-Telangiectasias
38) Scleroderma		
Si/Sx- **calcinosis** (calcium in soft tissue), **raynaud's** pnenomenon, **esophageal** dysmotility (lack peristaltic waves, ↓LES tone), **sclerodactyly** (thick, tight skin on fingers and toes), **telangiectasias.**	Dx- + RF, +ANA. • **Anti-Centromere** antibodies assoc with **CREST** syndrome. • **Anti-Scl-70 antibodies** for diffuse form. •**Anti-topoisomerase-I antibodies** in systemic sclerosis form.	Tx- **corticosteroids** for acute flares. **Ca-blockers** (nifedipine) for **Raynaud's phenomenon.** ACEIs when there is renal involvement.

Musculoskeletal

39) Systemic Lupus Erythematosus		
Multisystem autoimmune disorder => **antigen-antibody complexes** deposition. Risk factors: **African American women.** Si/Sx- fever, symmetric arthritis (non-deforming arthritis), joint pain, **"MALAR RASH,"** **discoid rash, oral ulcers,** photosensitivity, seizures, serositis.	Dx- +ANA (screening), **anti-dsDNA** and **anti-smith** antibodies (confirm diagnosis). **Pancytopenia** (↓RBC, ↓WBC and ↓platelets) **peripheral destruction** of blood cells.	Dx **Kidney biopsy** shows **immune complex-mediated** damage and ↓**serum C3**. Biospy is required for all new onset of lupus nephritis (class I-IV forms have different treatments).
40) Systemic Lupus Erythematosus		
Dx Drug SLE-**anti-histone** Neonatal-SLE- **anti-Ro** **Clinical PEARL:** **"SLE** assoc with **LSE"** **Libman-Sacks Endocarditis** non-infx vegetations on mitral valve. Assoc- SLE and **antiphospholipid syndrome.**	Tx- **NSAIDs, corticosteroids** for acute exacerbation. Use **corticosteroids** in thrombocytopenia, renal disease, CNS involvement, or hemolytic anemia.	Tx For severe cases use **hydroxychloroquine, cyclophosphamide,** and/or azathioprine instead of steroids. **Hydroxychloroquine** AE: retinopathy. **Cyclophosphamide** AE: hemorrhagic cystitis, bladder carcinoma.

Musculoskeletal

41) Lupus DOPAMINE RASH	42) Drugs that cause Lupus symps	43) APS
D- Discoid rash D- Oral ulcers P- Photosensitivity A- Arthritis M- Malar rash I- Immunologic N- Neurologic E- ↑ESR R- Renal A- ANA+ S- Serositis H- Hematologic	Drug SLE: • Isoniazid (INH) • Hydralazine • Methyldopa • Penicillamine • Procainamide • Chlorpromazine • Quinidine Dx- +anti-HISTONE antibodies. Tx- stop medication.	Antiphospholipid Antibody Syndrome Si/Sx- **arterial** and venous thromboses. Assoc- **spontaneous ABORTIONS.** Dx- thrombocytopenia, false +VDRL, ↑PTT. Tx- **LMWH** to avoid pregnancy loss.
44) Duchenne Dystrophy (XR)		**45) Becker Dystrophy (XR)**
Duchenne muscular dystrophy; deficiency of **DYSTROPHIN** (cytoskeletal protein). Si/Sx- clumsiness, fatigability, **MR** (common). It affects the **proximal and axial muscles.** Pts have difficulty walking; **GOWER's maneuver** (hands push off thighs when rising from floor), **pseudohypertrophy gastrocnemius muscle.** Dx- ↑CK, **NEG dystrophin immunostain.**	Dx- **Muscle biopsy** (confirms diagnosis) shows necrotic muscle fibers. Tx- physical therapy Comp- **cardiac failure** and respiratory failure. Poor prognosis with most pts in **wheelchair by 12yo.** **Clinical PEARL: Myotonic Muscular Dystrophy** (AD) Si/Sx-**inability to release** hand after "HANDSHAKE." Pt has +Gowers sign.	Becker muscular dystrophy: **"Like Duchenne muscular dystrophy"** Onset is LATER **5–15yrs** and life expectancy 30–40s. MR is uncommon. (DMD starts around 3–5yrs). Dx- western blot shows **dystrophin** levels are NORMAL, but **protein is abnormal.**

Musculoskeletal

46) Temporal Arteritis		47) Osgood-Schlatter Disease
Giant cell arteritis; subacute granulomatous inflammation of temporal artery.	Risk- **BLINDNESS** (occlusion of **central retinal artery**).	Overuse **apophysitis** of **tibial tubercle.**
Si/Sx- scalp pain, new HA, **TEMPORAL tenderness, JAW claudication, monocular blindness**.	Dx- ↑**ESR>50** (>100), **temporal artery biopsy.** Serial CXR for aortic aneurysms.	Si/Sx- **localized pain, knee pain,** at the front of the thigh.
	Tx- **HIGH-dose prednisone** to prevent ocular blindness.	Assoc- young very active boys and girls.
Assoc- **aortic aneurysms** (due to involvement of branches of aorta).		Tx- ↓activity for 2–3mos, brace for symptomatic relief.

48) Slipped Capital Femoral Epiphysis		
Separation of proximal femoral epiphysis => **displace femoral head.**	Risk- male, **OBESITY**, between 11–13yrs, AA, hypothyroidism.	Tx- **surgical pinning of the femoral head,** no weight bearing until after surgery.
Si/Sx- thigh or **knee pain** with **painful limp.** Inability to bear weight with limited internal rotation and **abduction of hip** (bilateral 50%).	Dx- XR both hips in the **AP and FROG-LEG lateral view.**	Comp- avascular necrosis (AVN).

49) Legg-Calve Perthes Disease		
Avascular Necrosis (AVN) of **femoral head**.	Si/Sx- hip has marked limitation of **internal rotation and abduction** at hip joint.	Tx- **observation** ONLY if full ROM.
Assoc- boys 4-10yo.		If ↓ROM consider brace, splints, or surgery.
Si/Sx- hip and knee pain with **limp.**	Dx-XR shows **wide articular space. MRI** much earlier to diagnosis than XR.	

Musculoskeletal

50) Limp STARTSS HOTT	51) Scoliosis	52) Nursemaid's Elbow
S- **Septic** joint T- **Tumor** A- **Avascular** necrosis R- **Rheumatoid**, JIA T- **Tuberculosis** S- **Sickle** cell disease S- **Slipped** capital femoral epiphysis H- **Henoch**-schonlein purpura O- **Osteomyelitis** T- **Trauma** T- **Toxic** synovitis	**Lateral curvature** of spine by >10 degrees. Types- **kyphosis, lordosis.** Si/Sx- accentuated by **forward bending test.** Dx- **XR** of the spine. Tx- close observation (<20 degrees). If severe spinal brace or surgical. Comp- **restrictive lung disease.**	**Radial head** dislocation from child **lifted or "PULLED by HAND."** Si/Sx- pt has refusal to bend elbow and keeps hand in a **pronated position.** Dx- clinical Tx- manual reduction by gentle passive **elbow flexion and forearm supination.**
53) Developmental Dysplasia of Hip		
Cx- **BREECH** presentation. Assoc- first-born **females in breech.** Si/Sx- flexed and adducted position, asymmetric skin folds. Flexion and abduction of lower extremities reveal a **palpable CLUNK.**	• **Allis' (Galeazzi's) sign** (knees unequal heights). • **Barlow's maneuver** (abducted thigh then adducted => **"clunk"**) • **Ortolani's maneuver** (abducted with anterior pressure=> **soft click**). Dx- clinical, early detection is critical.	Dx- **U/S scan of the hips** if inability to abduct the thigh. Radiographs at >4mos old (XR is unreliable until >4mos). Tx • **<6mos** splint with **Pavlik harness.** • **6–15mos-** hip **spica cast.** • **15–24mos** open reduction followed by cast.

11 CHAPTER
NEUROLOGY

Neurology

1) Headaches		2) Cluster Headache
When pts have HA it is important to R/O different causes. HA with following symps: • **Fever, rash** (meningitis) • **Jaw claudication** (temporal arteritis) • **Weight loss** (neoplastic)	• **Photophobia, nausea, vomiting** (migraine, SAH) • **Diplopia** (papilledema) Si/Sx- unilateral or bilateral HA. Dx- for **SAH** order **CT w/out contrast,** if CT is neg => **LP.** Tx- according to diagnosis.	MALE >F onset 25yrs. Si/Sx- excruciating, **UNILATERAL periorbital** HA last 30min–3hrs. **Clusters** HA are assoc with ipsilateral **eye LACRIMATION.** Dx- clinical, repeated attacks over a period of time. Tx- **high-flow O$_2$.**
3) Migraine Headache		**4) Tension Headache**
Female >M, 20s. Assoc- **SEROTONIN** **Triggers-** food, fasting, stress, **menses**, OCPs, **bright light**. Si/Sx- throbbing HA, **UNILATERAL,** >2hrs but <24hrs, nausea, vomiting, **photophobia,** visual **AURA.** Relieved by **sleep and darkness.** Tx- avoid triggers, **NSAIDs, sumatriptan.**	**Prophylaxis: beta-blockers** (propranolol, timolol), **TCAs** (amitriptyline), **CCB, anticonvulsant** (gabapentin, valproate, topiramate). **IV antiemetics: Chlorpromazine, prochlorperazine** or **metoclopramide** can also be used when pts have nausea and vomiting.	**Female >M,** most common type of HA. Assoc- **stress** and improves with relaxation. Si/Sx- **tight, "BANDLIKE" pain,** no nausea/vomit, or auras. Affects the **occipital,** frontal, and neck at the end of the day.

Neurology

5) Tension Headache	6) Partial Seizures	
Dx- diagnosis of exclusion. R/O giant cell arteritis >50yrs order **ESR**. Tx- avoid exacerbating factors, relaxation techniques, hot baths, massage. **NSAIDs** and **acetaminophen** (1st line). **Clinical PEARL: Papilledema** Si/Sx- morning HA, with **transient loss of vision** for few secs with change in **HEAD POSITION**. Dx- ophthalmologic exam; ↑intracranial pressure (ICP).	• **SIMPLE** Si/Sx- sensory, motor, or autonomic, **NO alter consciousness**. **"Simply no loss consicousness"** • **COMPLEX Temporal lobe (80%)** Si/Sx- spread bilateral, with **"LOSS of consciousness."** Pt may have lip smaking, chewing, or bit tongue. Pt have **postictal CONFUSION** (disorientation following episode) **or paralysis (Todd's paralysis)**.	Risk factors: stress, ↓sleep. Dx- **EEG**, R/O systemic cause by ordering CT or MRI. R/O **syncopal event** if pt rapidly returns to baseline with no confusion after episode. Tx-underlying cause, carbamazepine (tegretol), phenytoin, phenobarbital, valproic acid. In **children phenobarbital** (1st line).

Neurology

7) Tonic-Clonic (Grand Mal)		
Simple and complex partial can turn into general **tonic-clonic**. Si/Sx- **sudden LOSS of consciousness** with **tonic** extension of the back followed by 1–2min repetitive movements (**clonic**). Pts may have **tongue biting, incontinence,** and **slowly** regain consciousness, and may be **CONFUSED**.	Dx- **EEG** shows 10–Hz **tonic phase,** with slow waves during **clonic phase.** **Postictal lactic acidosis;** transient anion gap metabolic acidosis that **resolve in 60-90mins** of seizure. **Clinical PEARL: Sturge-Weber** Si/Sx- **seizures, MR, "PORT WINE" stain** along trigeminal nerve. Dx- skull XR shows gyriform intracranial **calcification tramlines**.	Tx- **protect airway** and give **phenytoin (1st-line).** Topiramate or lamotrigine (2nd line). **Clinical PEARL: Pseudoseizures** Si/Sx-stressful trigger seizure-like activity. Dx- order **prolactin level,** it **doubles** in a neurologic seizure, no change in prolactin level in pseudoseizure.
8) Absence (Petit Mal) Seizure		
Begin in **childhood,** familial. Si/Sx- **5–10sec unnoticeable impaired consciousness,** 100x per day.	Si/Sx Patient appears as if they are **staring or DAYDREAMING.** It is common to see **lip smacking** or eye fluttering in these pts.	Dx- **EEG** shows **"3-per-sec SPIKE and WAVE."** Tx- **ethosuximide (1st line)** or valproic acid (valproate).
9) Status Epilepticus		
Seizure for >10min "medical emergency" (convulsive or nonconvulsive). Cx- metabolic disturbance, infx, EtOH, sedative withdrawal, anoxic brain injury.	Dx- **obtain EEG, stat head CT** when pt is stable. Order LP in setting of fever or meningeal signs only after CT has been done. **Benzodiazepines** 1st-line tx (lorazepam).	Tx- **ABCs,** give **thiamine, glucose and naloxone.** Give **IV benzodiazepine + fosphenytoin.** If seizure continue, load **phenobarbital** and possibly intubate, EEG monitoring.

Neurology

10) Tx Status Epilepticus	11) Infantile Spasms	
First **ABCs**, Then Begin Giving Naloxone F- **Fosphenytoin** A- **ABCs** T- **Thiamine** B- **Benzodiazepine** G- **Glucose** N- **Naloxone**	Generalized epilepsy within **6mos of birth.** Si/Sx- bilateral, **tonic, jerks** of extremities, head, and trunk. Pts have **psychomotor development** arrest from age of seizure onset and MR. Ex- **colicy infant with muscle jerks** and a family member having the same problem.	Dx- **EEG hypsarrhythmia** (abnormal interictal pattern; high amplitude and irregular waves and spikes). Tx- **ACTH (1st-line),** prednisone, valproic acid, or clonazepam can also be used.
12) Cranial Nerves		
I- **Olfactory** (smell) II- **Optic** (sight) III- **Oculomotor** (eye movements, pupilary lens, **OPEN** eyelids) IV- **Trochlear** (movement of superior oblique muscle of eye) V- **Trigeminal** (mastication, face sensation) VI- **Abducens** (movement of lateral rectus muscle of eye)	**VII- Facial** (facial expressions, **taste anterior 2/3, salivation, CLOSE** eyelids) **VIII Vestibulocochlear** (hearing, balance) **IX- Glossopharyngeal (taste 1/3 posterior** tongue, **swallow,** salivation (parotid), carotid body and sinus chemoreceptors and baroreceptors).	**X- Vagus** (taste of epiglottic region, **swallow,** palatal elevation, **talk,** aortic arch chemo- and baroreceptors). **XI- Accessory** (turn head, shoulder shrugging) **XII- Hypoglossal** (tongue movements)

Neurology

13) Clinical Reflexes		
Reflexes: • **Achilles- S1, S2** • **Patella- L3, L4** • **Biceps- C5, C6** • **Triceps- C7, C8**	**Babinski sign:** Dorsiflexion of **BIG** toe and **FAN** other toes = **UMN lesion** (normal in the first year of life).	• **UMN** **Spactic, ↑DTRs,** +Babinski's sign. • **LMN** **Flaccid, ↓DTRs, atrophy, fasciculation.**
14) Facial Nerve Lesions		
• **UMN lesions** Contralateral **paralysis** **"LOWER face ONLY"** (forehead gets UMN innervation from **both sides** of the cortex).	• **LMN lesions** Cx- CN VII lesion. Ipsilateral paralysis of **"UPPER and LOWER face."**	**"Bell's palsy" CNVII** (LMN lesion) Assoc- **Lyme** disease, HSV, Epstein-Barr. Tx- oral **glucocorticoids** and eye lubricants to protect cornea drying.
15) Spinal Tract Functions		
CORTICOSPINAL Tract • **Function:** **"MOVEMENT"** • **Origin:** Motor cortex • **Decussation:** Pyramidal (at cervico**medullary** junction)	**SPINOTHALAMIC Tract** • **Function:** **"PAIN & TEMP"** • **Origin:** Nerve endings, pain fibers. • **Decussation:** Ventral **white commissure** (at **spinal cord** level)	**DORSAL COLUMN** • **Function:** Fine **touch, vibration, proprioception.** • **Origin:** Pacini's and Meissner's tactile discs, muscle spindles, and golgi tendon organ. **Decussation:** Arcuate fibers (at **medulla**)

Neurology

16) Spinal Cord Compression		17) Brown-Sequard Syndrome
↓Bone density and/or mineralization. Cx- disk herniation, **abscess** (IV drug use), trauma, **metastatic cancer to the SPINE**. Si/Sx- symmetric lower extremity weakness, hyperreflexia, possibly +Babinski sign. Dx- start **IV steroids**, then **MRI scan.**	Tx • **IV dexamethasone** (↓pressure on spinal column). • **Urgent surgery** for pts that have spinal cord compression syndrome. • **Urinary catheterization** to prevent bladder distention.	Si/Sx • Ipsilateral **spastic paralysis** (↓movement) • Ipsilateral **Babinski** (UMN damage) • Ipsilateral loss of **position and vibration** • Contralateral **LOSS of PAIN and TEMP**.
18) Spinal Cord Lesions		
• **Multiple Sclerosis** Si/Sx-triad: **nystagmus, scanning speech, intention tremor.** Dx- MRI shows cervical **white matter,** asymmetric, random **lesions.**	• **Amyotrophic Lateral Sclerosis** (Lou Gehrig's) **UMN and LMN with no sensory deficit.** Si/Sx- spacticity, fasciculation, atrophy, +**babinski's sign,** with ↑DTRs or ↓DTRs.	• **Poliomyelitis** **LMN** lesions 2nd to destruction of **ANTERIOR horn.** Si/Sx- flaccid paralysis.
19) Spinal Cord Lesions		
• **Ventral Artery Occlusion** Si/Sx- below level of lesion LOSS; - **Corticospinal tract** (movement) - **Spinothalamic tract** (pain & temp) - **"SPARES"** dorsal columns (fine touch, vibration, proprioception).	• **Tabes Dorsalis** (3rd syphilis) Degeneration of **DORSAL roots and columns.** Si/Sx- LOSS of **fine touch, vibration, proprioception.**	• **Acute Diffuse Encephalomyelitis** Assoc- vaccination, viral illness. Si/Sx- post viral, acute hemiparesis, cerebellar ataxia, neuropathies. Dx- **MRI shows diffuse demyelination of white matter** of brain and spinal cord.

Neurology

20) Spinal Cord Lesions		
• Vit B12 neuropathy & Friedreich's ataxia Demyelination of **all three tracts;** lateral corticospinal tract, spinocerebellar tract, and dorsal column. Si/Sx- **ataxia gait,** impaired position and vibration sense. **Clinical PEARL: Friedreich ataxia (AR)** • **Neurologic-** ataxia, dysarthria. • **Skeletal-** scoliosis, **FEET** deformities. • **Cardiac-** concentric hypertrophic.	• **Syringomyelia** Cross fibers of corticospinal tract. Cx-**"WHIPLASH"** from MVA. Si/Sx- post-traumatic whiplash symps mos-yrs later, **BILATERAL loss pain and temp.** Assoc- **Arnold-Chiari malformation** (congential cerebellar and medulla oblongata through foramen magnum)	• **Cervical Spondylosis** Si/Sx- **chronic neck pain,** limited neck rotation. Dx- XR shows **bony spurs** and sclerotic facet joints. Comp- **central cord syndrome (weak UPPER** > lower **extremities**, with loss of pain and temp).
21) Stroke Risk Factors	**22) Stroke**	
Modifiable: • **CAD** • **Obesity** • **Diabetes** • **Smoking** • **Hypertension** • **Hyper-cholesterolemia** • **Atrial Fibrillation** • **Carotid Stenosis** • **Drugs** (cocaine or IV drugs) **Non-modifiable:** Age >60yo, ethnicity (AA, Hispanic, Asian), male, FH of MI or stroke.	Cx- **Ischemic (80%),** hemorrhagic (20%). Risk factors: **atherosclerosis,** hypercholesterolemia, **HTN,** DM, A-Fib, male, endocarditis, **hypercoagulable,** >60yo, FH, ethnicity. **Clinical PEARL:** Child with hx of foreign body trauma to the **soft palate.** Gives risk of **internal carotid artery dissection** leading to **STROKE.**	Si/Sx • **TIA:** Si/Sx- **transient** neurologic deficit **<24hrs** (most <1hr). •**ACA:** Si/Sx- contralateral paresis and sensory **loss in LEGS, "PERSONALITY"** changes. • **PCA:** Si/Sx- **homonymous hemianopia, MEMORY** deficits, **dyslexia/alexia** (reading/words).

Neurology

23) Stroke

• Lacunar:	• Basilar artery:	• MCA:
Cx- **HTN**, diabetes.	Si/Sx- **"CN Palsies,"** apnea, visual symps, **drop attacks.**	Si/Sx- contralateral paresis and sensory loss **FACE and ARM, GAZE toward side lesion,** homonymous
Si/Sx- **PURE motor** or **PURE sensory,** dysarthria; **"CLUMSY HAND,"** ataxic hemiparesis.	**Sensory** loss **ipsilateral FACE and contralateral BODY**.	hemianopia, **aphasia, NEGLECT** (parietal lobe).
Dx- **non-contrast CT** looks normal due to the small size of the stroke in the **internal capsule,** small vessel hyalinosis.	Pts can also have **dysphagia, dysarthria, vertigo,** locked-in syndrome, coma.	Dx- **CT w/out contrast** determine ischemic vs hemorrhagic. **MRI, ECG and ECHO** if embolic. Possibly **carotid U/S scan,** MRA, angiography.

24) PCA Stroke	25) MCA Stroke	26) Subarachnoid Hemorrhage (SAH)
4D's: • **Dizziness**	• **Gaze TOWARD** lesion	Cx • **Marfan's syndrome** (mutation in fibrillin-1 gene)
• **Diplopia** (double vision)	• **Contralateral** paresis and sensory loss **FACE and ARMs.**	• **Kidney** (PCKD)
• **Dysarthria** (motor speech disorder)	• **Homonymous** hemianopia	• **Ehlers-Danlos syndrome** (hypermobile joints)
• **Dysphagia** (difficulty swallowing)	• **Aphasia**	• **Sickle cell anemia**
	• **Neglect**	• **Family History**

Neurology

27) Subarachnoid Hemorrhage (SAH)		
Cx- trauma, AVM, **BERRY Aneurysm.** Si/Sx- **abrupt,** painful **thunderclap HA, "WORST headache of my LIFE,"** neck stiffness, **CNIII palsy.** Comp- **communicating hydrocephalus** (dilation of ventricular system, enlargement of subarachnoid space) **Clinical PEARL: Intraventricular Hemorrhage** in premature infant can lead to SAH.	Dx • **CT without contrast** (look for bleed). • If CT is neg then order **LP** and look for **xanthochromia** (yellow CSF). • **4-Vessel Angiography** (after SAH confirmed). Tx • **Prevent rebleeding** (first 48hrs) by maintaining **systolic BP<150**.	Tx • **Prevent vasospasm** (5–7 days after SAH) with **Ca-blocker** (AE: peripheral edema). • Give **phenytoin** for seizure prophylaxis. • ↓**ICP** by raising the head of the bed, **hyper**ventilation (↓CO_2=> cerebral vasoconstriction), and/or mannitol. Can treat hydrocephalus with **serial LPs.** • **Surgical clipping** definitive tx for aneurysms.

Neurology

28) Treatment for ACUTE Stroke		29) Treatment for CHRONIC Stroke
ISCHEMIC Stroke (80%) • Give **tPA (tissue Plasminogen Activator)** if it can be administered **< 3HOURS of onset.** • **Thrombolytics** (streptokinase, urokinase, alteplase) can be used if it is given within **< 6HOURS of onset.** • In ischemic stroke allow HTN to prevent hypoperfusion. **If >220/120,** then give with **labetalol** or **nicardipine.**	**HEMORRHAGIC Stroke (20%)** Tx • **ICU admission** to monitor for possible ↑ICP and **herniation.** • **Serial CTs** should be ordered, **mannitol,** and **hyper**ventilation. Also treat **fever and hyperglycemia** (poor prognoses in acute stroke).	• **ASA, clopidogrel** 2nd to thrombosis. • **Carotid endarterectomy** if >70% stenosis. • **Anticoagulation** If new A-Fib or hypercoagulable state, **INR 2–3**. If prosthetic valve **INR 3–4**. • **Manage- HTN, atherosclerosis,** DM, and hycholesterolemia.
30) tPA Therapy Contraindications		**31) Intracerebral Hemorrhage**
• **MI** (recent) • **Stroke** <3mos • **GI bleed** <21days • **Surgery** <14days • **Prior hemorrhage** • **TIA (**transient ischemic attack)	• **Seizures** • **Low platelet**<100,000 • **Elevated BP**>185/110 • **Anticoagulation** INR>1.7	Risk factors: HTN, anticoagulation, vascular malformation (AVM), tumor, amyloid angiopathy. Si/Sx- **focal motor, sensory deficit** that gets worse with hematoma expands.

Neurology

32) Intracerebral Hemorrhage	33) Herniation	
Dx- immediate non-contrast head **CT**. Tx- similar to SAH; • Prevent rebleeding **systolic BP<150**. • Prevent vasospasm with **Ca-blocker** • Give **phenytoin** for seizure prophylaxis. • ↓ **ICP** by raising head of bed, mannitol. • Watch for possible **HERNIATION**.	• **UNCAL herniation** (transtentorial) Lesion in middle fossa. Si/Sx- **CNIII** "**Fixed and DILATED ipsilateral pupil,**" eye down and out, ipsilesional hemiparesis. • **Cingulate herniation** Lesion in **frontal lobe**. Si/Sx- asymp.	• **Transtentorial** Supratentorial mass push **midbrain** inferiorly. Si/Sx- rapid mental status change, **SMALL reactive pupils, "Cheyne-Stokes Resp."** • **Cerebellar tonsillar** Posterior fossa mass into foramen magnum. Si/Sx- **resp arrest**.
34) Subdural Hematoma		**35) Epidural Hematoma**
Cx- head trauma=> rupture **bridging vein**. Assoc- **alcoholics, elderly**. Si/Sx- HA, altered mental status. Can take several days to weeks for pt to have symps.	Dx- **CT scan** shows **CONCAVE, crescent shaped,** that does not cross **midline**. Tx- supportive, surgical evacuation if symptomatic.	Cx- lateral **skull fracture** => rupture of the **middle meningeal artery**. Si/Sx- severe **trauma,** loss of consciousness => **LUCID interval** (min–hrs) followed by gradual deterioration of consciousness.

Neurology

36) Epidural Hematoma

Comp: • Pt can get a **UNCAL herniation**=> that leads to coma with **BLOWN pupil** (fixed and dilated ipsilateral pupil). • **Diffuse axonal injury** from acceleration deceleration trauma. Dx- **CT** shows numerous **minute punctate hemorrhages** with blurring of **grey-white** interface.	Dx- **CT scan** shows **CONVEX, "LENS-shaped."** If pt has **normal CT scan** discharge home and have them return if pt develops any new symp (HA, confusion). Tx- **emergent** neurosurgical evacuation.	Remember: Any head trauma can cause spontaneous CSF leak; ↑**beta-2-transferrin** (CSF-specific marker). Could leak from nose or pts ear. **Clinical PEARL Cephalohematoma** Subperiosteal **hemorrhage** within few **hrs after birth** from scalp swelling. Reasorbs within 2wks-3mos.

37) Cavernous Sinus Thrombosis

Septic thrombosis of the cavernous sinus from orbit or nasal sinuses infx. Cx- **staph aureus** (most common), **mucor** (DM) or aspergillus. Si/Sx- pt appears ill with **fever** and **HA**. Pt may have diplopia, **red eye, ptosis,** orbital pain, and/or periorbital edema with **recent sinusitis or facial infx.**	Si/Sx- pts may have **lateral gaze palsy. CNIII, IV, V1, V2, and VI** all pass through cavernous sinus and can be affected. Comp- menigitis, sepsis. Dx- blood cultures, ↑**WBC**, CSF may show ↑protein. **CT or MRI with gadolinium** (confirms diagnosis).	Dx- possibly biopsy of paranasal sinuses for fungal infx. Tx- nafcillin or oxacillin + cefepime or ceftriaxone pending BCx. For anaerobic coverage use **metronidazole.** If MRSA is suspected add **vancomycin.** IV abxs should be given for at least 3-4wks.

Neurology

38) BPPV

Benign Paroxysmal Peripheral Vertigo **(BPPV)**; from dislodged **otolith** => disrupting **semicircular canal**. Si/Sx- episodic, **transient vertigo** **<1min** with nystagmus trigger by **HEAD POSITION** changes. Happens when pt **reaching over head or turning in bed.**	Dx- **Dix-Hallpike maneuver** (turn head 45 degrees R=>L while sitting to supine). Tx- most resolved with **Epley maneuver** (270-degree head rotation with Dix-Hallpike Maneuver).	**BPPV** **B- Benign** **otolith** disruption. **P- Paroxysmal** **sudden,** transient episodes lasting **<1min**. **P- Positional** starts with reaching overhead or **turning** in bed. **V- Vertigo** vertigo or **dizziness** is main symptom.

39) Meniere's Disease

Abnormal accumulation of **endolymph within the INNER EAR.** Si/Sx- **recurrent vertigo,** ear fullness, tinnitus, and **HEARING LOSS** for **hours–days,** with nausea, and vomiting,	Dx- clinically, **2 episodes that last at least 20mins** each with **hearing loss** that is diagnosed with audiometry.	Dx- R/O TIA or intracranial pathology. Tx- **low-sodium diet** and diuretic (1st line).

Neurology

40) Labyrithitis

Recent VIRAL infx=> now presenting with **VERTIGO** and vomiting. Si/Sx- acute onset with head-motion intolerance, **vertigo,** horizontal **nystagmus,** nausea, vomit, and unsteady gait **with hx of recent VIRAL illness.**	Dx- clinical, abnormal vestibulo-ocular reflex (VOR), horizontal nystagmus beat in opposite direction of lesion. **Diagnosis of exclusion,** may mimic; cerebellar stroke. **Clinical PEARL: Presbycusis** Sensorineural **hearing** loss occurs with **AGE.** Si/Sx- **bilateral hearing** loss, difficulty hearing in **noisy, crowded** environments.	Tx- **corticosteroids** <72hrs, can use **meclizine** for vestibular sedation, spontaneous resolves in wks–mos. **Clinical PEARL: Otosclerosis** Conductive hearing loss in **YOUNG** adults. Dx- **bone conduction > air conduction** on Rinne test.

41) Vestibular Migraine   42) Syncope (Neurocardiogenic)

41) Vestibular Migraine	42) Syncope (Neurocardiogenic)	
Recurrent **vertigo** in relation to migraine HA. Si/Sx- **recurrent episodes of vertigo** (min–days), dizziness, nausea, vomiting, and photophobia, but with **NO hearing loss.** Dx- **clinically** Tx- NSAIDs, triptans, or metoclopramide. Can also try antiemetics or benzodiazepines.	Cx- **VASOVAGAL** (most common), orthostatic hypotension (drop systolic ↓BP >20), basilar TIAs, arrhythmias, **situational syncope** (after urination). Si/Sx- dizziness, lightheadedness, weakness leading to **loss of consciousness and muscle tone <30sec** and recover (with no confusion) within **seconds.**	Triggers- valsalva maneuver, standing for a long time, fear of blood. Dx- **Upright tilt table testing** (confirm diagnosis). R/O TIA, seizure with **EEG (>30sec,** jerking, biting tongue) MI or arrhythmias with **ECG and cardiac enzymes.** Tx- underlying cause.

Neurology

43) Lambert-Eaton Myasthenic		
Antibodies against **presynaptic Ca2+** channels. Assoc- **SCLC**. Si/Sx- fatigability, weakness of the proximal muscles that **IMPROVES with USE!**	Spares: **extraocular** and respiratory muscles are **NOT affected.** Dx- **repetitive nerve stimulation** (pts will improve), **antibodies to presynaptic calcium** channels. Order **CT** for **lung neoplasm** (SCLC).	Tx- **pyridostigmine** (acetylcholinesterase inhibitor), guanidine, or 3,4-diaminopyridine. If severe **azathiprine or corticosteroids.** **SCLC** treatment may reverse symptoms.
44) Myasthenia Gravis		
Antibodies against **postsynaptic ACETYLCHOLINE (ACh) receptor.** Si/Sx- fatigable, muscle weak, **PTOSIS,** and **DOUBLE** vision. **"WORSE with USE,"** especially as the day progresses. Pt may have difficulty rising from chair, **brushing hair,** or climbing stairs. Comp: **Myasthenic CRISIS => respiratory** compromise.	Assoc- **THYMOMA, thyrotoxicosis.** Dx • **Tensilon test (edrophonium;** anticholinesterase) => rapid **improvement** for a few mins. • **Ice test** (ice eye for 5min resolves ptosis). • Abnormal **single-fiber EMG nerve stimulation** (confirm diagnosis).	Dx • **Ach antibodies** and anti-MuSK antibodies. • Order **CT chest** for possible **thymoma**. Tx- **neostigmine, pyridostigmine,** (anticholinesterases), and/or **prednisone.** Resection of **thymoma.** Severe (myasthenic crisis) cases use **IVIG or plasmapheresis.** **Avoid-** beta-blocker and aminoglycosides in these pts.

Neurology

45) NPH

Normal Pressure Hydrocephalus (NPH); impaired outflow CSF. Si/Sx- triad: • **Dementia** • **Gait apraxia** • **Urinary incontinence**	Dx- **Miller-Fisher test** LP- 30-50mL removal of CSF, if pt improves diagnostic and therapeutic.	Dx- CT or MRI shows **ventricular enlarged.** Tx- surgical; CSF shunting.

46) Amyotrophic Lateral Sclerosis

ALS/Lou Gehrig's	Si/Sx	Dx
Cx-unknown etiology. Si/Sx- asymmetric, degeneration of **UMN and LMNs**; with weakness of arms, legs, and diaphragm. Pt may have **fasciculations, and tongue atrophy.**	Disease progresses to **Respiratory failure** and death within five years of diagnosis. Ex- weakness on one side of body then fasciculations on the other side. Normal MRI. **Spares: EYE muscles** and **SPHINCTER tone.**	**Clinical,** involve tongue (CNXII), oropharyngeal (CNIX). R/O demyelinating disease with **EMG nerve conduction studies**. CT or MRI to R/O any sturctural lesions. **Normal MRI r/o MS, "Think ALS."** Tx- supportive.

47) Guillain-Barre Syndrome

Assoc- **viral infx,** influenza vaccination, **Campylobacter jejuni** (most common). Si/Sx- rapid progressiving **ascending paralysis** (distal to proximal), with areflexia and **respiratory muscles** involvement.	Dx- **EMG and nerve conduction studies** diffuse demyelination, ↑**CSF PROTEIN>55.**	Tx ICU for **respiratory** support. **Plasmapheresis or IVIG (1st line).** NO corticosteroids.

Neurology

48) Multiple Sclerosis (MS)		
"RELAPSING and REMITTING." multiple **neurologic complaints** that cannot be explained by single lesion. Si/Sx- **Optic neuritis** (↓ **COLOR vision,** ↓ visual acuity), limb weakness, paresthesias, diplopia, urinary retention, cognitive impairment with **unpredictable attacks lasting 6–8wks.**	Si/Sx Pts may also have depression, sexual dysfunction and bowel dysfunctions. **Triad:** • Scanning speech • Nystagmus • **Intranuclear ophthalmoplegia**	Dx **MRI** show **multiple, asymmetric, WHITE MATTER periventricular lesions** (Dawson's fingers) in corpus callosum. **MRI with gadolinium** may be used to enhance the lesions.

49) Multiple Sclerosis (MS)		
Dx **CSF** may show nonspecific **oligoclonal bands.** **Optic neuritis** may have normal funduscopic exam.	Tx **Corticosteroids** for acute exacerbations. **Mitoxantrone** for worse relapsing and remitting.	↓**RELAPSING- REMITTING** give: **"ABC"** **A-Avonex (Interferon-Beta 1a)** **B-Betaseron** (Interferon-Beta 1b) **C-Copaxone** (copolymer-1)

Neurology

50) Vascular Dementia		
Risk factors: Cardiovascular disease (CAD), **HTN, diabetes, age,** hx of **stroke.** Si/Sx- abrupt onset of dementia and focal neurologic symps.	Dx- **Dementia** +**2** of following: • **Abrupt onset** • **"STEPWISE dementia"** • **Focal neurologic** signs and symps • **Old infarct** or white matter changes on CT or MRI.	Tx- same protocols as **stroke.** **Clinical PEARL: Dissociative fugue** Si/Sx- **amnesia** after **traveling,** confusion about personal identity.

51) Alzheimer's		
Neuritic plaques, **neurofibrillary tangles** with **amyloid** deposits. Risk factors: FH, age, female, Down syndrome. Si/Sx- **AMNESIA** (memory loss) of **new information** is the first sign. Pt get **depression, agitation**, and may have language deficits.	**5A's of dementia:** • **Amnesia** (memory loss) • **Agnosia** (loss of ability to recognize) • **Apraxia** (skilled movements) • **Abstract** thinking and though process is lost. • **Aphasia** (speechless)	Dx- **diagnosis of exclusion,** definitive diagnosis on autopsy. MRI or CT may **show atrophy.** Tx- **supportive,** treat depression, agitation, delusions, and sleep disorder. Prevent progression: Cholinesterase inhibitors (1st-line); **donepezil, tacrine, galantamine, rivastigmine.**

Neurology

52) Creutzfeldt-Jakob		53) Fronto-Temporal PICK's
PRION disease, which is a very **rare** form of **dementia.** Si/Sx- **"RAPID" declining** subacute dementia of **WEEKS-MONTHS.** Pts may have **ataxia and/or myoclonic JERKs.**	Dx- clinical, **EEG** shows **pyramidal signs and periodic SHARP waves.** Tx- **none,** death within 1yr of onset of symps.	**Frontotemporal dementia** with **PICK bodies** on pathology. Si/Sx- **behavior and personality** changes early in disease. Dx- atrophy of **frontal and temporal** lobes on CT or MRI. **PICK bodies** are classic pathologic finding. Tx- symps only.
54) Huntington's (AD)		
HD gene on chrom 4 has multiple abnormal **CAG triplet repeats.** Assoc- **anticipation** (multiple CAG repeats expand with each generation). Si/Sx- Pts have alterated **behavior, dementia, depression,** and may have antisocial behavior.	Si/Sx- pt show signs of **"CHOREA,"** purposeless, **dancelike movements** (from excess ↑dopamine). Dx- clinical, confirm with **genetics.** CT or MRI may show **cerebral atrophy of CAUDATE** and putamen.	There may be a FH of **ANTICIPATION** with each generation. Tx- no cure, control movements with dopamine blockers; **haloperidol, risperidone, reserpine, olanzapine, tetrabenazine. SSRIs** for depression.

Neurology

55) Parkinson's (Lewy dementia)		
↓**DOPAMINE in basal ganglia, substantia nigra,** with **LEWY bodies** (intraneuronal eosinophilic inclusions). Cx- idiopathic, trauma, MPTP (designer drug), viral encephalitis.	Si/Sx **Masked facies, micrographia** (abnormally small handwriting), **MEMORY loss,** postural instability, bradykinesia, and **resting tremors**. **LEWY body dementia;** fluctuating cognition, visual **hallucinations,** with motor features of parkinsonism.	Dx- clinical. **Tetrad:** • **Rigidity** (cogwheeling) • **Postural** instability • **Bradykinesia** (slow movements) • **Resting tremor** Affects one or both hands (**pill roll**) while at **rest and improve with activity**.
56) Parkinson's Treatment		
Tx • **Levodopa and carbidopa** (dopamine precursors). AE: confusion, hallucinations, dyskinesia. • **Ropinirole, bromocriptine, pramipexole** (dopamine agonists). AE: dry mouth, urinary retention, blurred vision, constipation. **Pramipexole** AE: ↑**gambling risk**.	• **Entacapone** or tol**capone** (COMT inhib) AE: confusion, hallucinations. • **Selegiline** (MAO-B inhib) neuroprotective. AE: insomnia, confusion.	• **Amantadine** (mild antiparkinsonian activity, improve rigidity and tremor) AE: livedo reticularis (purplish mottled skin), ankle edema. **Clinical PEARL: Essential Tremor** Si/Sx- suppressed at rest and exacerbated **with action.** Tx- **propranolol** (1st-line).

Neurology

57) Open-Angle Glaucoma

↑**Flow aqueous humor** => ↑**IOP**. Risk factors: **Diabetes, African American** (AA), >40yo, myopia. Si/Sx- asymp, gradual loss of **peripheral vision** over years and eventual **tunnel vision.**	Si/Sx Pts have **bilateral "FREQUENT LENS"** changes. Dx- **tonometry, "CUPPING" of optic nerve** on funduscopic exam. **Screening-** annual eye exams in high-risk populations.	Tx- **timolol** eye drops (1st-line). Can also use **betaxolol (**topical beta-blockers) to ↓aqueous humor production or **pilocarpine** to ↑aqueous outflow. If severe **laser trabeculoplasty.**

58) Closed-Angle Glaucoma

↑Pressure in **posterior chamber pushes iris forward** blocking the angle. **Risk factors:** older age, FH, prolonged dilation, lens dislocation, uveitis. Si/Sx- **unilateral HARD, RED, eye pain** with **blurry vision** leading to a **dilated and non-reactive pupil** to light. Pt may also have HA, nausea, vomiting. Dx- clinical, HA (triggered by dark light).	Tx- **medical emergency** that can cause blindness. ↓IOP with eye drops: **timolol, pilocarpine, apraclonidine**. Systemic meds: **acetazolamide, mannitol**. Avoid mydriatic agents like atropine. If severe **laser peripheral iridotomy** (hole in peripheral iris).	**Clinical PEARL: Cataracts** Progressive **thickening of lens**. Si/Sx- blurred vision and **"GLARE,"** worse at night. Painless loss of vision. Dx- ophthalmoscopic exam. Tx-surgery, excision of opacified lens and insertion of lens implant.

Neurology

59) Age-Macular Degeneration		
Most common cause of permanent bilateral blindness in **elderly** in the U.S. Risk factor: smoking. Si/Sx- **painless loss of "CENTRAL vision." Drusen** (tiny yellow, white accumulations) and pigmentary changes.	**Types:** • **Atrophic** (dry) gradual (80%). • **Neovascualar** (wet) rapid, rare (20%). Dx **Funduscopy** shows **pigmentary** and atrophic changes. **GRID test** of parallel vertical and horizontal lines look **"BENT, WAVY or CURVED."**	Tx • **Atrophic-** Vit C, E, beta-carotene, zinc, may slow disease. • **Exudative** ranib**izumab**, or bevac**izumab** (improve vision), **pegaptanib** (slow visual loss). **Clinical PEARL: Presbyopia** Age-related $\downarrow$ **LENS elasticity**, difficulty with near vision. Si/Sx- elderly pt hold books at **arms length to read.** Tx- reading glasses.
60) Strabismus		**61) Pseudostrabismus**
Misalignment of eyes. Si/Sx-pupil turns inward on lateral gaze, and corneal light reflex **"ASSYMETRIC."** Dx- lateral gaze shows **assymetric** light reflex. Tx- **cover NORMAL eye.**	**Vision screening** children 0-5yo. Complication if pts is not treated: **Amblyopia** reduction in central visual acquity due to sensory deprivation.	Si/Sx- pupil turns inward on lateral gaze, and corneal light reflex **SYMMETRIC.** Assoc- **flat nasal bridge,** flat epicanthal fold. Dx- lateral gaze shows **symmetric** light reflex. Tx- **reassure parents** child is normal.

Neurology

62) Retinal Detachment		
Separation of LAYERS of retina. Assoc- 40-70yo, cataract surgery. Si/Sx- Sudden loss of vision **curtain falling down over eyes.**	Si/Sx **FLASHES of light** (photopsia) with new **FLOATERS,** and blurred vision. Dx- ophthalmoscopic exam shows **grey, elevated retina.**	Tx- **laser therapy** and cryotherapy connect the neurosensory retina, retinal pigment epithelium, and choroid.

63) Amaurosis Fugax		
Cx- **retinal emboli** from carotid artery bifurcation. Si/Sx- monocular, **transient** visual loss, **like a curtain falling down.**	Dx- ophthalmoscopy shows **zone of whitened, edematous** retina **following retinal arterioles**.	Dx **Duplex U/S** scan of carotids for degree of carotid artery stenosis. Tx- important to reduce risk of stroke by treating atherosclerosis.

64) Retinal Artery Occlusion		
Cx- central **retinal artery occlusion**. Si/Sx- sudden **painless,** unilateral blindness, **pupil is sluggish** to react to direct light.	Dx- Funduscopic exam shows pallor of optic disk, **CHERRY-RED spot** on fovea, and **BOXCAR segmentation** of blood in retinal veins.	Tx- **ocular massage** and **high-FLOW O2** (1st-line). Intra-arterial thrombolysis of ophthalmic artery **within 8hrs** onset, or IV **acetazolamide**.

Neurology

65) Retinal VEIN Occlusion

Cx- **central retinal vein occlusion**.

Si/Sx- sudden **painless vision loss**.

Dx- funduscopic exam shows **"Blood and THUNDER."**

Dx- funduscopic exam shows also shows **swollen optic disk**, retinal **hemorrhages**, dilated veins, and **"COTTON-WOOL spots,"** with edema of macula.

Tx- **laser photocoagulation**.

Clinical PEARL: External Hordeolum Cx- staph abscess of eyelid (**stye**). Tx- warm compresses.

66) Metastatic Brain Tumor

Cx- metastatic tumors from **lung, GI, breast, renal, skin cancers.**

Si/Sx- hx of cancer, HA, ↑**ICP**, seizures, nausea, vomiting, diplopia, intracranial hemorrhage.

Dx- **contrast CT or MRI** with or without **gadolinium** shows multiple discrete nodule in **"GRAY-WHITE" junction**.

Clinical PEARL: Cushing's Reflex HTN and bradycardia due to intracranial pressure from brain tumor, death is imminent.

67) Metastatic Brain Tumor Treatment

Tx- palliative care, **corticosteroid** to ↓ICP.

• **Solitary** brain metastasis; **surgical resection** followed by **whole brain radiation is standard.**

• **Multiple** brain metastases are best treated with **palliative whole brain radiation**.

• Radiation and chemotherapy have varying results.

• Chemotherapy induced nausea and vomiting give **serotonin antagonists; Ondansetron** (block 5HT3 receptors, 1st-line).

68) Pseudotumor Cerebri

Si/Sx- HA, blurry vision, papilledema, nausea, vomiting.

Assoc- **OBESE women, OCP, Vit A.**

Dx- MRI shows **EMPTY sella and slit-like ventricles.**

Diagnosis of exclusion. LP reveals **normal CSF with ↑ opening pressure.**

Neurology

69) Astrocytoma	70) Schwannoma	71) Glioblastoma Multiforme (adults)
Most common posterior fossa tumor in **children**. Arise from brain parenchyma. Si/Sx- HA, focal deficits, **seizures**. Dx- contrast CT or MRI. Prognostic factors are age of pt and **tumor grade I-IV**. Tx- surgical resection and radiation.	**Acoustic Neuroma** Cx- **schwann cells** Si/Sx- ipsilateral **HEARING loss, tinnitus**, and **vertigo**. Assoc: **Neurofibromatosis-2** (bilateral acoustic neuromas). Dx- **contrast CT** or MRI. Tx- surgical resection.	Grade IV **astrocytoma**. Si/Sx- nausea, papilledema, seizure, focal deficits, HA. Dx- MRI shows **ring-enhancing lesions** with classic **"BUTTERFLY" appearance** of GBM. Poor prognosis <1yr. Tx- surgical resection, possibly radiation and chemotherapy.
72) Medulloblastoma		
Second most common brain tumor in **children**. Cx- primitive neuroectodermal tumor that arises from **Cerebellar VERMIS**.	Si/Sx- HA, **trunk dystaxia, unbalanced gait**, papilledema, horizontal nystagmus.	Dx- **contrast CT** or MRI. Tx- surgical resection with chemotherapy and radiation.

Neurology

73) Neurofibromatosis	74) NF1 von Recklinghausen	75) NF2
Neurocutaneous disorder. **Type:** **NF1** (von Recklinghausen) and **NF2**. Dx- **MRI with gadolinium** of brain and spine. Also obtain an dermatologic, auditory, and ophthalmologic exam. Tx- no cure, treat symps; debulking tumors, resection of **optic gliomas and acoustic neuromas.**	Cx- AD, chrom 17. Si/Sx • **6 café au lait spots** >5mm child, >15mm adults. • **Freckle in axillary, and/or inguinal area.** • **Lisch nodule** (pigment iris hamartomas) • **OPTIC glioma** • Neurofibromas (two or more) • 1st degree relative with NFl.	Cx- AD, chrom 22. Si/Sx • **Bilateral Acoustic Neuromas** • **Cafe au lait spots** • **Seizures** • Skin nodules • Neurofibromas, gliomas, meningiomas, or schwannoma. • 1st degree relative with NF2. **Clinical PEARL:** **McCune-Albright** also has "**cafe au lait spots**" **3P's: Precocious** puberty, **Pigmentation** (cafe au lait spots), **Polyostotic** fibrous dysplasia (multiple bone defects).

Neurology

76) Tuberous Sclerosis (AD)		
Si/Sx- **seizures, skin lesions, and MR.** The following my be seen; • **Infantile spasms** (convulsive **seizures**) • **Mental Retardation** • **Hypopigmented "ASH-LEAF" lesions** on trunk. • **Renal;** hamartomas angiomyolipomas.	• **SHAGREEN patch** (rough papule in lumbosacral) • **Sebaceous adenomas** (small **red nodules** on cheeks, nose in **shape of butterfly**) • **Retinal** lesions; **mulberry tumors, phakomas** (gray, flat, round lesions in retina) • **CHF (rhabdomyoma)**	Dx- clinical, **wood's UV light** for skin lesions. • **Head CT** may show **calcified tubers** in cerebrum. • **ECG** evaluate for **rhabdomyoma.** **Renal U/S** may reveal mass. Tx- **infantile spasms** give **ACTH** or vigabatrin. **Seizures** give carbamazepine or lamotrigine.
77) Broca's (motor) **Aphasia**	**78) Wernicke's** (sensory) **Aphasia**	**79) B12 Deficiency** (Cyanocobalamin)
Damage to **posterior inferior frontal gyrus** secondary to left **MCA stroke.** Si/Sx- **BROKEN speech;** impair repetition. Pt shows **frustration** because they are **aware of deficit.** Tx- speech therapy.	Disorder with **comprehension** secondary to left side **MCA stroke.** Si/Sx- **"WORD SALAD," neologisms** (made-up words). Pt has **lack of awareness of the deficit.** Tx- speech therapy. "**BRO**ca's is **BRO**ken speech and **W**ernicke's is **W**ord salad."	Subacute degeneration of posterior and lateral columns. Cx- **pernicious anemia** (most common), Ileal/GI resection (Crohn's disease), malnutrition, strict vegetarians. Si/Sx- **"STOCKING GLOVE" symmetric paresthesias,** sensory neuropathy. Pt may have spasticity, paraplegia, **smooth tongue,** dementia, bowel and/or bladder dysfunction.

Neurology

80) B12 Deficiency (Cyanocobalamin)	81) Folate Deficiency	
Dx- megaloblastic anemia, **MCV>100**, multisegmented nuclei. Elevation in: • ↑**Homocysteine** • ↑**Methylmalonic acid (MMA).** Tx- **Vit B12 injections** or PO Vit B12. Comp- pts with pernicious anemia have ↑risk of **gastric cancer**.	Cx- **alcoholics,** malnutrition. Si/Sx- irritability, personality changes, confusion, anemia, glossitis, but **NO neurologic symptoms.** Risk- fetal **neural tube defects (NTD).**	Dx- megaloblastic anemia, **MCV>100**, multisegmented nuclei, check **folate level**. Elevation in: • ↑**Homocysteine** • **NORMAL Methylmalonic acid** (MMA). Tx- folate replacement.
82) Thiamine Deficiency (Vit B1)		
Cx- **alcoholics,** starvation, dialysis, HIV/AIDS, high-dose glucose administration. Tx- **thiamine administration.** If given early almost immediately reversal of symptoms.	• **WERNICKE'S Encephalopathy** Si/Sx- triad: • **Ataxia** • **Encephalopathy** • **Ophthalmoplegia** (nystagmus) Tx- replace **thiamine** (always give **thiamine before glucose**).	• **KORSAKOFF'S** Si/Sx- same as Wernicke's + antrograde and retrograde **AMNESIA, confabulations.** Tx- irreversible if thiamine treatment is late.

Neurology

83) Coma

Cx	Si/Sx- neurologic exam, **glasgow coma scale (GCS).** Also ask if pt is on any **sedatives.**	Dx-check electrolytes, complete medical hx, **head CT w/out contrast, LP, EEG.**
• **Diffuse hypoxic** • Axonal injury • Hemorrhage • Infarction • Herniation • Infxs • Toxins • Seizure • Endocrine • Metabolic	On exam may also R/O brain death by doing **DOLL's EYE maneuver, corneal reflex, cold-water caloric test,** gag reflex, pupillary response. R/O **"Locked-IN" syndrome** (awake, moving eye and eyelids).	Tx- **ABCs** and **DON'T** forget: • **D**- **D**extrose • **O**- **O₂** • **N**- **N**aloxone • **T**- **T**hiamine **Coma**- pt have a **resp drive.** (brain dead pts have NO resp drive).

84) Glasgow Coma Scale (GCS)

| **"4 Eyes** (see), **Jackson-5** (verbal), **V6 Engine** (motor)"

4 EYES open
4 spontaneously
3 on command
2 open to pain
1 no response | **VERBAL**
"Jackson 5"
5 alert, oriented
4 confused
3 inappropriate
2 incomprehensive
1 no response

Glasgow Coma Scale (GCS)- endotracheal intubation is warranted with **GCS<8.** | **MOTOR**
"V6 Engine"
6 follows direction
5 localize pain
4 withdraws to pain
3 decorticate (flexed)
2 decerebrate (extended)
1 no response |

12 CHAPTER
OBSTETRICS

Obstetrics

1) Pregnancy Terms		2) Prenatal Nutrition
• **Gravidity** (number of pregnancies) • **Parity** (births beyond 20wk) • **Gestational Age (GA)** Is number of wks and days from **last menstrual period (LMP).** Can also determined with fundal height, fetal heart tones, fetal movements, U/S crown-rump length (CRL). **U/S scan at 5–12wk** is the most reliable.	**U/S for GA** is most reliable during the **first trimester.** **Nagele's Rule** (due date)= LMP + 9mos + 7days. • **1st trimester** (2–14wk) • **2nd trimester (14–28wk)** • **3rd trimester** (28–40wks)	• **Exercise-30min daily** at moderate intensity. • **Iron-** 30mg/day • **Ca-** <19yo give 1300mg/day, >19yo give 1000mg/day • **Vit D-** 10ug or 400IU/day • **Vit B12-** 2ug/day • **Folic Acid 0.4mg/day,** if pt has hx of NTD give **4mg/day**.
3) Beta-hCG		
Beta-hCG is secreted by **syncytiotrophoblast** and is responsible for preservation of **corpus luteum** in pregnancy. **Beta-hCG double every 48hrs in early preg.** It is reduced by placenta and peaks 100,000 at 10wks of gestation. It starts to ↓**2nd Tri** (14–28wk).	**Beta-hCG** is used to determine: • **Diagnose** pregnancy • **Ectopic** pregnancy • **Monitor trophoblastic** • **Screen for fetal aneuploidy**	**Clinical PEARL: Pseudocyesis** Rare psychiatric condition in which pt has all Si/Sx of pregnany, but has a **normal endometrial stripe** and **NEG preg test.** "Pt is NOT preg."

Obstetrics

4) PAPP-A	5) Prenatal Schedule & Testing	6) NORMAL Pregnacy Changes
PAPP-A = Pregnancy Associated Plasma Protein-A.	**Wks 0–28:** every 4wk **Wks 29–35:** every 2wk **Wks 36–birth:** wkly	**THYROID** • ↑TBG
Diagnose: 85% Down syndrome, 98% trisomy 18.	**Initial Visit:** • **Heme-** CBC, Rh, blood type screen.	• ↑TOTAL T4, T3
Recommendation at **9–14wks**: **PAPP-A + B-hCG + U/S scan** (to determine **nuchal transparency**; fluid in fetal neck).	• **Infx-** U/A, culture, rubella antibody, HBsAg, **RPR/VDRL**, cervical gonorrhea, chlamydia, PPD, HIV, pap smear.	• **Normal TSH** • Normal FREE T4, T3 **GI** • ↑Gastric emptying
Less invasive than **chorionic villus sampling** (CVS in wks 10-12).	• **Possibly-** HbA1c, sickle cell screen. • **Genetic screen** Tay-Sachs, CF.	• ↓Sphincter tone

7) NORMAL Pregnacy Changes		
CARDIOVASCULAR • ↑**Heart rate** (20%) • ↑Stroke volume (max 19wks) • ↑Cardiac output (20%) • ↑Peripheral venous distention (to term) • ↓**Blood pressure** (10%) • ↓Peripheral vascular resistance (to term)	**PULMONARY** • ↑**Tidal volume** (30-40%) • ↑Respiratory minute volume (40%) • ↓Expiratory reserve • **Respiratory rate unchanged** • Vital capacity unchanged • **Respiratory Alkalosis** (effect progesterone on medullary resp center)	**BLOOD** • ↑**Volume** (50%) • ↑**Fibrinogen** • ↓Hematocrit • Electrolytes unchanged

Obstetrics

8) Prenatal Schedule & Testing		
• **9–14wk** PAPP-A + nuchal transparency + free beta-hCG. • **15–20wk MSAFP or Quad screen** (AFP, estriol, B-hCG, inhibin A) +/-amniocentesis. • **18–20wk U/S scan** full anatomic screen.	• **24–28wk OGTT- 1hr 50gram oral glucose challenge test** for gestational diabetes screening. If **>140mg/dL,** then order 3hr OGTT. • **28–30wk RhoGAM** for **Rh- neg** mother.	• **35–37wk** (2-3wk prior to delivery) **Screen GBS (S. agalactiae)** with culture vagina/rectum, and repeat CBC. • **34–40wk** Cervical chlamydia and gonorrhea culture, if high-risk HIV, RPR.

9) Quad Screening		
Quad screening: • Estriol • B-hCG • Inhibin A • MS-**AFP** (maternal serum **alpha-fetoprotein**) **Trisomy 18** **All four are ↓** ↓AFP, ↓Estriol, ↓Beta-hCG, ↓Inhibin A	**Trisomy 21** **2up, 2 DOWN** ↓AFP, ↓Estriol, ↑Beta-hCG, ↑inhibin A • **↑MSAFP** (>2.5MoMs) Assoc- **neural tube defects** (spina bifida, anencephaly), multiple gestation, **inaccurate dating** (most common), placental abruption.	• ↓MSAFP (<0.5MoMs) Assoc- trisomy 21 and trisomy 18, fetal demise, **incorrect dating** (most common). Dx- **U/S scan** confirm GA, incorrect dating, detect fetal anomalies, multiple gestation, confirm viable preg.

Obstetrics

10) Chorionic Villus Sample (10-12wks)	11) Amniocentesis (15-20wks)	
Recommended at **10–12wks (1st tri)** of transabdominal or transcervical **aspiration of placental "TISSUE"** (chorionic villi). • **Advantages:** Diagnosis accuracy. • **Disadvantage:** Risk **fetal loss (1–2%)**, cannot detect NTD. **<10wks GA** has greater risk of limb reduction defects.	Recommended at **15–20wks (2nd tri)** of transabdominal **aspiration amniotic "FLUID"** (U/S guided, fetal cells and genetic studies). **Amniotic fluid index:** • **AFI >20cm** polyhdramnios • **AFI <5cm** oligohydramnios Risk- postterm pregnancies >42wks (monitor for 2x wkly).	Indications for amniocentesis: • **>35 yo** • **Abn quad screen** • **Rh-sensitized mom** • **Evaluate lung maturity via lecithin-to-sphingomyelin ratio >2.5.** **Clinical PEARL: Amniotic Fluid Embolism (AFE)** Risk of amniocentesis Si/Sx- sudden respiratory failure, cardiogenic shock, purpuric rash. Tx- intubation.

12) Amniocentesis (15-20wks)	13) FDA Pregnancy Drug Risk	
• **Advantages** Detects; **neural tube defects** (80%), Down syndrome (85%), and Trisomy 18 (60%). • **Disadvantages** Risk premature rupture of membranes (PROM), **fetal loss** (0.5%).	**A- NO RISK. Vit B6, folic acid.** **B:** No well-controlled studies. Ampicillin, acetaminophen, bupropion. **C:** animal studies adverse effects, but not studies in women. Diphenhydramine, rifampin, **zidovudine (AZT).**	**D:** acceptable despite risk. Alcohol, tetracycline, phenytoin. **X: RISK** outweighs possible benefit. **Isotretinoin, warfarin,** thalidomide.

Obstetrics

14) Teratogenic Agents		
• **ACEIs** AE- **renal failure, IUGR.** • **Alcohol** AE- microcephaly, cardiac defects, renal defects, growth restriction, MR. **Fetal alcohol syndrome;** midfacial hypoplasia, short palpebral fissures, MR, **smooth philtrum, thin upper lip.** • **Androgen** AE- female **virilization.** • **Carbamazepine** AE- NTD/IUGR, fingernail hypoplasia, microcephaly.	• **Cocaine** AE- IUGR, bowel atresia, congenital malformation of limbs, face, GU, and heart. **Newborn** maybe SGA, be irritable, inconsolable, have **HIGH-pitched CRY, excessive SUCKING,** tremors, and/or tachy. • **Opiates (heroin, methadone)** AE: Neonatal **HIGH-pitched CRY,** poor sleep, tremors, seizures, sweating, **"SNEEZING,"** tachypnea, poor feeding, vomiting, and diarrhea.	• **Diethylstibestrol** AE- **vaginal CLEAR cell adenocarcinoma.** • **Lead** AE- spontaneous abortion (SAB) • **Lithium** AE- **Ebstein's anomaly** (tricuspid valve displaced into right ventricle of heart) • **Methotrexate** AE- spontaneous abortion (SAB) • **Mercury** AE- cerebral atrophy, MR, microcephaly, seizures, spasticity, blindness.

Obstetrics

15) Teratogenic Agents

• **Phenytoin**
AE- IUGR, microcephaly, **digital hypoplasia, fingernail hypoplasia**, hirsutism, **cleft palate**.

• **Radiation**
(safe if <0.05 Gy)
AE- microcephaly, MR

• **Streptomycin**
AE- **hearing loss,** CN VIII damage.

• **Tetracycline**
AE- **brown TEETH**.

• **Thalidomide**
(In 1950's was used to tx morning sickness)
AE- bilateral **LIMB deficiencies,** anotia (no ears), cardiac and GI anomalies.

• **Trimethadione**
AE- cleft lip or palate, MR, cardiac defects, microcephaly.

• **Valproic acid**
AE- **NTD** (spina bifida), craniofacial defects.

• **Vit A**
AE- spontaneous abortion (SAB), cardiovascular defects, craniofacial, MR, thymic agenesis, cleft lip or palate.

• **Warfarin**
AE- IUGR, nasal hypoplasia, **stippled bone epiphyses,** ophthalmologic abnormalities.

• **Isotretinoin**
"Strict contraception"
AE- craniofacial dysmorphism, heart defects, deafness.

Obstetrics

16) TORCHHS

T-TOXOPLASMOSIS	O- OTHER	C- CMV
Cx- Toxoplasma gondii Assoc- **raw meat, cat feces** (avoid in pregnancy), goat's milk. Si/Sx- classic triad: • **Chorioretinitis** • **Hydrocephalus** • **Intracranial Ca** Dx- serologic testing, **head CT may show ring-enhance lesion.** Tx- **TMP-SMX,** prophylaxis **spiramycin** in 3rd trimester.	Parvovirus, varicella, TB, malaria, listeria, fungi. **R- RUBELLA** Si/Sx- **"blueberry muffin" rash, cataracts, hearing loss,** patent ductus arteriosus **(PDA)**, MR. Dx- serologic testing. Tx- immunize before pregnancy, **vaccinate MMR** before delivery if serologic neg.	Si/Sx- **PETECHIAL RASH,** periventricular calcifications. Dx- urine culture, PCR of amniotic fluid. Tx- postpartum **ganciclovir.** **TORCHS** (all) Si/Sx- microcephaly, hepatosplenomegaly, chorioretinitis, deafness, thrombocytopenia.

17) TORCHHS

H-HIV	H-HERPES (HSV)	S-SYPHILIS
Si/Sx- asymp, transmission in utero and through **breast milk.** Dx- **ELISA** (screen), **western blot** (confirm). Tx- **zidovudine (AZT) or nevirapine** in HIV pregnancy. Infant give prophylactic **zidovudine (AZT),** and **no breast-feeding**.	Si/Sx- **active lesions** can lead to infant infx on skin, mouth, eyes, and CNS infects. Dx serologic testing. Tx- **acyclovir,** if **lesions** are present at delivery than do **C-section.**	Si/Sx- rash, rhinorrhea, **"SNIFFLES,"** **ulcerative** lesions on **palms and soles.** Later pts get saddle nose, saber shins. **Hutchinson's triad:** peg-shaped **incisors, deafness,** and interstitial **keratits.** Dx- **dark-field microscopy** (shows spirochetes), **VDRL/RPR** (screen), **FTA-ABS** (confirm). Tx- **penicillin**

Obstetrics

18) Normal Labor and Delivery	19) Bishop Score	
Leopold's maneuvers • **Fetal lie** (long or transverse) • **Presentation** (breech or cephalic) **Cervical exam:** Dilation, effacement, station, consistency, position. Sterile speculum exam if rupture of membranes (ROM).	Score each from left to right with 0, 1, 2, or 3pt • **Dilation** closed, 1–2, 3–4, 5+ • **Effacement** 0–30, 40–50, 60–70, 80+ • **Station** -2, -1, +1, +2 • **Consistency** firm, medium, soft • **Position** posterior, mid, anterior	**Bishop score:** • **0–4-** give **prostaglandins** for induction. • **5–9-** give **pitocin** for induction. • **10–13-** high probability for success.
20) Fetal Heart Rate (FHR)		**21) Variability**
Normal FHR (110–160bpm) • **FHR <110** Cx- hypoxia due to **uterine hyper-stimulation,** cord prolapse, or rapid fetal descent. • **FHR >160** Cx- hypoxia, fetal anemia, maternal fever. **Variability** (normal 6–25bpm) used to detect fetal distress.	**If pt has no complications** Do FHR tracing every **30min** in 1st stage of labor, and every **15min** in 2nd stage. **If pt has complications review** FHR tracing every **15min** in 1st stage, and every **5min** in 2nd stage.	**Accelerations** (reassuring) ↑FHR peak in <30sec. = **REASSURING.** **Decelerations:** • **EARLY** Decelerations (**mirrors contractions**) Cx- **HEAD Compression.** • **VARIABLE** Decelerations Cx-**UMBILICAL cord compression.** Tx- administer O2 and change maternal position.

Obstetrics

22) Variability	23) Nonstress Test (NST)	
Decelerations: • **LATE Decelerations** (after the peak contraction) Cx- **hypoxemia, utero-placental insufficiency.** Tx- indication for **emergent cesarean** section.	If ↓ fetal movements: order **Nonstress Test (NST)** which is FHR monitoring for uterine contractions. **Normal fetal movements** is 10 movements in 20mins at **32–42wks** (if pt has risk factors check at 26–28wk).	• **Reactive NST** 2 accelerations of >15bpm for at least 15sec over 20mins. • **Nonreactive NST:** < 2 accelerations over 20mins => then order **biophysical profile (BPP).** Nonreactive Cx: GA<32wk, sleeping, sedative, narcotics.
24) Biophysical Profile (BPP)		**25) Contraction Stress Test (CST)**
BPP: • Fetal **tone** • Fetal **breathing** • Fetal **movement** • **Amniotic fluid vol** • **Nonstress test (NST)** Each assessment is graded either **0 or 2pts,** then added up to yield number between **0 and 10.**	• **8—10pts: normal fetal well being.** • **6pts:** considered equivocal, **order CST.** • **4pts:** consider **steroids,** and **BPP within next 24hrs.** • **< 4pts:** extremely worrisome, **deliver fetus if >26wks** gestational age.	**FHR** is monitored while pt is in **lateral recumbent position.** • **Neg CST** "Fetal well-being" No late or variable decelerations in 10mins. • **Positive CST** **LATE decelerations,** possible **fetal compromise=> delivery.**
26) Stages of Labor		
1st STAGE: • **LATENT** **(3–4cm dilation)** Prim 6-11hrs Multi 4–8hrs (Prim= primigravida, Multi= multigravida)	• **ACTIVE** **(4–10cm dilation)** Prim 4–6hrs Muti 2–3hrs	**Failure to progress in STAGE 1** Tx- **AMNIOTOMY** (artificial rupture of membranes), then possibly **oxytocin.** C-section if cephalopelvic disproportion.

Obstetrics

27) Stages of Labor		
2nd STAGE: **Complete dilation** to **delivery** of infant. Prim 0.5–3hrs Multi 5–30mins **3rd STAGE:** **Delivery** of the **placenta.** Prim 0–0.5hrs Multi 0–0.5hrs	**Failure to progress in STAGE 2** Tx- **lower epidural rate** and continue **oxytocin.** Consider forceps, vaccum, or C-section.	**Clinical PEARL:** **Arrest Disorders** **3P's:** • **Power** (contractions) • **Passenger** (baby) • **Passage** (pelvis)
28) Rupture of Membranes (ROM)		
• **Spont ROM** ROM **>1hr** before onset of labor. • **PROM** **Prolonged** ROM, rupture **>18hr prior delivery.** • **PPROM** **Preterm Premature** Rupture Of Membrane **<37wks.**	Si/Sx- **GUSH clear** or blood-ting **amniotic fluid.** **Clinical PEARL:** **Chorioamnionitis** (intraamniotic infx) Si/Sx- maternal fever, uterine tenderness. Risk- **PPROM <37wks** Tx- broad-spectrum abxs and **immediate delivery.**	Dx- 1st STEP: • **Sterile speculum exam** check for pooling of amniotic fluid in vaginal vault. • **+ Nitrazine paper test** (turn **blue,** alkaline pH amniotic fluid). • **+ Fern test** (amniotic fluid dries on glass slide in a **ferning pattern**). 2nd STEP: **U/S scan** to assess amniotic volume. **Do not perform a digital vaginal exam.**

Obstetrics

29) Rupture of Membranes (ROM)		
Tx • **Term-** check **GBS** (S. agalactiae) and **induce labor**. • **>34–36wks-** consider induction of labor.	• **<32wks- BED REST betamethasone or dexamethasone** x 48hr (promote fetal lung maturity). • If signs of **infx or fetal distress** give **ampicillin + gentamicin** and induce labor.	**Clinical PEARL: False Labor** Si/Sx- **absent cervical changes,** contractions **do not shorten** or increase in intensity, every 10-20mins, **relieved by sedation**. Tx- reassurance.

30) PRETERM Labor 20–37wks		
Si/Sx- menstrual like cramps, **low back pain,** new vaginal discharge or bleeding between **20-37wks gestation.** Dx- **regular uterine contractions** (>3 of 30sec over 30min) and **CERVICAL changes.** **Sterile speculum exam,** and **U/S scan** to R/O uterine anomalies. Assess if there are any contraindications to **tocolysis.**	Tx- hydration, bed rest and **TOCOLYTIC** (anti-contraction meds or labour repressants); indomethacin (NSAIDs). • **Magnesium sulfate** therapy or **Beta-agonists**; terbutaline, ritodrine (supress premature labor). • **Betamethasone** (fetal lung maturity).	Tx Also give **penicillin** or **ampicillin** for **GBS** prophylaxis. For penicillin allergy use **cefazolin.** If severe allergy to penicillin use **vancomycin.** Risk- **germinal matrix hemorrhage** (hypoxic insults). **Clinical PEARL: Unknown GBS Status** give prophylaxis if: • **Delivery <37wks** • **ROM >18hrs** • **GBS bacteriuria** at any point in pregnancy • **Prior hx GBS sepsis**

Obstetrics

31) Fetal Malpresentation		32) Multiple Gestations
• VERTEX Head closest to birth canal, considered **normal** presentation (most common). • **Frank breech** (50–75%) thighs flexed, knees extended. Tx- >37wks GA can attempt **external cephalic version** (breech into cephalic).	• **Footling breech** 1or 2 legs extended below buttock. • **Complete breech** (rare) thighs and knees flexed. Tx- most spont go to **VERTEX by 38wk.**	• **Monozygotic Identical** twins. • **Dizygotic Non-identical** twins (fraternal twins). Si/Sx- rapid uterine growth, more fetal parts on Leopold's maneuvers.

33) Multiple Gestations	34) Shoulder Dystocia	
Dx- **U/S, hCG, and MSAFP** are elevated for gestational age (GA). Tx- multifetal reduction, close observation due to higher risk pregnancy. Comp- **risk of being hospitalized with** preeclampsia, preterm labor, PPROM, placental abruption.	Risk- **obesity, diabetes,** prior shoulder dystocia or prior macrosomic infant. Dx- prolonged **2nd stage labor.** Tx- help mother to reposition.	• **McRoberts Maneuver** Hyperflex mother's legs to abdomen. • **Episiotomy** Incision on perineum. • **Wood's screw** Enter vagina with attempt to rotation. • Last can try to reach for fetal arm.

193

Obstetrics

35) Spontaneous Abortion		
Loss of products of concept (POC) **<20WEEKS**. Cx- **chrom abn,** ↑age, infx, **antiphospholipid antibodies** (SLE), DM, tobacco, alcohol, cervical incompetence.	Dx-↓ **hCG levels,** **U/S scan**. Tx- give **RhoGAM** to **Rh neg** mother.	**Clinical PEARL:** **Septic Abortion** Si/Sx- fever, chills, abd pain, bloody/purulent discharge. Tx- **cervical cultures and blood cultures** followed by **IV abxs** and gentle suction **curettage.**
36) Types of Spont Abortions		
• **Complete abortion** Si/Sx- POC (products of conception) expelled, **closed Os.** U/S shows **EMPTY uterus.** • **Incomplete abortion** Si/Sx- **some POC** expelled, **OPEN Os.** • **Threatened abortion** Si/Sx- no POC expelled, **BLEEDING,** +/- abd pain, **closed Os.** Tx- reassurance, outpt follow-up, U/S in 1wk.	• **Inevitable abortion** Si/Sx- no POC expelled, **bleeding,** cramp, **OPEN Os** +/- ROM. • **Missed abortion** Si/Sx-**no POC expelled,** no fetal cardiac motion, no bleed. **Closed Os, no fetal tissue on U/S.** Tx- remove POC with **dilation and curettage** or with vaginal **misoprostol**.	• **Intrauterine fetal demise (IUFD)** absence of fetal cardiac activity; **no FHT or movement on U/S.** Risk of DIC. Tx- **induction of labor.** Lactation suppression with **tight fitting bras and ice packs.**

Obstetrics

37) Elective Abortion		
1st TRIMESTER: • **>1mo** (up to 49 day) Tx- **Methotrexate** + misoprostol or **mifepristone** + misoprostol. • **2mos** (up to 56 days) Tx- **Misoprostol** (3 doses). • **3mos** (up to 13wks) Tx- surgical with **D&C** (dilation and curettage) with vacuum.	**2nd TRIMESTER:** (13–24wk) • **Obstetric** treatment Induction labor with **prostaglandins, amniotomy** (artificial rupture of membranes, AROM), and **oxytocin.** • **Surgical** treatment **D&E** (dilation and evacuation).	**Clinical PEARL:** **Methotrexate** is used in early ectopic pregnancy, but is contraindicated in missed abortions.

38) Rhesus Isoimmunization		
RhoGAM (anti-D gamma globulin) administer to all pts who do not have **alloantibodies at 28wks gestation.**	**Fetomaternal Hemorrhage** Tx- if suspect **fetomaternal hemorrhage** perform **E-Rosette test** (microscope shows RBCs that form cluster that looks like a flower). If **NEG E-Rosette test** treat with standard **300-ug dose IM.**	If **E-Rosette test** is positive order **Kleihauer-Betke stain** (estimate fetal cells in maternal blood). **For every 15mL** of fetal blood in maternal give **300-ug IM** with **max of 5 shots.**

Obstetrics

39) Hyperemesis Gravidarum

Cx-↑ **beta-hCG levels,** ↑estradiol. Si/Sx- **morning sickness,** and **persistent vomiting** that persists **AFTER 1st trimester**; onset between **weeks 4-10** and resolve by week 20. Dx- R/O **molor pregnancy** with checking B-hCG levels and doing an U/S.	Dx- Pts may have **metabolic alkalosis** with possibly respiratory compensation. Labs; **ketonuria,** ↑AST, ↑ALT, ↑lipase, ↑amylase. Tx- **Vit B6 (1st line), doxylamine** (antihistamine). If dehydrated give IV fluids, dimenhydrinate or promethazine.	If severe give **ondansetron, metoclopramide,** promethazine, or prochlorperazine. **Clinical PEARL:** Chemotherapy-induced nausea and vomiting. Tx- **serotonin antagonist** (5HT3 antagonist).

40) Anesthesia and Analgesia

• **Opioids** Tx- PAIN AE- ↓fetal heart rate (FHR). • **Epidural** Tx- most effective **PAIN relief.** AE- **hypotension** (from blood venous pooling).	• **Lidocaine** Tx- **repair lacerations.** AE: hypotension, seizures, cardiac arrhythmias, **asystole.**	• **General Anesthesia** Tx- **emergent C-section delivery.** AE- maternal **aspiration,** neonatal depression.

Obstetrics

41) Gestational DM		
Diabetes that is **first diagnosed during pregnancy**. Si/Sx- **asymp**, may have polyhydramnios, **large for GA** infant (>90%). Dx- **OGTT, 1hr 50g** glucose challenge test **(24–28wks),** value >140mg/dL abnormal. Confirm with **OGTT 3hr (100g) oral glucose tolerance test:** 1hr>180, 2hr >155, **3hr >140mg/dL.**	**Risks to fetus;** macrosomia, hypocalcemia, **hypoglycemia, hyperviscosity** (due to polycythemia), congestive heart failure. Tx- DM diet, exercise, **strict glucose monitoring** (4xday), **fasting <100** (goal fasting 75-90), postprandial <150.	Tx- **add insulin** if diet does not control blood sugar. **Periodic fetus NSTs and U/S.** Comp- 50% of pts go on to **develop DM2.** **Clinical PEARL: Klumpke's Paralysis** (brachial palsy). From excessive traction on arm during birth of newborn. Si/Sx- **hand paralysis** and **ipsilateral Horner's** syndrome (ptosis and miosis).
42) Pre-Gestational DM		
Diabetes **before <20wks** gestation. Si/Sx- asymp. Dx- think pregestational DM when **U/A shows glycosuria in <20wks.**	**"1st Trimester Hyperglycemia."** Tx- **strict glucose control;** diet, exercise, insulin, and frequent monitoring.	Tx **Goal:** • Fasting morning **glucose <90**mg/dL. • 2hr postprandial **glucose <120**mg/dL

Obstetrics

43) Gestational Hypertension		44) Preeclampsia
Hypertension that starts **after 20wks** gestation. Si/Sx- **asymp HTN, >20wks** gestation. Dx- **hypertension without** proteinuria. • **Gestational HTN** AFTER **20wk.** • **Chronic HTN <20wk** (this is not gestational HTN).	Tx- monitor BP closely and give **methyldopa, labetalol** (beta-blocker), or **nifedipine.** **Do NOT give ACEIs, ARBs** or diuretics (tetrogenic)!	Si/Sx- **HTN, HA,** edema, **proteinuria.** Dx- **new** onset **HTN >140/90** and **proteinuria >300mg** in 24hrs, **>20wks gestation.** Tx- bed rest if far from term. If close to term, induce labor with **IV oxytocin, prostaglandin, or amniotomy** (artificial rupture of membranes).
45) Severe Preeclampsia	**46) Preeclampsia**	**47) Eclampsia**
Si/Sx- HTN, HA, blurred vision, epigastric pain, RUQ pain (stretching of hepatic, Glisson's capsule), hyperactive reflexes. Assoc- **HELLP** (hemolytic anemia, elevated liver enzymes, low platelets). Dx- **BP >160/110, proteinuria >5g/24hrs.** Tx- control BP with **labetalol** and/or **hydralazine.** Give **Mg sulfate** drip to prevent further seizures. Deliver by induction or C-section. If pt gets Mg toxicity give **Ca gluconate.**	• Preeclampsia "It's not just HyPE" **H- Hypertension** **Y** **P- Proteinuria** **E- Edema** • Severe preeclampsia **HELLP syndrome** **H- Hemolytic** anemia **E- Elevated** **L- Liver** enzymes **L- Low** **P- Platelets** Tx- only cure is delivery. **Clinical PEARL:** **Magnesium toxicity** Si/Sx-↓**DTR,** respiratory depression. Tx- **calcium gluconate.**	Si/Sx- new onset grand-mal **SEIZURES with preeclampsia.** Dx- HTN, proteinuria, and **seizures.** Tx- ABCs, **Mg sulfate** to prevent further seizures, and **induce delivery.** If pt has recurrent seizures give IV diazepam. Control BP with **labetalol** and/or **hydralazine.**

Obstetrics

48) Antepartum Hemorrhage		49) Placental Abruption
Si/Sx- **ANY bleeding after >20wks** (if <20wks bleeding it is a threatened abortion). Cx • **Placental Abruption** • **Placenta Previa** • **Vasa Previa** Dx- clinical Tx- underlying cause.	**Clinical PEARL** **Vasa Previa** Rare condition in which **fetal blood vessels traverse** between baby and cervical os. Si/Sx **fetal HR from tachy to brady** to sinusoidal pattern suddenly **after ROM**. Normal maternal vital signs. Tx-**"Crash C-section"**	**Premature separation** of implanted **placenta**. Risk factors: **HTN** (most common), **MVA/trauma,** tobacco, **cocaine,** prior abruption.
50) Placental Abruption		
Si/Sx- **"PAINFUL," DARK red bleed** (absence of blood does not r/o, blood in 80%) in third trimester, >20wks). Pts may also have abd pain, back pain, HTN, with **no change in fetal station**. Dx- clinical. Comp- **feto-maternal hemorrhage,** fetal hypoxia.	Tx- stabilize pt, **hospitalize,** with fetal monitoring and bed rest. If severe immediate delivery. Correct the dose of **anti-D immune globulin** for **Rh NEG** mother with blood loss using the **Kleihauer-Betke stain**.	**Clinical PEARL:** **Uterine Rupture** Si/Sx- **intense** abd pain, vaginal **bleeding,** change in **fetal station.** **Hypovolemia and SHOCK** are common in uterine rupture. Assoc- **Uterine SCAR** from prior caesarian section. Tx- emergent C-section delivery.

Obstetrics

51) Placenta Previa

Cx- abnormal placental implantation that **covers cervical Os.** **Types:** • **Low lying-** placenta close to os. • **Marginal-** placenta to margin of os. • **Total-** placenta covers cervical os.	Risk factors: **Prior C-section** (low transverse), advanced age, smoking, multiple gestations, prior placenta previa. Si/Sx- **"PAINLESS," BRIGHT red blood in** third trimester (>20wks). Dx- transabdominal or **transvaginal U/S scan** high sensitivity (95%).	Tx- **No vaginal exam!** Stabilize pt with premature fetus and give **tocolytics, serial U/S, and betamethasone** (for fetal lung maturity). **Scheduled cesarean section.** Emergency deliver by **C-section** if: life-threaten bleeding, **>36wks,** or there is **fetal distress.**

52) Ectopic Pregnancy

Si/Sx- amenorrhea, abd pain, +/- vaginal spotting or bleeding. Dx- **+preg test** and empty uterus and **adnexal sac** on **transvaginal U/S scan** (more accurate than transabdominal U/S).	Dx- **Serial hCG** (confirms diagnosis) **without** appropriate **doubling of hCG** for pregnancy. Once B-HCG is >1,500 repeat transvaginal U/S.	Tx- **methotrexate** (if small), surgical with **salpingectomy** or salpingostomy with laparoscopy or laparotomy. Comp- **tubal rupture, hemoperitoneum** (blood in peritoneal cavity) medical emergency.

Obstetrics

53) IUGR		
Intrauterine growth restriction (IUGR); **EFW <10%**. Risk factors: • **SYMMETRIC growth restriction** (fetal factors) Head and body lag behind dates. Cx- **chrom,** congenital anomalies, **infxs (TORCH).**	Risk factors: • **ASYMMETRIC growth restriction** (maternal factors) Normal head size, reduced abdominal. Cx- **hypoxemia, HTN, smoking** (most common), preeclampsia. Si/Sx- HTN, anemia, or intrauterine infx. Dx- **abdominal circumference** is most effective parameter for estimating fetal growth restriction (FGR).	Dx- **serial U/S** for fundal **height and EFW** (est fetal weight). Tx- underlying etiology, give **betamethasone** (for fetal lung maturity). Fetal monitoring with **NST, CST, and BPP.** If nonreassuring and near term then delivery.

54) Rh Isoimmunization		
Fetal RBCs into maternal circulation => **maternal anti-Rh IgG antibody.** In 2nd pregnancy maternal anti-Rh IgG cause 2nd trimester **hemolysis of fetal Rh RBCs** leading to **erythroblastosis fetalis.**	Risk factors: **Rh NEG** mother, Rh positive baby. Dx- Rh neg mothers with **titer >1:16 should be closely monitor** for fetal hemolysis.	Tx Prevention: give **RhoGAM** to Rh NEG mother at **28wks.** Comp- **hydrops fatalis** occurs when fetal Hg drop <7g/dL.

Obstetrics

55) Gestational Trophoblastic		
• **Complete mole (46XX)** empty ovum. • **Incomplete/partial mole (69XXY)** normal ovum, 2 sperm.	Si/Sx- **1st trimester uterine BLEEDING** (most common), uterine size greater than dates, with nausea and vomiting. Risk- **folate def** or **beta-carotene def.** Dx- no fetal heart beat, ↑ **beta-hCG >100,000.**	Dx- U/S shows **SNOWSTORM** with no gestational sac. **"GRAPELIKE" molar clusters** into vagina. Tx- eval uterus and **Beta-hCG wkly.** Comp: **Choriocarcinoma** (↑Beta-hCG).
56) Choriocarcinoma		
Choriocarcinoma is a form of **gestational trophoblastic disease (GTD).** Assoc- **after molar pregnancy,** normal gestation, abortion, or ectopic pregnancy.	Si/Sx- irregular vaginal **bleeding, enlarged uterus**, pelvic pain or discomfort. Irregular vaginal **bleeding >8wks post-partum** is abn, and should raise suspicion of **GTD.**	Dx- quantitative **beta-HCG.** Comp- **metastatic spread to lungs.** These pts may have pulm symps of chest pain, dyspnea, hemoptysis.

Obstetrics

57) Postpartum Hemorrhage		58) Sheehan's Syndrome
Loss of blood during delivery of: • >500mL in vaginal delivery. • >1000mL in C-section delivery. Si/Sx- anemia, tachycardia, SOB. Risk- Uterine ATONY is the most common (soft, enlarged, BOGGY uterus).	Tx- uterine massage (1st-line), oxytocin, methergine, or prostaglandin. Comp- Sheehan's syndrome (pituitary ischemia and necrosis) leading to failure to lactate.	Postpartum pituitary necrosis from massive blood loss. Si/Sx- weakness, lethargy, amenorrhea (↓LH, ↓FSH), inability to lactate (↓prolactin). Dx- ↓prolactin levels and MRI of pituitary. Tx- replace hormones.
59) Postpartum Infections		
FEVER two or more of the 10 days postpartum days, but not within the first 24hrs. Si/Sx- FEVER >38C within 36hrs postop, uterine tenderness, malodorous lochia.	Risk factors: emergency C-section, PROM, prolonged labor, prolonged ruptured membranes, postpartum endometritis. Tx- if endometritis, give IV clindamycin and gentamicin until afebrile for 48hrs.	Tx If pt does not improve on abxs R/O septic pelvic thrombophlebitis. Clinical PEARL: Endometritis Cx- polymicrobial infx. Si/Sx- fever, uterine tenderness, foul-smelling lochia. Tx- clindamycin and gentamicin.

Obstetrics

60) Mastitis

Cellulitis by nipple trauma. Si/Sx- **2–4wks postpartum, unilateral** breast tenderness, edema, warmth, nipple drainage. Pts may also have fever and chills.	Dx- **+breast milk culture, ↑WBCs.** Tx- analgesics, abxs and **continuation of breastfeeding** or using a **breast pump** (if no longer breastfeeding) to prevent accumulation of infx material.	Tx Possibly start PO abxs of **amoxicillin/ clavulanate,** dicloxacillin, azithromycin, or clindamycin.

61) 6 W's of Postpartum Fever

• **Wind** (Atelectasis, day 1-2) **Prevent-** pain control, **incentive spirometry,** elevate head of the bed (↑lungs functional residual capacity >20%).	• **Water** (UTI, day 3-4) • **Womb** (Endomyometritis, day 4–5) Tx- **clindamycin** and **gentamicin**.	• **Wound** (incision, day 5–6) • **Walking** (DVT, PE, day 7–8) • **W-Weaning** (breast engorgement, day 7–21)

14 CHAPTER
GYNECOLOGY

Gynecology

1) Fibrocystic Change (FCC)		2) Fibroadenoma
Most common **benign breast growth, 30-50yo** Si/Sx- **CYCLIC bilateral PAIN** and swelling, **just before menstruation.** Rapid **fluctuation** in size, bumpy and irregular like; **"oatmeal with raisins."** **"Cyclic** for fibro**Cystic"**	Dx- mammography is of limited use. **U/S scan** helps differentiate **cystic from solid.** If no fluid or blood is obtained by **FNA** do a **excisional biopsy.** Tx- **OCPs**, use **danazol** (↓estradiol) for severe pain.	**Benign,** slow-growing breast tumor. Most common **<30yr.** Si/Sx- **round, RUBBERY,** solitary, mobile, **NON-TENDER** mass that is **1–3cm. NO change with cycle.**

3) Fibroadenoma	4) Breast Cancer	
Dx- **breast U/S scan** to differentiate cystic from solid and also a **FNA or needle biopsy.** If pathologic exam remains uncertain do an **excision biopsy.** Tx- **excision** (recurrence is common).	Breast cancer is the most common cancer in women. Risk factors: **BRCA1, BRCA2,** 1st degree relative, >age, high-fat, low-fiber diet. ↑**ESTROGEN**; nulliparity, early menarche, late menopause, and/or 1st pregnancy >35yo.	**Palpable breast abn:** • **<30yo-** U/S scan; simple cyst needle aspiration, complex cyst order core biopsy. • **>30yo-Mammogram and U/S**; suspicious for malignancy order core biopsy.

Gynecology

5) Breast Cancer		
Si/Sx- **upper OUTER quadrant,** single, nontender, firm mass, with ill-defined margins. Breast may have **skin retraction,** axillary lymphadenopathy, and back pain (mets). • **Intraductal Papilloma** Si/Sx- **"bloody"** nipple discharge.	• **Paget's disease of nipple** Si/Sx- eczematous, ulcerating, **itchy rash,** scaling erosion of nipple for prolonged time. Assoc- underlying **adenocarcinoma.** Dx- biopsy shows large cells surrounded by clear halos.	Dx 90% found by pt. **Screening by mammograms** every 2yrs starting at 50yo. • **Premenopausal** U/S (solid vs cyst). • **Postmenopausal** Order **mammography.** If papilloma is small in size, **galactogram** may be helpful.
6) Breast Cancer		
Dx Check tumor markers: **CEA, CA 27-29, CA15-3, ER, PR** (estrogen receptor and progesterone receptor), **HER2/neu.**	Look for possible metastatic disease: ↑ESR, ↑Ca, ↑AlkPh. Possibly order CXR, CT, and/or bone scan. **Clinical PEARL:** **Pubertal gynecomastia in boys** are most often **benign.** Tx-observation.	**Clinical PEARL:** **Breast Fat Necrosis** Si/Sx appears similar to breast cancer, skin and nipple retraction and **calcifications on mammography.** Dx- biopsy of mass reveals **fat globules** and **foamy macrophages.**

Gynecology

7) Breast Cancer Treatment

Prognosis:
TNM stage I–IV
(Tumor, Node,
Metastasis). This is the
**single most important
prognostic factor** when
determining treatment.

Surgery:
• <4cm- **lumpectomy**
+ axillary dissection
then **radiation**.

• >4cm- **radical
mastectomy**.

Hormone Receptor:
• If positive (+ER,
+PR) use **tamoxifen.**

• If **ER receptor is neg**
use chemotherapy.

Hormone Receptor:
• For **+HER2/neu**
receptors use
**trastuzumab
(HER**ceptin).

Trastuzumab
AE: **cardiotoxicity**
(pts should have
ECHO before starting
treatment).

8) Menopause

Average onset 51yo, or
premature menopause
under the age of <40yo.

Si/Sx- **"HAVOC"**
H- **Hot** flashes

A- **Atrophy** of

V- **Vagina**

O- **Osteoporosis**

C- **Coronary** artery
disease

Dx- ↑**FSH,** later on
there will be an ↑**LH.**

Dx- check for
osteoporosis with
DEXA scan and
order lipid profile
(↑cholesterol ↓HDL).

Tx
• **HRT** (comb estrogen
and progestin).
AE: ↑CVA, **breast CA,
endometrial CA,**
thromboembolism,
hypertriglyceridemia.

• ↓**Hot flashes**
Tx- **venlafaxine** or
clonidine (AE- rebound
HTN in cessation).

Tx
• **Vaginal atrophy**
Tx- **estradiol** vaginal
ring or cream.

• **Osteoporosis**
Tx-**calcium,
bisphosphonates**.

**Clinical PEARL:
Primary
Ovarian Failure**
Dx- ↓Estrogen,
↑**FSH,** ↑**LH,**
FSH/LH >1.0.

Gynecology

9) Contraceptives >99%		
• **Implanon (lasts 3yrs) Progestin only implant.** Fertility with removal, safe with breastfeeding. AE- spotting, weight gain, depression.	• **IUD- Progestin** (mirena, lasts **5yrs**) Fertility with removal, safe with breastfeeding. AE-spotting, acne. • **Surgical sterilization** Vasectomy or tubal ligation.	• **IUD- ParaGard (COPPER T-380A,** lasts **10YRS)** Fertility with removal, safe with breastfeeding. AE- cramping and bleeding.
10) Contraceptives 90–99%		
• **Oral Contraceptives** (estrogen and progestin) Fertility upon cessation. **OCP** AE: **Hypertension**, MI, thromboembolism, ↑triglyceride, stroke, ↑cholestasis, DM, **hepatic adenoma. NO weight gain assoc**. **OCP Protective: ovarian CA,** endometrial CA, dysmenorrhea.	• **Progestin-ONLY "minipills" SAFE with breastfeeding** used in lactating mothers who want contraception**. • **Depo-provera (IM 3mos)** (medroxy-progesterone) Safe with breastfeeding. AE-irregular bleeding, weight gain, **delayed fertility.**	• **Ortho evra patch (wkly)** Low-dose progestin and estrogen. Make period more regular. • **NuvaRing** (vaginal ring of progestin and estrogen) 3wks on and one wk without ring.
11) Contraceptives 75–90%		**12) Emergency Contraceptives**
• **Male condoms ONLY method** effectively protecting against pregnancy, **STDs, and HIV.** • **Diaphragm with spermicide-** some protection from STDs (fitted by provider).	**Clinical PEARL: Adolescents** without parental consent; **contraception, prenatal care, STDs, or substance abuse** and are entitled to strict pt confidentiality. **68–74%** • Withdrawal, and/or spermicide.	• **Levonorgestrel ("Plan B")** **Use within 120hours** of sex. • **Copper-T IUD** use within 7 days of unprotected sex (99% effective).

Gynecology

13) Contraception Contraindications		14) Pediatric Vaginal Discharge
• **OCPs, Nuva ring, and Patch** C/I- pregnancy, hx CAD, DVT, breast cancer, tobacco use. • **Mirena Alone** C/I- breast cancer, liver disease, +BRCA, levonorgestrel allergy.	• **Copper-T IUDs** C/I- preg, PID, **vaginal bleeding**, cervicitis, cervical or uterine CA, abn PAP, valve replacement. • **Copper T alone** C/I- Wilson disease (↑↑copper).	• **Foreign Objects (most common)** Si/Sx- malodorous, yellow-green discharge. Tx- **irrigation with warm fluid.** If unsuccessful remove with sedation.
15) Pediatric Vaginal Discharge	**16) Precocious Puberty <8yrs**	
• **Infectious vulvovaginitis** Si/Sx- malodorous, yellow-green discharge. Cx-Group A Strep (GAS). Dx- r/o **STDs**. • **Candidal infection** Assoc with diabetes. • **Sarcoma botryoides** Cx-rhabdomyosarcoma Si/Sx- "**Bunches of GRAPES**" in vagina.	Cx • **Central** Hypothalamic **GnRH**. Early activation of hypothalamic-pituitary-ovarian axis. • **Peripheral** Non-hypothalamic GnRH. Si/Sx- **before the age of 8 years old**; breast development, vaginal bleed, pubic hair growth, ↑clitoris, and ↑body odor.	• ↑**Estrogen** (breast development, vaginal bleed)=> r/o **ovarian** cysts or tumors. • ↑**Androgens** (pubic hair growth, ↑clitoris, ↑body odor) => r/o **Adrenal** tumors or congenital **Adrenal** hyperplasia (CAH).

Gynecology

17) Precocious Puberty <8yrs		
Dx • **Central** ↑**FSH,**↑**LH** (GnRH activation) •**Peripheral** ↓FSH,↓LH (gonadal or adrenal) Dx- **accelerated bone growth** and advanced bone age (common). R/O when **bone age** is within one yr of **chronological age** (**puberty** not started).	**GnRH agonist** (leuprolide) **stim test:** • **Central** If +↑**LH response** => then order cranial **MRI** (R/O CNS tumor). • **Peripheral** If **NEG LH** => order **U/S of ovaries and adrenals** to look for cysts/tumors.	**Source:** • If ↑**Estradiol** possibly **ovarian** cysts or tumors. • If ↑**Androgens** (**DHEA, DHEAS;** dehydroepi-androsterone sulfate) possibly **adrenals**. • ↑**17-OH progesterone;** screen bone age, possibly **CAH.**
18) Precocious Puberty <8yrs		
Central tx: • **Leuprolide** (1st-line, GnRH agonist), to prevent premature fusion of epiphyseal plates. **Peripheral** tx: • **Ovarian cysts** (will regress). • **CAH** give glucocorticoids.	**Peripheral** tx: • **McCune-Albright 3P's Precocious** puberty, **Pigmentation, Polyostotic** fibrous dysplasia of bones. Give **tamoxifen, ketoconazole, testolactone** (↓estrogen).	**Clinical PEARL:** **Tamoxifen** is mixed agonist/antagonist; ↓**risk of breast CA** (antagonist) and ↓osteoporosis, but ↑**risk endometrial CA** (agonist).

Gynecology

19) Primary Amenorrhea		
Absence **secondary sexual** characteristics by **14 years old** or **absence MENSES by age 16 years old.** Si/Sx- **no menses by 16yo,** or secondary sex characteristics by **14yo.**	Cx • **Turner's** (ovarian dysgenesis, ↑FSH). • **Kallmann's syndrome (46XX,** assoc with **anosmia-** lack smell). • **Imperforate hymen** • **Androgen insensitivity syndrome** (46XY, MIF) • **Mullerian agenesis**	Dx- if **no breast** development by **14yo order FSH.** If ↓FSH order MRI of pituitary. ↑FSH do karyotyping. **Clinical PEARL: Mullerian agenesis** (genotype XX) **Blind ended vaginal pouch,** little or **no uterine tissue.**
20) Primary Amenorrhea		**21) Androgen Insensitivity**
Dx- first order **pregnancy test,** then R/O following: • **Constitutional growth delay** (most common) by checking bone age. • **Hypothalamic or pituitary-** ↓GnRH, ↓LH/FSH, ↓E/P (estrogen/progesterone). • **PCOS** ↑GnRH, ↑LH/FSH, ↑E/↑P.	Tx- **hypogonadism** give **estrogen** low-dose then twelve months later, begin cyclic **estrogen/ progesterone.**	46XY, ↑mullerian inhibiting factor **(**MIF). Si/Sx- **normal** breast, axillary and pubic hair. **No upper vagina,** uterus, fallopian tubes. Dx- ↑ **testosterone** undescended testes, **MIF**; inhibits **uterus, fallopian tubes, upper portion of vagina**. Tx- testicular resection at puberty and creation of neo vagina.

Gynecology

22) Secondary Amenorrhea		
Absence menses for >6mos with menarche in the past. Si/Sx- **amenorrhea;** lack menarche for **>6mos**. Pt has had menarche in the past. Dx- first R/O preg with **pregnancy test.**	Dx **If NEG B-hCG** (neg preg test) then order **TSH and Prolactin**: • ↑**TSH** r/o Hypothyroidism. • ↑**prolactin** (inhib LH, FSH) r/o pituitary adenoma. Next order **Progestin Challenge Test;** give 10days of progestin and see if pt has **withdrawal bleeding.**	Dx • **Positive Progestin challenge test** (bleeding) => check LH. If ↑↑**LH**=> **PCOS.** • **NEG Progestin challenge test** (no bleeding) => check FSH. If ↑**FSH**=> **ovarian failure** (↑FSH, ↑LH, ↓estrogen)**.**
23) Secondary Amenorrhea		
Dexamethasone suppression test (ACTH antagonist) can be done to r/o CAH, Cushing's, Addison's syndrome, or ectopic ACTH syndrome.	**Dexamethasone suppression test** (ACTH antagonist)**:** • **Normal-** ↓cortisol with low dose dexa. • **Cushing's-** ↓cortisol with high dose dexa. • **Ectopic ACTH syndrome-** if no supression with low or high dose dexa.	Tx- underlying cause. • **Prolactinomas** Tx-**cabergoline,** or **bromocriptine** (both dopamine agonist). • **Premature ovarian failure** (<40y) Dx- **FSH/LH >1.0** Tx-estrogen + progestin. **In vitro fertilization** in women who desire pregnancy.

Gynecology

24) Primary Dysmenorrhea

Menstrual PAIN assoc with ovulatory cycles (↑**prostaglandins**; PGF2-alpha). Si/Sx-lower abd pain that is midline and radiates to back or thighs, assoc **ovulatory cycle, menstrual pain.**	Dx- exclusion. Tx- **NSAIDs, OCP,** Mirena IUD, and/or heating pads.	**Clinical PEARL: Mittelschmerz** (midcycle pain) Si/Sx- regular menstrual periods, **lower abd pain about two weeks** after LMP.

25) Secondary Dysmenorrhea

Menstrual PAIN secondary to **other underline pathology**. Cx- **endometriosis,** adenomyosis, fibroids, PID, polyps, tumors, or adhesions.	Si/Sx- **lower abd pelvic pain,** menstrual cramping, radiates to back or thighs.	Dx- **B-hCG** r/o ectopic preg, **U/A** to r/o UTI, STDs (gonococcal, chlamydial), PID. Tx- etiology specific.

26) Endometriosis

Endometrial tissue **"OUTSIDE"** the uterus. Si/Sx- **CYCLICAL** menstrual pelvic pain. Comp- **infertility.**	Si/Sx- **"3D's"** • **Dyspareunia** (pain with sexual intercourse) • **Dysmenorrhea** (pain with menstruation) • **Dyschezia** (pain with defecation)	Dx **LAPAROSCOPY,** ovaries may have **CHOCOLATE cysts.** Tx- **OCPs (1st line),** **leuprolide** (GnRH analog) and **danazol.** If severe surgical lysis of adhesions.

Gynecology

27) Adenomyosis

Endometrial tissue **"INSIDE"** the myometrium.	Comp- endometrial cancer (**rare**).	Dx- **U/S scan** shows **enlarged symmetrical uterus.**
Si/Sx- **NON-CYCLICAL lower, midline, pelvic** abd pain, dysmenorrhea, menorrhagia.	Tx- **NSAIDs (1st line)** + OCPs or progestins. If severe surgery resection using hysteroscopy.	

28) Dysfunctional Uterine Bleeding

• **Menorrhagia** ↑Amount of flow, heavy periods, lasting **>7days or >80mL.**	• **Metrorrhagia Bleeding between cycles,** breakthrough bleeding or spotting.	**Clinical PEARL: Cessation of menstrual cycles (>6mos)** => pt is now having abnormal uterine bleeding. **"think CANCER."**
• **Oligomenorrhea** ↑Length between menses, >35day intervals between periods, only 4-9 periods in a year.	• **Menometrorrhagia** ↑Bleeding and irregular bleeding. • **Dysmenorrhea** PAINFUL cycle.	

29) Dysfunctional Uterine Bleeding

Dx • **B-hCG** r/o ectopic preg.	Dx • **CBC** r/o anemia.	Dx • **Anovulation** Common in **first two years of menarche,** may have menorrhagia.
• **U/S scan** of ovaries, uterus, endometrium. If endometrium **>4mm** in **postmenopausal woman** order biopsy.	• **Platelet, BT, PT/PTT** r/o von Willebrand's disease, bleeding disorders.	Dx- ovulation can be tested by measuring **midluteal phase progesterone** level.
• **PAP** r/o cervical cancer.	• **TFTs** r/o hyper- or hypothyroidism and hyperprolactinemia.	Tx- **NSAIDs** (1st line), OCPs or mirena IUD.

Gynecology

30) Dysfunctional Uterine Bleeding

Dx	Tx	Tx
If >35yo with DUB (dysfunctional uterine bleeding) is indication for endometrial biopsy. Endometrial biopsy should also be done in pts <35yo with HTN, diabetes, or obesity.	Bleeding disorder give desmopressin (↑von Willebrand's and VIII). Anovulatory bleeding give progestins for 10days to stimulate withdrawal bleeding (convert proliferative endometrium to secretory).	If severe HEAVY bleeding give high-dose ESTROGEN IV (promote endometrial growth). If cannot control bleeding with estrogen within 12–24hr D&C.

31) CAH

Congenital Adrenal Hyperplasia (CAH) Cx- 21-hydroxylase deficiency, CYP21 genotype. Si/Sx- salt wasting, ambiguous genitalia, hirsutism, virilization, clitoromegaly, acne, amenorrhea, abnormal uterine bleeding, infertility.	Si/Sx Newborn female with ambiguous genitalia, life-threatening salt wasting. Dx ↑17-OH progesterone => CAH. • ↑Testosterone r/o ovarian tumor. • ↑DHEAS r/o adrenal tumor.	Tx- prednisone (glucocorticoids). Clinical PEARL: Aromatase def Si/Sx normal internal genitalia with ambiguous external genitalia, clitoral hypertrophy. Dx- ↑FSH, ↑LH, ↓estrogen.

Gynecology

32) Polycystic Ovarian Syndrome

PCOS is also called **Stein-Leventhal syndrome**.

Si/Sx- **hirsutism, acne, obesity (BMI>30), HTN, DM,** acanthosis nigricans, irregular menses, anovulation, **infertility.**

HAIR-AN:
H- Hyper-
A- Androgenism
I- Insulin
R- Resistance
A- Acanthosis
N-Nigricans

Comp- **infertility, DM2,** metabolic syndrome (obesity, insulin resistance, HTN, dyslipidemia).

Dx- ↑ **testosterone, OGTT, U/S scan** shows polycystic ovaries **"PEARL necklace sign"** (ovarian cysts lined up in a row).

R/O other cx; order TSH, prolactin, 17-OH progesterone (CAH).

Tx- **clomiphene citrate** (estrogen analog) to induce ovulation for pregnancy. **Metformin** helps prevent DM2.

Risk- **endometrial carcinoma** (↑estrogen).

33) Causes of Hyperandrogenism

• **PCOS**
Si/Sx- HTN, hirsutism, obesity, irregular menses.
Dx- **U/S cystic ovaries**.

• **21-Hydroxylase def**
Si/Sx- severe hirsutism, **salt wasting,** family hx CAH.
Dx-↑**17-OH progesterone**.

• **Hypothyroidism**
Si/Sx- fatigue, weight gain, constipation, cold intolerance, hyperprolactinemia (due to ↑TRH).
Dx- ↑**TSH, ↓T4.**

• **Hyperprolactinemia**
Si/Sx- amenorrhea, **galactorrhea** (spont milk flow from the breast), infertility.
Dx- ↑**prolactin** level.

• **Cushing's syndrome**
Si/Sx- **HTN,** truncal obesity, buffalo hump, purple striae.
Dx- **dexamethasone suppress test** (check cortisol level after dose of dexamethasone; ACTH antagonist).
Cushing's- ↓cortisol with high dose dexa.

Gynecology

34) TOTAL Incontinence		
Cx- **involuntary LOSS of URINE** due to **loss sphincteric** muscle control. Si/Sx- uncontrolled **LOSS "all the times."**	Assoc- nerve damage, previous surgery, cancer. Dx- **U/A and UCx** to exclude UTI. Have pt make a **voiding diary.**	Dx- order BUN/Cr to r/o renal dysfunction. Possibly **urodynamic studies** including **cystometry.** Tx- surgery.

35) STRESS Incontinence		
Cx- laxity of **PELVIC FLOOR muscle**=> urethral sphincter insufficiency. Si/Sx- loss of urine when **COUGHING, SNEEZING, or lifting.**	Assoc- pelvic surgery, multiparous women. Dx- clinical, U/A, UCx, urodynamic studies.	Tx- **kegal exercise (1st-line), pessary** (plastic device that is held in place by pelvic floor muscles). **Urethropexy** vaginal vault suspension surgery for severe pts.

36) OVERFLOW Incontinence		
Detrusor inactivity and prevent urinary sphincter relaxation. Cx • **Autonomic neuropathy** (denervated bladder, detrusor weakness). • **Bladder outlet obstruction.** • MEDS; **anti-cholinergics** (diphenhydramine, chlorpheniramine, hydroxyzine, doxepin), **TCAs,** sedatives, antipsychotics.	Chronic **urinary RETENTION=> distended bladder=>** small amount of urine **dribbles out.** Assoc- **epidural anesthesia,** tumor, stricture, lesion, meds. Si/Sx- **distended bladder,** small amounts of urine **"DRIBBLES"** out.	Dx-clinical, U/A, UCx, urodynamic studies. Tx- place **intermitent urethral catheter** shows large residual volume. Have pts **void every few hrs** and treat underlying disease or cause. Can also give **cholinergic meds** like **bethanechol.**

Gynecology

37) URGE Incontinence		38) Vaginitis
Cx- **DETRUSOR hyperreflexia;** detrusor muscle **contracts too frequently=>** unexpected urge to void. Si/Sx- **strong URGE** to void. Assoc- neurogenic bladder, inflammatory condition.	Dx- clinical, U/A, UCx, urodynamic studies. Tx- **behavioral training**; frequent voiding (every 1-2hrs), **Kegel exercises**. Can also use **anticholinergic or TCA**.	Si/Sx- abnormal malodor discharge, **pruritus, burning,** irritation, swelling, dyspareunia, dysuria. Cx • **Bacterial vaginosis** ("FISHY" discharge) • **Trichomonas** (GREEN, motility) • **Yeast** (cottage cheese)
39) Bacterial Vaginosis		
"Gray-Fishy-Clue" Cx- gardnerella vaginalis. Si/Sx- **GRAY-white** discharge with **"FISHY" odor.** With NO pruritus.	**Dx- CLUE cells** (epithelial cells coated with bacteria), vaginal **pH >4.5.** KOH prep **+WHIFF test** (fishy).	Tx- metro**nidazole** or ti**nidazole** (1st-line), clindamycin (2nd-line). Both safe in pregnancy.
40) Trichomonas "Green and motile"		
Cx- **trichomonas vaginalis (STD)** Si/Sx- vaginal pruritus, dysuria, dyspareunia, with **GREEN-yellow,** frothy, discharge.	Si/Sx- pts may have **"STRAWBERRY"** petechiae on cervix (rare). Dx- wet mount test shows **MOTILE trichomonads** (pear-shaped flagellated organism, 3-5 flagella). Vaginal pH 5-6.	Tx- metro**nidazole** or ti**nidazole**. **Both partners** should be treated to prevent recurrent infxs.

Gynecology

41) Yeast	42) Cervicitis	
"No odor"		
Cx- **candida albicans** Risk factors: **DM,** OCP, IUD, broad-spectrum abxs, **corticosteroids,** HIV. Si/Sx- burning, pruritus, no odor, **thick white** **"COTTAGE cheese."** Dx- KOH shows **pseudo-hyphae.** Tx- PO **fluconazole** or topical azole (avoid oral azoles in preg).	**Inflammation** of the uterine **CERVIX.** Cx- **chlamydia** (most common), gonococcus, HPV, HSV, trichomonas. Si/Sx- **cervical motion** **tenderness,** yellow- green mucopurulent discharge.	Dx- U/A, UCx. Tx- underlying infx. **Clinical PEARL:** **Physiologic** **Leukorrhea** Si/Sx- no pruritus, no burning, with **white yellow** **discharge.**

43) Pelvic Inflam Disease (PID)		
Infx of **upper genital** **tract.** Assoc- **chlamydia,** **gonorrhoeae.** Risk factors- multiple sex partners, prior STD or PID, smoking. Si/Sx- fever, lower abd pain, adnexal tenderness and **"CHANDELIER"** **sign** (pain as if pt is going to jump up to chandelier), cervical motion tenderness.	Dx- order **B-hCG and** **U/S scan** to R/O pregnancy. **Hysterosalpingogram** (identify structural abn in fallopian tubes). **Criteria for diagnosis:** • Fever >38C • WBC >10,000 • ↑ESR • Pelvic pain • Uterine or adnexal tenderness. • Cervical motion tenderness.	Tx- **ofloxacin** or levo**floxacin** 14days +/- metronidazole. In hospital; **Cefoxitin/** **Doxycycline,** Cefotetan/ Doxycycline, or Clindamycin/ gentamicin (all IV). **Tx partner if possible.** Comp- **ectopic** **pregnancy, infertility,** **Fitz-Hugh-Curtis** **syndrome** (PID with RUQ pain, and abn LFTs).

Gynecology

44) Toxic Shock Syndrome (TSS)		
Cx- **staph aureus toxin** (exotoxin; TSST-1), tampons. Si/Sx- **Abrupt FEVER (102F), hypotension,** diffuse macular erythematous **RASH, desquamation** (skin peeling) of the **palms and soles.**	Si/Sx- strawberry tongue, and conjunctival hyperemia. Pts may have vomiting, watery diarrhea, conjunctivitis. Dx- **neg BCx** because symps are from **TOXIN not organism.**	Tx- **rehydration, nafcillin or oxacillin** (anti-staphylococcal), possibly steroids. If penicillin allergy use vancomycin. Comp- hypotension, ARDS, DIC.

45) Uterine Leiomyoma (fibroid)		
Benign smooth muscle neoplasm (most common neoplasm of female genital tract). Assoc- estrogen and progesterone sensitive (↑in pregnancy, ↓menopause).	Si/Sx- asymp, anemia due to long **heavy periods,** with pelvic pain and pressure. Comp- transform to **leiomyosarcoma** (rare). Dx- **CBC** for anemia, U/S may show **uterine myomas**, can r/o ovarian mass.	Tx- **NSAIDs + OCPs.** Medroxyprogesterone or danazol to ↓bleeding. **Leuprolide, nafarelin** (GnRH) to ↓myomas and ↓further growth. **Surgery**-if torsion consider myomectomy or hysteroscopy.

Gynecology

46) Endometrial Cancer		
Atypical **endometrial hyperplasia.** Si/Sx- **vaginal bleeding,** pain, and possibly metabolic syndrome. Dx- endometrial and endocervical **biopsy. U/S scan** shows **thick endometrial tissue.**	Dx • **Type I (**most): **Unopposed estrogen** (from **tamoxifen,** or exogenous estrogen). • **Type II:** **p53 mutation** (unrelated to estrogen) Tx- premenopausal women with simple or complex hyperplasia **without atypia** give **cyclic progestins (1st-line)** with repeat biopsy in 3-6mos.	Premenopausal with complex hyperplasia and **ATYPIA** needs a **total hysterectomy** (1st-line). **Type I** give **high-dose progestins,** TAH/BSO +/- radiation for postmenopausal. **Type II** TAH/BSO + chemo for advanced. stage cancer.
47) CERVICAL Cancer		
HPV DNA is found in 99% of all cervical cancers. • **HPV16** (squamous cell) • **HPV18** (adenocarcinoma)	Risk factors: STDs, smoking, immunosuppression, HIV, OCP. Si/Sx- **metrorrhagia** (abn bleeding), **postcoital spotting,** and cervical ulcerations.	Prevention- **gardasil vaccine** (9-26yo). **Screen-** start at 21yrs, **PAP smear** yrly. If pt is >30yo with normal PAP => every 3yrs.

Gynecology

48) CERVICAL Cancer		
Dx Atypical glandular cells (AGC): • **AGC <35yo:** proceed with obtain **colposcopy, endocervical** curettage, and **HPV DNA testing.** • **AGC >35yo:** abn bleeding with endometrial cancer factors => **biopsy.**	**LSIL** Low-grade squamous intraepithelial lesion. **HSIL** High-grade squamous intraepithelial lesions. • **LSIL** <21: repeat pap **12mos** >21: **immediate COLPOSCOPY** with targeted biopsy, **HPV DNA testing,** and repeat **pap 6mos.**	• **HSIL** immediate **colposcopy ALL.** If biopsy is neg, a second biopsy is recommended in 6-8wks. If preg it should be done 6-8wks after delivery.
49) CERVICAL Cancer Dx and Tx		
Cervical Intraepithelial Neoplasia **(CIN).** **CIN I:** 60% will regress, follow with **close observation.** Pap 6–12mos or HPV DNA testing at 12mos. Positive result of either one require repeat **colposcopy.**	**Persistent CIN I** => **ablation** (cryotherapy or laser ablation) or excisional with **LEEP.** **CIN II, III:** 40% regress. Should be treated with **ablative** and excisional with **LEEP.** **Recurrent CIN II or III- hysterectomy** +/- chemotherapy.	**Clinical PEARL: Cervical Insufficiency** Risk factors: **cervical LEEP** or cone biopsy, DES exposure, multiple gestation, second-trimester pregnancy loss. Dx- **transvaginal U/S (1st-line);** normal length should be >25mm at 24wks. Cervical length <10% for GA is a short cervix.

Gynecology

50) VULVAR Cancer		
Risk factor- **HPV (types 16, 18, 31)** Si/Sx- pruritus, painful, ulcers or nodular raised, and pigmented=> white, **"CAULIFLOWER"** like lesion. **Clinical PEARL: Bartholin's Gland Abscess** Si/Sx- painful **unilateral labial swelling,** pain with walking, sitting and sexual intercourse. Dx- clinical Tx- **incision and drainage.**	Dx- vulvar **punch biopsy.** **Vulvar Intraepithelial Neoplasia (VIN).** **VINI and II:** Mild dysplasia. **VINIII:** Carcinoma in situ. Tx- topical **betamethasone or clobetasol** and **crotamiton** for pruritus.	**VIN high grade** give topical chemotherapy, laser ablation, and wide local excision. **Clinical PEARL: Lichen Sclerosus** Premalignant lesion. Si/Sx- **porcelain-white atrophy.** Dx- vulvar punch **biopsy** r/o vulvar SCC. Tx- topical **corticosteroid (1st-line).**
51) VAGINAL Cancer		
Cx- **squamous cell CA, adenocarcinoma.** Assoc: postmenopausal women. Risk factors: multiple sexual partners, immunosuppression, radiation for cervical CA, **diethylstilbestrol (DES).**	Si/Sx- **abn vaginal bleeding,** discharge, postcoital bleed. Dx- cytology, colposcopy, and **biopsy.** Tx- **local excision,** invasive disease requires radiation.	Tx- **radiation** is excellent alternative for pts that are poor surgical candidates. **Clinical PEARL: Clear Cell Adenocarcinoma** of vagina and cervix. Risk- **diethylstilbestrol (DES)** (used in in the past for tx of threatened abortion).

Gynecology

52) OVARIAN Cancer

Risk factors: **BRCA1, BRCA2, HNPCC (**Lynch II syndrome), **↑age,** low parity, delay childbear, +FH, Lower Risk- **OCPs.** **Clinical PEARL Lynch II Syndrome** (HNPCC) ↑risk of colon, ovarian, endometrial, and breast cancer.	Si/Sx- **asymp,** pelvic pain or pressure, urinary frequency, urgency, pain, adnexal fullness, non-specific GI symps. Most pts present with **advanced malignant disease** because most pts are asymp. Comp- pleural effusion from **metastatic spread to pleura.**	**No screening** is recommended for pts with an average risk. Dx-**↑CA-125** to determine progression and recurrence. **U/S scan** screening for **high-risk pts.** Pt with **BRCAI** should be **screened annually** with U/S, and CA-125. Also giving **OCP** will **lower the risk.**

53) OVARIAN Cancer

Tx- if palpable mass **surgery and chemotherapy** is routine. **Clinical PEARL: Granulosa Cell Tumor** (malignant ovarian) Assoc- precocious puberty in young child and postmenopausal bleeding elderly pts. Dx- **↑ESTROGEN.**	Tx • **Premenopausal** **<8–10cm** most regress, **>8–10cm** surgical. • **Postmenopausal** Unilateral simple cysts **<5cm** and normal CA-125 **closely follow** with serial **U/S.**	**Clinical PEARL: Cystic Teratomas** (**benign** ovarian tumor) **Struma ovarii** (50% of teratoma is **thyroid tissue**) and is assoc with **↓TSH, ↑T4** (hyperthyroidism). There is risk of malignancy so teratoma should be removed.

15 CHAPTER
PEDIATRICS

Pediatrics		
1) Developmental Milestones: 2 mos	**2) 4 mos**	**3) 6 mos**
GM- **lifts HEAD** FM- tracks past midline Lang- ooo/aah Social- **SMILE** (GM- gross motor, FM- fine motor)	GM- **ROLLS front to back** FM- grasps rattle Lang- orients to voice Social- looks around, **LAUGHS**	GM- **SITS unassisted** FM- transfers objects, feeds self, reaches, and pulls to sit. Lang- **babbles** Social- **STRANGER anxiety,** sleeps all night
4) 9 mos	**5) 12 mos**	**6) 15 mos**
GM- **CRAWLS, pulls to stand** FM- **3-finger PINCER grasp** Lang- says **"Mama, Dada"** (nonspecific) Social- **wave bye,** pat-a-cake	GM- **WALKS alone,** cruises FM- **2-finger PINCER grasp** Lang- Says **"Mama, Dada"** (**Specific**) Social- **SEPARATION anxiety,** imitates actions	GM- walks backward FM- **uses CUP, SCRIBBLES** Lang- 4–6 words Social- **temper tantrums,** plays ball with examiner
7) 18 mos	**8) 24 mos**	**9) 3 yrs**
GM- **RUNS,** kicks ball FM- builds **tower 2–4 CUBES**, drinks from cup Lang- names common objects Social- **starts toilet training**	GM- **walks up/down steps** with help, jumps FM- **6 -CUBE tower** Lang- **2-word phrases, 200 WORDS** Social- follows **two-step commands,** removes garment	GM- ride **TRICYCLE,** climbs stairs alternating feet FM- copies **CIRCLE,** uses **spoon/fork** Lang- **3-word sentence, 300 words** Social- **brushes teeth** with help, washes/dries hands

Pediatrics

10) Developmental Milestones: 4 yrs	11) 5 yrs	12) Transposition Great Vessel
GM- hops FM- copies **SQUARE** Lang- knows **COLORS, NUMBERS** Social- **COOPERATIVE play**, plays board games, dresses with no help	GM- **skips, walks backward** for a long distance FM- **TIES shoes,** knows left and right, **prints letters** Lang- 5-word sentences Social- domestic role playing, **plays dress-up**	Most common cause of **cyanotic NEWBORN.** Cx- aorta connected to right ventricle and pulmonary artery to left ventricle (two arteries switched). Assoc- CATCH 22 (DiGeorge syndrome)
13) Transposition Great Vessel		
Si/Sx- **extreme CYANOSIS at birth,** hypoxemia, tachypnea with severe illness in **NEWBORN.**	Si/Sx- pt may have **single S2** and signs of **CHF.** Dx- CXR **egg-shaped heart,** may show ↑pulm vascular markings, **ECHO** (confirms diagnosis).	Tx- **PGE1 keep PDA oPEn.** (incompatible with life without a PDA). Surgical correction.
14) Tetralogy of Fallot		
Most common **cyanotic** heart disease in **CHILDREN <4yo.** **Tetralogy of Fallot:** • **Pulmonary** stenosis • **RVH** • **Overriding** aorta • **VSD** Si/Sx **"Squat for relief"** Tell spell= cyanosis, panic, squat posture.	Si/Sx-dyspnea, fatigability, tachypnea, **CHILD** will **squat for relief, "tet spells"** (squat cause L=>R shunt, helps ↑systemic vascular resistance). **Pansystolic murmur** at left upper sternal border, **right ventricular heave,** and **single S2.** Risk factor- DiGeorge syndrome.	Dx- CXR shows **"boot-shaped"** heart, may show ↑pulm vascular markings. Echo and catheterization (confirms diagnosis). Tx- **PGE1** to keep PDA **oPEn,** support with fluids, O2, morphine, propranolol, phenylephrine, **knee-chest position.** Surgical correction.

Pediatrics

15) Ventricular Septal Defect

VSD is the **most common** congenital heart defect.

Assoc:
Down syndrome, trisomies 13 and 18, **tricuspid atresia,** fetal alcohol syndrome, TORCH syndrome, **Apert's syndrome** (fusion of digits and cranial deformities).

Clinical PEARL: Tricuspid Atresia
Si/Sx- cyanosis early in life, left axis deviation. Assoc- **VSD.**

Si/Sx- **asymp,** if it is a small defect. If large defect pts may have **freq resp infxs, dyspnea,** failure to thrive, and CHF.

Exam reveals **harsh holosystolic murmur** heard best at **LOWER LEFT sternal border,** with mid-diastolic **apical rumble,** and narrow S2.

Dx- **ECG, CXR** may show LVH, ↑pulm vascular markings, **ECHO** (diagnostic).

Tx- monitor by ECHO, most **small VSDs will close spont. Surgical repair** if pt has symps and have failed medical manangement.

Tx CHF with diuretics **(furosemide), inotropes.**

16) Atrial Septal Defect (ASD)

Cx- **ostium secundum defect** (most common), or ostium primum defect that causes an **opening in atrial septum**=> L-to-R shunt.

Assoc:
Down syndrome, fetal alcohol syndrome, Holt-Oram syndrome.

Si/Sx- asymp, fatigability, frequent resp infxs in **LATE childhood.**

Exam reveals a **"FIXED WIDE"** split S2, systolic ejection murmur or **mid-diastolic** rumble at **LEFT** sternal border.

Dx- **ECG** shows RVH, **CXR** may show cardiomegaly and ↑pulm vascular markings. **ECHO** (diagnostic).

Eisenmenger's syndrome L=>R shunt lead to pulm HTN and **shunt reversal** (R=>L).

Pediatrics

17) Patent Ductus Arteriosus (PDA)

Cx- failure of ductus arteriosus closer=> leading to L-to-R shunt (aorta to pulmonary artery).

Risk factor: **Rubella infx** in 1st-trimester.

VSD, ASD, PDA
"Don't go the right way"
L=>R shunts

TGV, TOF
"**Truly** the right way"
R=>L shunts

Si/Sx- asymp, recurrent resp infxs, **bounding peripheral pulses,** clubbing, CHF. On exam **WIDE pulse pressure,** thrill.

Systolic murmur that spills into diastole; **CONTINUOUS "machinery murmur"** at **2nd LEFT** intercostal space radiates to **clavicle.**

Dx- **ECG** may show LVH and **CXR** shows cardiomegaly. **ECHO** with color flow doppler (diagosis).

Tx- **IND**omethacin to **END** the PDA. Keep o**PE**n use PE1 (Prostaglandin E1).

Surgical closure with **ligation** if failed medical management.

18) Coarctation of Aorta

Constriction of portion of aorta.

Assoc- **Turner's syndrome,** bicuspid aortic valve, berry aneurysms.

Si/Sx- asymp HTN in **child, ↑ BP upper** extremities, ↓ **BP lower** extremities, "**WEAK femoral pulses."**

Dx- **ECG** shows LVH. CXR may show **"3" SIGN** and **"RIB notching."**

ECHO with color flow doppler (diagnostic).

For Turner's syndrome confirm by karyotype analysis.

Tx- keep PDA o**PE**n with Prostaglandin **E1** (PGE1).

19) DiGeorge Syndrome

Si/Sx- **CATCH 22:**

C- **Cardiac** abn

A- **Abnormal** facies (low-set ears, micrognathia; small jaw)

T- **Thymic** aplasia

C- **Cleft** palate

H- **Hypocalcemia** (hypoparathyroidism, prolonged QT)

22- **22q11** deletion

Pediatrics

20) Ebstein's Anomaly	21) Down Syndrome (21)	
Tricuspid valve displaced into right ventricle. Cx- **LITHIUM** Si/Sx- cyanosis, tricuspid regurgitation. Risk-SVTs, WPW, a-fib Dx- ECG shows left axis deviation and ↓pulmonary blood flow.	Cx- **trisomy 21 (most common)**, robertsonian translocation. Si/Sx- MR, flat facial profile, **epicanthal folds, "brushfield spots"** (speckled irises), hypotonia, **simian crease palms.** **Clinical PEARL: Jejunal Atresia** Si/Sx- bilious vomiting, abdominal distention. Dx- Abd XR shows **"triple bubble,"** and gasless lower abd.	Assoc- **duodenal atresia, ASD, VSD** due to **endocardial cushion defects, Hirschsprung's dz.** Risk- **ALL**, early **Alzheimer's** disease, **Atlantoaxial** instability (atlas C1 and axis C2). Dx- screening with **CVS, amniocentesis** during pregnancy.
22) Edward's Syndrome	**23) Patau's Syndrome**	**24) Klinefelter's Syndrome**
Cx- **trisomy 18.** Assoc- **ASD** Si/Sx- LBW, severe MR, low-set ears, **ROCKER-BOTTOM FEET,** micrognathia (small jaw). **"CLENCHED" hands** (closed fists) with 3rd and 5th digit overlapping 4th. Dx- screening with **CVS, amniocentesis** during pregnancy. Tx- none, death within first year of life.	Cx- **trisomy 13.** Si/Sx- severe MR, **CLEFT lip, CLEFT palate,** microcephaly (small head), microphthalmia (small eyes), holoprosencephaly (one eye). **POLYDACTYLY** (>5 fingers or toes). Dx- screening with **CVS, amniocentesis** during pregnancy. Tx- none, death. within one year of life.	Cx- **45, XYY.** Si/Sx- **TALL stature, LONG extremities,** hypogonadism (testicular atrophy), and **gynecomastia.** Dx- karyotyping, **Barr body.** Tx- testosterone. [Genetic diseases: Down, Edwards, Patau's, Klinefelter's, Turner's, Fragile X, Phenylketonuria.]

Pediatrics

25) Fragile X Syndrome	26) Phenylketonuria	27) Tay-Sachs Disease (AR)
X-link defect that affects **methylation** and **FMR1 gene.**	Phenylalanine hydroxylase deficiency =>↑ **phenylalanine.**	HeXosaminidase A deficiency => ↑ **GM2 ganglioside.**
Si/Sx- everything is **"eXXXtra"** large; large JAW, large EARS, **macroorchidism,** long face, MR, and **AUTISM** spectrum behaviors.	Si/Sx- **BLOND** hair, **BLUE** eyed, FAIR skin, eczema, and **"MUSTY or MOUSY"** urine odor, MR.	Assoc- Jews. Si/Sx- child is normal until **3–6mos,** then pt **starts to regresses.** Hyperacusis (over-senstivity to sounds), MR, seizures.
Dx- karyotyping, **CGG trinucleotide repeats** that may show anticipation.	Comp- heart disease. **Dx- GUTHRIE test** is a qualitative (coloration) test that detects **phenylalanine in urine.** Screen at birth.	**Dx- ophthalmoscope** shows shows **"CHERRY-RED"** spot in macula.
Can do **amniocentesis** in 2nd trimester to determine in pregnancy (CVS not reliable).	Tx- ↓ **phenylalanine** and ↑ **tyrosine diet.**	Tx- none, death by 3–4yo.

Pediatrics

28) Metachromatic Leukodystrophy AR	29) Hurler's (AR)	30) HUNTER'S (XR)
Arylsulfatase A deficiency => ↑**sulfatide** in brain, liver, kidney, and peripheral nerves. Si/Sx- **muscle rigidity,** developmental delays, paralysis, dementia. Tx- none, death by 5yo **[Lysosomal storage diseases:** Tay-Sachs, ML, Hurler's, Hunter's, Niemann-Pick, Gaucher's, Krabbe's, Fabry's. **Most are AR]**	**Alpha-L-iduronidase** deficiency => glycosaminoglycans buildup, heparan sulfate and dermatan sulfate buildup. Si/Sx- **"CORNEAL clouding"** and **MR**. Dx- genetic counseling, urine test for mucopolysaccharides excreted in urine. Tx- enzyme replacement.	**Iduronate sulfatase** deficiency Si/Sx-**"mild Hurler's,"** mild MR. **Hunter's SEE** so **"no corneal clouding,"** and aim for the **X** (X-link). Dx- ↓**iduronate sulfatase** enzyme activity, urine test for mucopolysaccharides, also known as glycosaminoglycans. Tx- enzyme replacement.
31) Fabry's Disease (XR)	**32) Krabbe's Disease** (AR)	**33) Niemann-PICK Disease** (AR)
Alpha-galactosidase A deficiency => ↑**ceramide trihexoside** in brain, heart, kidney. Si/Sx- renal failure, risk of stroke and MI. Dx- blood test measure ↓**alpha-galactosidase** activity. Tx- enzyme replacement therapies.	**Galactosylceramidase** deficiency => ↑**galactocerebroside** accum in brain. Si/Sx- **spasticity, optic atrophy,** early death. Tx- no cure, BMT has been shown to benefit.	"**PICKs** his nose with his **sphinger.**" **Sphingomyelinase** deficiency => ↑**sphingomyelin** cholesterol in tissue. Si/Sx- hypotonia, **unsteady gait, protruding belly,** hepatosplenomegaly, **lymphadenopathy,** regression of developmental milestones. Dx↓sphingomyelinase, **"CHERRY-RED spot,"** in macula (also in Tay-Sachs). Tx- supportive

Pediatrics

34) Gaucher's Disease (AR)

Acid beta-glucosidase deficiency (lysosomal enzyme) => ↑**glucocerebroside** in liver, spleen, brain, and BM. Assoc- Ashkenazi Jews. Si/Sx- chronic **fatigue, easy bruisability, bone pain,** and pathological fractures, hepatomegaly, splenomegaly.	Dx- **anemia, pancytopenia, thrombocytopenia.** **Genetic testing** for sequencing beta-glucosidase gene. Radiologic study may show **erlenyeyer flask deformity** of distal femur.	Dx Bone marrow studies shows **Gaucher cells** with "**CRINKLED paper,**" enlarge cytoplasm (confirms diagnosis). Tx- enzyme replacement tx with IV **glucocerebrosidase.**

35) Cystic Fibrosis (AR)

AR disorder caused by a mutation in **CFTR gene, chrom 7 (gene deletion).** Assoc- **Meconium Ileus** (ground glass appearance on abd XR), bilateral **nasal polyps, pseudomonas** pulm infxs.	Si/Sx- **failure to thrive, sinopulmonary disease,** clubbing, wheezing, hemoptysis. Pulm infxs esp with **PSEUDOMONAS.**	Si/Sx- skin has a "**SALTY TASTE**" (due to abn chloride channel). GI symps, rectal prolapse, steatorrhea, lack absorption of **fat-soluble vit def KADE.** (Vit K, A, D, E), DM2.

Pediatrics

36) Cystic Fibrosis (AR)

Dx- **sweat chloride test >60mEq/L** (gold standard), DNA probe test. Tx- **corticosteroids, abxs, bronchodilators,** DNase, pancreatic enzymes with **fat soluble Vits KADE,** high calorie/protein diet.	Tx- offer nutritional counseling and support. Pseudomonas infx give **cefepime, piperacillin-tazobactam, or ceftazidime and gentamicin.**	**Clinical PEARL: Celiac Disease** Si/Sx- **malabsorption** and **iron def anemia,** think "Celiac Disease." Assoc- **dermatitis herpetiformis** (herpes like). Dx- **anti-endomysial** antibodies. Serological studies with ELISA for IgA antibodies to **gliadin, endomysium,** tissue transglutaminase.

37) Intussusception

TELESCOPES of one part of bowel into adjacent bowel. Assoc- **Meckel's** diverticulum, **Henoch-Schonlein purpura** (palpable purpura, hematuria, abd pain), **Cystic Fibrosis (CF),** celiac disease.	Si/Sx- child with **ABRUPT colicky,** abd pain with **flexed knees** and vomiting. RUQ abd **"SAUSAGE shaped"** palpable mass with **"CURRANT JELLY"** stools.	Dx- **AIR contrast barium enema** is both diagnostic and curative.

38) Pyloric Stenosis

Hypertrophy of pyloric sphincter=> obstruction. Assoc- **FIRST BORN MALE,** tracheo-esophageal fistula.	Si/Sx- **NON-bilious "PROJECTILE"** emesis after all feedings, in a **3wk old.** Pt may have a palpable **"OLIVE shaped"** non-tender, epigastric mass.	Dx- **U/S scan** shows hypertrophic pylorus. **Barium studies** show narrow pyloric channel. Labs: **hypo**chloremia, **hypo**kalemic, **metabolic alkalosis** (due emesis of HCl). Tx- surgical **pyloromyotomy.**

Pediatrics

39) Hirschsprung's Disease

Lack of ganglion cells in distal colon. Si/Sx- **failure to pass meconium** within the first **48hrs of BIRTH.** Bilious vomiting and **"CONSTIPATION."** Assoc- **Down's syndrome.**	Dx- **Barium enema** (performed first) is imaging study of choice; shows narrowed distal colon with dilation of the proximal colon.	Dx- full-thickness rectal **biopsy** (confirms); absence **myenteric** (auerbach's) and **submucosal** (meissner's) plexus. Tx- **Surgical repair** with colostomy followed by connecting remaining colon to rectum in several weeks.

40) Meckel's Diverticulum

Failure of **omphalomesenteric (or vitelline) duct** to obliterate in the small intestine. Si/Sx- asymp, sudden **"PAINLESS" rectal bleeding** (black stools or melena).	Dx- Meckel's scintigraphy scan; **technetium-99m pertechnetate** ↑uptake if ectopic **gastric mucosa** is present in Meckel's diverticulum (diagnostic). Tx- surgical **excision of diverticulum.**	**Rules of 2's:** • **< 2yo** (most common) • **2:1 M:F** • **2 types** of tissue: pancreatic, gastric. • **2 inch** long • **2 feet** from ileocecal • **2%** of pop

41) Necrotizing Enterocolitis (NEC)

Bowel necrosis of part of the bowel. Assoc-**PREMATURE infants**, or low birth weight infant (LBW). Si/Sx- **premature infant** with fever, vomiting, ↓bowel sounds.	Si/Sx- ↑**gastric residual volume,** abd distension, **bloody stools** and **pneumatosis intestinalis.** Dx- AXR shows **DILATED bowel loops,** intermural **AIR bubbles;** pneumatosis intestinalis.	Dx- **Serial AXR** should be done every 6hrs. Tx- NPO, orogastric tube for **gastric decompression.** Consider IV abxs and TPN.

Pediatrics

42) Malrotation and Volvulus		
Congenital **malrotation of MIDGUT** leads to abn positioning of small intestines. Si/Sx- **bilious vomiting, abdominal distention,** and **passage of BLOODY stool** in newborn period (<1month old).	Risk factors: postsurgical **adhesions** can lead to volvulus. Dx- **upper GI study** (study of choice) shows **corkscrew-shaped duodenum** abnormally located in right abdomen.	Dx- **AXR** may shows absence of intestinal gas. Tx- **IV fluid** hydration, **NG tube** to decompress intestine, and possibly surgical repair.

43) Immuno-deficiencies		
• **B cell** deficiency **AFTER >6mos old.** • **T cell** deficiency **In the FIRST 1–3mos,** with **fungal,** viral, and intracellular bacteria infxs.	• **Phagocyte** deficiency **Catalase positive** organisms (staph aureus), fungi, and gram neg enteric infxs. • **Complement** deficiency **Encapsulated** organisms.	[**Immunodeficiency diseases:** MAC def, Hereditary angioedema, CGD, Chediak-Higashi, Leukocyte adhesion, Wiskott-Aldrich, SCID, Ataxia-telangiectasia, DiGeorge, IgA def, Bruton's, Common variable]

44) Bruton's (Boys)		
Bruton's Agamma-globulinemia (**X-link**); **B cell deficiency**=> panhypo-gamma-globulinemia in **BOYS** only.	Si/Sx- infxs **AFTER >6mos** with strep, haemophilus, encapsulated (strep and H. influenzae) and Giarrdia infxs (IgA def).	Dx- **ABSENT B cells,** ↓IgG, ↓IgA, ↓IgM, ↓IgD, and **absent TONSILS.** Tx- **IVIG**

Pediatrics

45) Ataxia-Telangiectasia	46) Hereditary Telangiectasia (AD)	47) SCID
Cx-**DNA repair defect.** Risk factors: gastric CA, non-Hodgkin's lymphoma, leukemia. Si/Sx • **Cerebellar ATAXIA** • Oculocutaneous **Telangiectasias** Tx- if severe **IVIG**	**Osler-Weber-Rendu** Si/Sx- recurrent **epistaxis,** blanching lesions, hemoptysis, **pulm AVMs** (arteriovenous shunting). Dx- recurrent nose bleeds, **polycythemia.**	Severe Combined Immunodeficiency (SCID). Cx- lack **B and T cells.** Si/Sx- severe, **frequent bacterial** infxs, chronic **candidiasis,** and opportunistic infxs. **ABSENT** lymph nodes, **tonsils, and thymic.**

48) SCID	49) Wiskott-Aldrich Syndrome (X-link)	
Dx- flow cytometic analysis shows **ABSENT B cells and T cells.** Absent lymph nodes and tonsils. CXR **absent thymic shadow.** Tx- **BMT,** IVIG, abxs, and **PCP prophylaxis.**	**MILD** B and T cell dysfunction. Si/Sx- **triad:** • **ECZEMA** • **Thrombocytopenia** • **Recurrent infxs;** otitis media, bacteria, viruses, fungi, and PCP. Comp- atopic disorders, infxs, **lymphoma,** and leukemias.	Dx- ↑ IgE ↑ IgA, ↓ IgM, ↓ platelets (quite small). Tx- **IVIG,** abxs, if severe tx with BMT. Severe disease die by age 15yo.

Pediatrics

50) CVI		51) IgA Deficiency
Common Variable Immunodeficiency (CVI) Cx- **defect in B and T cells.** Si/Sx- decrease immunoglobulin leading to upper and lower resp infxs in **20–30yo.**	Comp- lymphoma and autoimmune diseases. Dx- low levels of immunoglobulins in serum: ↓IgA, ↓IgD, ↓IgE, ↓IgG, ↓IgM. Tx- **IVIG** and prophylacitc abxs.	**IgA deficiency** is the **most common** immunodeficiency disease. Si/Sx- asymp, **recurrent GI and sinopulmonary infxs.** Dx- ↓IgA serum. Tx- abxs, **Do NOT give immunoglobulins** (risk of anti-IgA antibodies).
52) Chronic Granulomatous		
Chronic Granulomatous Disease (X-link, or AR). **Defect in NADPH oxidase** => lack ability for phagocytes to make the **reactive oxygen species** and radicals. Risk- **+Catalase** infxs: **aspergillus,** Klebsiella, **S. aureus,** Serratia, Burkholderia.	Si/Sx- anemia, lymphadenopathy, hepatitis, osteomyelitis. **"CATALASE" positive** infxs; chronic skin, pulm, GI, and UTI infxs.	Dx- gram stain shows **neutrophils filled with bacteria.** Absolute neutrophil count with neutrophil assays. **NITROBLUE tetrazolium test** (diagnostic). Tx- **TMP-SMX,** IFN-gamma, BMT, gene therapy.

Pediatrics

53) DiGeorge Syndrome		
Cx- **22q11** deletion. Si/Sx- **TETANY in first days of life** (hypocalcemia). ↑Infxs with fungi, PCP, and **THYMIC aplasia.**	Assoc- **CATCH 22:** C- Cardiac A- Abn facies T- Thymic aplasia C- Cleft palate H- Hypocalcemia 22- 22q11 deletion	Dx- absolute lymphocyte count. Tx- **IVIG, PCP prophylaxis,** BMT, consider thymus transplantation.

54) Hereditary Angioedema (AD)	55) Terminal Complement Def	56) Leukocyte Adhesion Def
C1-Esterase deficiency. Si/Sx- **recurrent ANGIOEDEMA** provoked by stress or trauma. Risk- life-threatening **airway edema.** Dx- **C1 esterase deficiency, CH50** complement. Tx- C1 esterase, FFP.	**Deficiency C5-C9** => inability to form **membrane attack complex (MAC).** Si/Sx- recurrent **gonococcal and meningococcal** infxs. Tx- **meningococcal vaccine,** abxs.	Leukocytes defect in **chemotaxis.** Si/Sx- recurrent skin, mucosal, and pulm infxs. **Delayed separation of UMBILICAL CORD. "NO PUS"** within infected wounds. Dx- **no pus,** ↑WBCs. Tx- BMT curative.

Pediatrics

57) Chediak-Higashi Syndrome (AR)	58) Congenital Hypothyroidism	
Defect in **neutrophil chemotaxis** and **microtubule** polymerization. Cx- **ALBINISM, neutropenia** with neuropathy. Infxs with strep pyogenses, staph aureus, and pseudomonas. Dx- **GIANT granules in neutrophils.** Tx- BMT	T4 is crucial in first 2yrs life for **BRAIN development.** Cx- **thyroid dysgenesis** (most common cause in the U.S, 85% of cases) Si/Sx- **hypotonia,** sluggish movement, abd bloating, COARSE facial features, large **protruding tongue, umbilical HERNIA.**	Dx-↓T4, ↑TSH, ↑indirect bilirubin. **Manditory newborn screening.** If diagnosis is delayed >6wks pt will have **severe MR.** Tx- **thyroxine/** levothyroxine.

59) Ewing's Sarcoma		
Sarcoma, derived from **neuroectoderm.** Assoc- **chrom 11:22 translocation.** Sx- Local pain, swelling, and possibly fever. Often in **midshaft of long bone.** Seen in femur, pelvis, fibula, or humerus.	**Clinical PEARL: Child Growth BONE PAIN** Si/Sx- poorly localized leg pain that wakes child from sleep. Dx- normal labs, normal XR. Tx- reassurance to parents.	Dx: leukocytosis, ↑**ESR, XR** shows lytic bone lesion with **periosteal "ONION SKIN"** appearance. Tx- local excision, chemo, and radiation. R/O **Langerhans histiocytosis** which is solitary, painful, lytic long bone lesion with hypercalcemia.

60) Osteosarcoma		
Most common primary malignancy of the bone. Si/Sx- persistent bone pain that may be worse at night. Pain begins after trauma; **knee pain with swelling.**	Si/Sx **Metaphyses** of long bones of **distal femur, proximal tibia**, or proximal humerus. Dx- **normal ESR,** ↑**AlkPh.**	Dx- plain XR shows **SUNBURST lytic lesions** and **periosteal** elevation; "**Codman's triangle.**" Order chest CT to r/o pulm met. Tx- local excision, chemotherapy.

Pediatrics

61) Henoch Schonlein Purpura (IgA)		62) Kawasaki
Assoc- Berger's disease. Sx- following an URI, classic tetrad: • **Palpable purpura, RASH** on legs and buttocks. • **Arthralgias** • **Abd pain** (intussusception) • **Renal** disease; **hematuria**	Risk- **intussusception**. Dx- ↑**IgA,** ↑**CRP**. Biopsy of the skin shows **leukocytoclastic vasculitis with IgA** deposition. Kidney biopsy shows by immunofluorescence microscopy. Tx- **NSAIDs**.	Assoc- **<5yo,** Asians. Si/Sx-**FEVER for 5 days** => followed by **conjunctivitis,** cervical lymphadenopathy, **strawberry tongue,** erythema of **palms and soles.** Comp- **coronary artery aneurysms**. Tx- high-dose **ASA + IVIG.**

63) Kawasaki	64) Acute Otitis Media	
Dx **"BURN and CRASH"** **BURN:** Fever >5 days **CRASH:** **C- Conjunctivitis** (bulbar), **Cervical** lymphadenopathy. **R- Rash** palms and soles **A- Aneurysms** coronary **S- Strawberry tongue,** with chapped lips. **H- High ESR**	Cx- **Strep pneumoniae (most common),** H. influenzae, moraxella catarrhalis. Si/Sx- ear pressure, ear pain, **fever,** ↓hearing, ↓ **mobility of tympanic membrane.** Pts may have yellow ear discharge, or postnasal drip. Child may tug at their ear, or have difficulty feeding.	Dx- **otoscopic exam** shows bulging or retraction of TM, ↓**TM mobility** (hallmark). Tx- **amoxicillin** for 10days. Resistant cases can give ceftriaxone, cefuroxime axetil, or amoxicillin/clavulanic acid (2nd-line). Comp: **Nasopharyngeal CA** (assoc-EBV).

Pediatrics

65) Acute Otitis Media	66) Pertussis (<3mos) "whooPing"	
Clinical PEARL: Cholesteatomas Middle ear disease Si/Sx- new hearing loss, **chronic ear drainage** despite abx therapy. Dx- **otoscopy** reveals tympanic membrane with **granulation tissue and skin debris.**	Cx- **bordetella pertussis** (gram neg bacillus, whooping cough) Si/Sx- STAGES: • **Catarrhal** URI several weeks => • **Paroxysomal** "WHOOPING cough" • **Convalescent** Symps slowly improve.	Dx- ↑WBC, culture (gold standard). Tx- **erythromycin** (macrolides), hospitalize if <6mos. ALL close contacts give **erythromycin for 14 days**, relardless of age or immunizations. Prevent- **DTaP vaccine** (early childhood)

67) Croup"BARK" (3mos - 3yrs)		
Laryngo-tracheobronchitis; inflammation in larynx and **subglottis** airway. Cx- **parainfluenza** (most common), RSV, adenovirus.	Si/Sx- hx URI symp, wheezing, rales, airtrapping, tachypnea. Pts have hoarse voice **SEAL-like** **"BARKING" cough, inspiratory stridor,** that is worse at night.	Dx- neck XR shows **STEEPLE sign** from **subglottis narrowing.** Tx: fluids, O_2, corticosteroids. If severe try **racemic epinephrine,** decreases the need for intubation.

Pediatrics

68) Bronchiolitis (<2yrs)	69) Epiglottitis (3-7yr)	
Inflam of small airways in **children <2yo.** Cx-**RSV** (most common), influenza. Sx- fever, cough, rhinorrhea, **tachypnea, wheezing,** crackles, **nasal flar.** Comp- **asthma** later in life. Dx- **clinical,** nasopharyngeal aspirate, CXR r/o pneumonia. Tx- **supportive,** O_2 as needed, possibly bronchodilators.	Cx- **H. influenzae,** Streptococcus pyogenes Si/Sx- high FEVER, **muffled voice,** inspiratory stridor, **DROOLING, leaning forward.** Pt may have **neck hyperextended;** **"SNIFFING Dog "** position. Dx- clinical, endoscopy **cherry-red epiglottitis.** CXR shows **"THUMBPRINT" sign.**	Dx It is important to have **anesthesiologist or otolaryngologist** present to examine the throat. Tx- E-Epiglottitis is a **medical E-Emergency!!!** Examine pt in OR, intubate as needed, and give IV **ceftriaxone.**
70) ToRCHHS	**71)T-Toxoplasmosis**	**72) R-Rubella**
Si/Sx- fever and poor feeding, **chorioretinitis, microcephaly, and cerebral calcifications.** Pt may have petechial rash and hepato-splenomegaly. Assoc- eye problems, MR, autism, and loss of hearing. Dx- serologic testing	Cx-poorly **cooked meat, cat feces.** Dx- serologic testing. Tx- **pyrimethamine + sulfadiazine. Spiramycin** prophylaxis 3rd trimester.	Cx-**1st trimester** infx (80%). Si/Sx- low grade fever, **cataracts, deafness, "BLUEBERRY" muffin rash,** and lymphadenopathy. Assoc- **PDA,** ASD. Dx- serologic testing Tx- immunize before pregnancy.

Pediatrics

73) C-CMV	74) H-HIV	75) H-HSV
#1 congenital infection. Si/Sx- **retinitis**. Dx-urine culture, PCR amniotic fluid. Tx-postpartum **ganciclovir.**	Dx- ELISA (screening), Western blot (confirm). Tx- **Zidovudine (AZT)** or nevirapine. C-section if viral load >1000. Infant should have prophylacitc with **Zidovudine (AZT)** and mother should **avoid breastfeeding.**	**Herpes Simplex Virus** Si/Sx- painful lesions on lips and/or genital mucosa. Solitary or grouped vesicles. Dx- serologic testing. Tx-**acyclovir,** if vaginal **LESION present** schedule a **C-section** delivery.

76) S-Syphilis	77) Meningitis	
Si/Sx- **SNUFFLES,** saddle **nose,** osteochondritis, **Hutchinson teeth, saber shins.** Dx- dark-field microscopy, **VDRL/RPR** (screen), **FTA-ABS** (confirm). Tx- **Penicillin.** Pregnancy with penicillin allergies treat with **penicillin desensitization.**	Cx- Strep. pneumoniae, Neisseria meningitis, E. coli, enteroviruses. • **<3mos- GBS** (S. agalactiae), Listeria, E. Coli. • **>3mos-** N meningitis, S. pneumonia, influenzae. Si/Sx- HA, fever, **nuchal rigidity**. **Kernig's sign** (pain with hip flex), **Brudzinski's sign** (pain with neck flexion).	Si/Sx- **meningococcal** meningitis has **petechiae** and purpura **RASH** or skin lesions. Dx- perform **LP,** if ↑ICP then **start abxs** and then order **head CT.** Tx- empiric **ceftriaxone + vancomycin,** and possibly add **ampicillin**. Add acyclovir if concern for herpes encephalitis.

Pediatrics

78) Erythema Infectiosum		
Fifth Disease= Erythema Infectiosum. Cx- **parvovirus B19** (parvovirus B19 is also assoc with viral arthritis). Si/Sx- **"SLAPPED" cheek rash**, pruritic rash **starts on arms** and spreads to trunk and legs. Rash gets **worse with fever or sun exposure.**	Comp- **aplastic crisis** (sickle cell anemia), hereditary spherocytosis. Dx-clinical. Tx- **self-limiting,** oral analgesics and antihistamines, or topical antipruritics.	[**Viral Exanthems:** Erythema infectiosum (Fifth disease), Hand-Foot-Mouth dz, Rubella, Roseola infantum, Measles, Varicella]

79) Hand-Foot-Mouth Disease	80) Rubella (German measles)	
Cx- **Coxsackie A** Si/Sx- **FEVER =>** then **RASH on HANDS and FEET, ORAL ulcers,** rash clears in one week. Infx is contagious by contact. Dx- clinical Tx- self-limiting, resolves in 1week.	Cx- **togavirus** Si/Sx- pt does not appearing ill, but does have: • **Lymphadenopathy** (sub-occipital and posterior auricular) • **RASH for 5 days** starts on **FACE=>** spreads distally • **Fever** (low grade)	Dx-serologic testing; **rubella virus specific IgM antibodies** (positive test persists over years so should be done near time of rash). Tx- **immunize with MMR** before pregnancy.

Pediatrics

81) Measles		82) Roseola Infantum
Cx- **paramyxovirus** Si/Sx- low-grade fever, **3 C's** • **Cough** • **Coryza** • **Conjunctivitis** • **Koplik's spots** (red spots) on **buccal** after 1–2 days. **Rash starts head** => spreads toward feet.	Risk- otitis media, pneumonia. Dx- clinical. Tx- supportive. **Clinical PEARL:** **Vit-A** has been shown to reduce morbidity and mortality in **measles**.	Cx- **HHV-6** Sx- abrupt **HIGH FEVER 1–5 days** => then "**ROSE-PINK**" macular RASH on **TRUNK** => spread to **face and extremities**, rash last <24hr. Comp- **febrile seizure** (due to rapid fever).

83) Roseola Infantum	84) Varicella	
Dx-clinical Tx- self-limiting, **acetaminophen or ibuprofen** to reduce their temp. Avoid aspirin, due to **Reye's** syndrome (AMS, ↑ammonia, ↑LFTs, fulminant hepatic failure).	Cx- **varicella-zoster virus** (VZV) Sx- mild fever, pruritic, **TEARDROP rash in "different STAGES"** of healing. Lesions contagious until they crusted over.	Dx- clinical; lesions in **different stages** of healing. Tx- **valacyclovir (1st-line),** or acyclovir. **Acyclovir** AE: **crystalline nephropathy**; renal tubular obstruction. Avoid with adequate hydration.

85) Zoster		
Cx- **reactivation of varicella** in pts that are immunocompromised, or elderly pts. Si/Sx- **pain** along sensory nerve and **rash** in **DERMATOMAL** distribution.	Tx- **valacyclovir** (1st-line), or **acyclovir.** **TCA** (desipramine, amitriptyline, or nortriptyline) for pts with **postherpetic neuralgia**.	Comp- **herpes zoster ophthalmicus**; dendriform corneal ulcers and vesicular rash in trigeminal distribution.

Pediatrics

86) Newborn Jaundice		
Cx- elevated serum **bilirubin >5mg/dL** due to ↑hemolysis or ↓excretion. Si/Sx- **jaundice,** lethargy, poor feeding. Pt with **jaundice in <24hrs** need detailed evaluation. **Clinical PEARL: Physiological jaundice AFTER >24hrs** of birth in second or third day of life and **resolves within first few weeks** (normal most of the time).	**UN-CONJUGATED** (insoluble in water) • **Hemolytic anemia:** Spherocytosis, G6PD, pyruvate kinase def. • **Acquired:** ABO/Rh, infxs, drugs, twin-twin transfusion, maternal diabetes, fetal hypoxia.	• **UDP Glucuronyl Transferase deficiency**: **Crigler-Najjar Type I** (**SEVERE** jaundice, **Kernicterus,** Indirect bilirubin 20-25mg/dL. **Crigler-Najjar TypeII** Dx- **Milder,** indirect bilirubin **<20mg/dL.** **Gilbert's** Dx- **MILD** unconjugated hyperbilirubinemia **<3mg/dL.**
87) Newborn Jaundice		
CONJUGATED (water soluble) • **Metabolic:** Galactosemia, Alpha-1 antitrypsin deficiency (cirrhosis and panacinar emphysema). • **Infection:** Sepsis, ToRSH, syphilis, hepatitis.	• **Congenital: Dubin-Johnson** Dx- ↑coproporphyrin I, liver biopsy shows dark granular pigment in hepatocytes, **"BLACK liver".** **Rotor syndrome** (hematuria, excreted in urine, conjugated bilirubin is soluble in water) **Extrahepatic biliary atresia.**	**Clinical PEARL: Galactosemia Galactose-1-phosphate uridyl transferase deficiency** Si/Sx- jaundice, failure to thrive, **bilateral cataracts,** and **hypoglycemia.**

Pediatrics

88) Newborn Jaundice	89) Breastfeeding Failure Jaundice	90) Breast MILK Jaundice
Dx- CBC, **Coombs Test and bilirubin levels.** U/S scan to r/o hepatic obstruction. HIDA scan for possibly cholestatic disease. Tx- **phototherapy,** and/or exchange transfusion if above >20mg/dL.	Cx- ↓intake and ↑enterohepatic circulation. Si/Sx- jaundice within **"FIRST WEEK"** of life. Dx- ↑**unconjugated bilirubin** in first few days after birth. Tx- ↑**feeding to 15-20mins every 2hrs.**	Cx- glucuronyl transferase inhibitor present in breast milk. Si/Sx- jaundice more than >**1-3 WEEKS of birth.** Tx-temporarily stop breastfeeding if ↑↑bilirubin.

91) Kernicterus		
Cx- **hyperbilirubinemia deposit** in basal ganglia, pons, cerebellum. Si/Sx- **jaundice, lethargy, HIGH PITCHED CRY, hypertonicity,** seizures.	Risk factors: sepsis, prematurity, asphyxia. Dx- CBC, blood smear, **Coombs test** and >**25–30 unconjugated bilirubin levels.**	Tx- **phototherapy** and/or **exchange transfusion** if >20mg/dL.

Pediatrics

92) Aseptic Avascular Necrosis		93) Slipped Capital Femoral Epiphysis
• **Legg-Calve-Perthes** necrosis of **head of femur**. • **Osgood-Schlatter** (traction apophysitis) necrosis of **tibial tubercle**. • **Kohler's Bone** necrosis of **navicular bone of foot**.	Si/Sx- afebrile, with **localized pain**. Dx- normal WBC and ERS. **XR shows** sclerosis in affected area, ↓ **uptake epiphysis**.	Si/Sx- **OBESE**, adolescent with dull pain in knee or hip. Dx- XR shows femoral head separating that looks like **ICE-CREAM scoop falling off cone**. Tx-no weight bearing, surgery with pins into femoral head.

94) Toxic synovitis	95) Septic arthritis	96) Osteomyelitis
Si/Sx- **post-viral URI** with pain in the joint. Dx- **normal WBC** and **normal ESR**, ↑uptake epiphysis. Tx- no weightbearing, **analgesia (ibuprofen), and rest**.	Cx- **staph** aureus. Si/Sx- red, warm, tender, painful joint. Dx-↑**WBC and** ↑**ESR, aspiration** (diagnostic). Tx- septic joint in child is a **surgical EMERGENCY** and needs **immediate surgical drainage**, IV abxs and analgesia.	Cx- **staph,** strep. Si/Sx- pain and tenderness in the affected extremity. Dx- **MRI** (gold standard). Tx- **prolonged abxs**, and possibly surgical debridement.

Pediatrics

97) APGAR Score (1 and 5mins of birth)	98) Duodenal Atresia	
A- Appearance (blue, pink trunk, all pink) P- Pulse (0, <100, >100) G- Grimace (0, grimace, cough) A- Activity (0, some, active) R- Resp (0, irregular, regular) Score each as: 0, 1, or 2. Best score is 10/10.	Complete or partial failure of duodenal lumen to recanalize during 8–10wks gestation. Si/Sx- **BILIOUS emesis** within hrs after **FIRST FEEDING.** Assoc- **Down syndrome,** malrotation, annular pancreas, **imperforate anus.**	Dx- AXR may show **"DOUBLE bubble" sign** (air bubbles in stomach and duodenum), proximal to the atresia. Tx- surgical repair.
99) Tracheo-Esophageal Fistula		
Tract between trachea and esophagus. Assoc- **esophageal atresia.** Si/Sx- drooling saliva, **"CHOKING" on first feed,** gagging, resp distress, and **aspiration pneumonia**.	Dx- CXR shows **COILED NG tube, air in GI tract,** Confirm diagnosis with **bronchoscopy.** Tx- surgical repair	**Tracheo-esophageal fistula** is associated with several defects: **VACTERL** • **Vertebral** abn • **Anal** abn • **Cardiac** abn • **Tracheal-** • **Esophageal** fistula • **Renal** disease • **Limb** abn

Pediatrics

100) Diaphragmatic Hernia		
GI tract segments that herniates into the thorax. Si/Sx- resp distress from pulm hypoplasia, pulm HTN, sunken abdomen, **bowel sounds in LEFT hemithorax.** Dx- **CXR shows intestines** in the thoracic cavity.	Dx- **Barium swallow or CT scan** with oral contrast can also be used. **NG tube** in pulm cavity is diagnostic. Tx- high-freq ventilation, O_2, and **surgical repair.**	**Clinical PEARL: Mechanically Ventilated** Respiratory quotient (RQ) is used for weaning pts off ventilation. RQ for **Glucose** 6CO2/6O2=1.0, **Protein 0.8**, **Fatty acids 0.7.** Excessive CO2 with carbohydrates makes weaning difficult.
101) Omphalocele (into sac)		**102) Gastroschisis** (no sac)
Herniation of **abd viscera** through umbilicus **into SAC.** Si/Sx- **premature,** polyhdramnios in utero. Assoc- **Beckwith-Wiedemann**. Dx- clinical. Tx- keep sac covered with **petroleum and gauze, NG suction** to prevent abd distention.	**Clinical PEARL: Beckwith-Wiedemann** Si/Sx- macrosomia, microcephaly (small head), macroglossia, visceromegaly, **omphalocele,** hypoglycemia, **hyper**insulinemia.	Herniation of **intestine only** through abd wall next to the umbilicus with **NO SAC.** Si/Sx- often infant is **premature**, and has polyhdramnios in utero. Dx- clinical Tx- **immediately wrap** exposed bowel in **sterile saline and plastic wrap** to minimize heat and fluid losses. **Surgical** repair.

Pediatrics

103) Respiratory Distress Syndrome

RDS (also called hyaline membrane disease) is the most common cause of resp failure in **preterm infants.**

Surfactant deficiency => alveolar collapse, atelectasis.

Risk- **prematurity,** ↓GA, C-section, **maternal DIABETES.**

Si/Sx- hypoxemia, cyanosis in **first 48–72hrs of life, RR>60, nasal flaring.**

Dx- ABGs, CBC, BCx, CXR shows **"GROUND-GLASS"** appearance with diffuse atelectasis.

Tx- **CPAP** or intubation with mech ventilation, artificial **surfactant** can lower the mortality.

Pretreat mother that will have **delivery <30wks** give **corticosteroids.**

If preterm delivery **(<30wks)** monitor fetal lung maturity with **L/S ratio; lecithin-to-sphingomyelin <2.0** (prematurity) and presence of **phosphatidylglycerol** in amniotic fluid.

L/S ratio <2:1 Need maternal **glucocorticoid adm** (between 24-34wks).

Weaning off intubation- low RR, the better, RR/TV <100.

104) Cerebral Palsy

Movement and posture disorders secondary to perinatal neurologic insult.

Cx- **cerebral anoxia** (most common).

Risk factors: prematurity, LBW, maternal infx, neonatal cerebral hemorrhage, trauma.

Si/Sx **SPASTIC paresis** of all limbs, hypotonia, hyperactive DTR, **MR, toe walking, scissor gait,** seizures.

Dx- clinical, **U/S or CT** to identify possible intracranial hemorrhage.

Tx- no cure.

105) Febrile Seizures

Si/Sx- rapid **acute high FEVER** that gives rise to a **SEIZURE.**

Dx- No labs if consistent with febrile seizures. LP if signs of CNS infx, but r/o ↑ICP first. Possibly CBC, U/A, BCx, UCx, CSF culture to r/o other cx.

Tx- **acetaminophen,** but **avoid ASA (Reye's syndrome).** If seizure is >15mins **diazepam or phenobarbital** as needed.

Pediatrics

106) Lead Poisoning

Cx- child exposure to **lead household "PAINT"** (screen at 12–24mos). Si/Sx- irritability, hyperactivity, anorexia, **abd pain, peripheral neuropathy**; wrist or foot drop.	Si/Sx- pts may also have hx of living in **old house or new job**. Dx- ↑**LEAD levels,** >10 ug/dL intervention is needed (fingersticks may have false positive, so do blood draw).	Dx- CBC with peripheral blood smear may show **basophilic stippling.** Tx- **EDTA** or oral **succimer**.

107) Neuroblastoma

Embryonal tumor of **neural crest** origin. Assoc- **N-myc**, Hirschsprung's disease, neurofibromatosis. Most common sites: **abdomen > thoracic > cervical**.	Si/Sx- anemia, fever, **HTN, non-tender abdominal mass,** Horner's syndrome. If there is **metastasis** pt may have proptosis, subcutaneous nodules, myoclonus, or hepatomegaly.	Dx- ↑serum and urine **catecholamines (VMA and HVA).** CT guided FNA of tumor; **"BLUE tumor cells with ROSETTE pattern."** Tx- local excision, chemotherapy and/or radiation.

108) Wilm's Tumor

Cx- **RENAL tumor**. Assoc- **Beckwith-Wiedemann** syndrome, neurofibromatosis. **Beckwith-Wiedemann** Si/Sx- macrosomia, microcephaly, macroglossia, omphalocele, **hypo**glycemia, **hyper**insulinemia.	Si/Sx- asymp, child 2–5yo with **smooth, non-tender abd mass, aniridia** (absent iris), MR, HTN, hematuria. Dx- CBC, BUN/Cr, **U/A, and Abd U/S.** CT scan can be done to detect metastases.	**WAGR** • **Wilm's tumor** • **Aniridia** (absent iris) • **Genitourinary** abn • Mental **Retardation** Tx- local resection and nephrectomy.

Pediatrics

109) Choanal Atresia		
Obliteration or **blockage** of **posterior nasal aperture.** Si/Sx- **cyanosis,** worsens during feeding and **improves when infant CRYING.**	Dx- **insert catheter through nose** (best initial step). **CT with intranasal contrast** (confirms diagnosis). Tx- intubation via oropharynx (immediate relief), surgery for definitive correction.	Assoc: **CHARGE** • **C- Colobomas** (key-hole shaped defect of the eye) • **H- Heart defects** • **R- Retardation** (growth and/or mental) • **G- Genitourinary** abnormalities • **E- Ear anomalies**
110) Esophageal Atresia		
Most common esophageal anomaly is esophageal atresia with **tracheoesophageal fistula.** Si/Sx- **newborn chokes,** regurgitates and coughs during **first feeding.**	Si/Sx- excessive drooling, frothy **bubbles in mouth, rattling breath sounds** with abd distention. **Pneumonitis and atelectasis** from aspiration of food.	Dx- **inability to pass feeding tube into stomach** is suggestive of esophageal atresia. **CXR shows bilateral atelectasis and gastric distension.** Tx- surgical correction.
111) SIDS		
Sudden **I**nfant **D**eath **S**yndrome (SIDS) Si/Sx- sudden or **unexpected death** of infant 1-12mos of age.	Death remains unexplained after **detailed medical hx, and complete autopsy.** Dx- diagnosis of exclusion. Eye exam may show **retinal hemorrhages.**	Dx- autopsy may show **intrathoracic petechiae or pulmonary edema.** Tx- prevent by putting infant **"BACK to bed"** (baby on back, **supine position**).

Pediatrics

112) Vaccine Types

• **Live**: **MMR,** polio (sabin), **yellow fever,** influenza (spray). • **Killed:** cholera, HAV, polio (Sal**K**), influenza (injection), rabies (**BATS** are major reservoir for rabies virus).	• **Toxoid** (inactivated): diphtheria, tetanus. • **Conjugate:** Hib, strep pneumoniae. • **Subunit:** HBV, pertussis, strep pneumoniae, HPV, meningococcus.	**Clinical PEARL: Pertussis Vaccine** If pt gets **seizure** after they are given **DTaP vaccine,** it is attributed to **pertussis.** Pt should instead be given **DT alone.**

113) Immunization Schedule

• **Newborn-** Hep B. • **2mos** Hep B, RV, DTaP, Hib, PCV, IPV. • **4mos** RV, DTaP, Hib, PCV, IVP. • **6mos** Hep B, RV, DTaP, Hib, PCV, IVP, Influenza (>6mos yrly).	• **12mos-** Hib, PCV, MMR (not before 1yr), varicella, Hep A. • **15mos-** DTaP, Hep A. • **4–6yr** DTaP, IVP, MMR. • **11–12yr-** varicella, MMR (if 2nd not given) **Preterm** immunization use **chronologic age** (not gestational age).	Number = total # shots: **Hep B-** Hepatitis B (3) **RV-** Rotavirus (3) **DTaP-** Diphtheria, Tetanus, Pertussis (5) **Hib-** Haemophilus influenzae type b (4) **PCV-**Pneumococcal(4) **IPV-** Inactivated poliovirus (4) **MMR-** Measles, Mumps, Rubella (2) **Hep A-**Hepatitis A (2) **Varicella** (2)

16 CHAPTER
PSYCHIATRY

Psychiatry

1) Schizophrenia

↑**DOPAMINE** leading to=> limbic **hyper**activity and frontal **hypo**activity. Pt will also have ↑ventricular size on CT. Si/Sx- >**6mos** of delusions, hallucinations, behavioral disturbances, disordered thoughts.	**Subtypes:** • **Disorganized** Speech and behavior that is disorganized. Tx- **risperidone** (1st-line). • **Paranoid** Delusions and hallucinations. • **Catatonic** Mutism, ↓motor, flat affect.	Dx- **two of following for >6mos:** • **+ Symp:** bizarre behavior, hallucinations (auditory), delusions, disorganized speech, and thought disorders. • **Neg Symp:** flat affect, ↓emotional reactivity, ↓speech, anhedonia (inability to experience pleasure).

2) Schizophrenia	3) Other Types of Schizo- Disorders	
Tx- **antipsychotics**, supportive psychotherapy. **Antipsychotics block dopamine** activity along the tuberoinfundibular pathway. **Antipsychotics AE:** extrapyramidal symptoms (EPS), ↑prolactin.	• Schizo**phreniform** < **6 MONTHS.** • Schizo**affective** Schizophrenia + **major affective disorder** (major depressive or bipolar).	• **Brief Psychotic Disorder** >**1 DAY - 1 MONTH** Hallucinations, disorganized speech, and/or behavior. • **Delusional Disorder NON-bizarre delusion** (fixed, false belief), but no hallucinations, disorganized thoughts. **Folie a' deux-** shared non-bizarre delusion (two individuals).

Psychiatry

4) Extrapyramidal Symptoms (EPS)		
AE from antipsychotics **Extrapyramidal Symptoms (EPS):** • 4 hrs-**Acute dystonia** • 4 days- **Akinesia** • 4 wks- **Dyskinesia** • 4 mos- **Tardive dyskinesia**	**• 4 HRS** **Acute dystonia** Si/Sx- muscle spasm; neck, jaw, tongue, eyes, entire body. Tx- **benztropine, trihexyphenidyl** (anticholinergics), or **diphenhydramine** (antihistamine).	**• 4 DAYS** **Akathiasia** Si/Sx- restlessness. Tx- **propranolol** (beta-blockers).
5) Extrapyramidal Symptoms (EPS)		
• 4 WKS **Dyskinesia** Si/Sx- cogwheel rigidity, shuffling gait, pseudoparkinsonism. Tx- **benztropine, trihexyphenidyl** (anticholinergic), or **amantadine** (↑dopamine).	**• 4 MOS** **Tardive dyskinesia** (irreversible) Si/Sx- tongue protrusion, lip smacking, neck torticollis, grunting noises, limb twisting. Tx- ↓ **dose** or stop med, change to **risperidone** or clozapine.	**Clinical PEARL: Anticholinergic toxicity** Cx- **benztropine, trihexyphenidyl.** AE: flushing, dry mucous membranes, sweating, pupillary dilation, urinary retention, and delirium. **"Red** as a beet, **dry** as a bone, **hot** as a hare, **blind** as a bat, **mad** as a hatter, and **full** as a flask."

Psychiatry

6) Typical Antipsychotics	7) Typical Antipsychotics AE's	
Haloperidol, droperidol, fluphenazine, thioridazine, chlorpromazine (all block dopamine D2 receptors). Tx: **positive psychotic disorders** (block D2 dopamine), acute mania, and Tourette's. **Compliance issues** use depot forms: **haloperidol** decanoate, **fluphenazine** decanoate, **risperidone** depot, **paliperidone** depot.	Typical antipsychotics AE: • **Extrapyramidal Symptoms (EPS)** Acute dystonia, akathiasia, akinesia, dyskinesia, tardive dyskinesia. • **Hyperprolactinemia** (due to ↓dopamine) • **Anticholinergic** Urine retention, dry mouth, constipation. • **Hypothermia** (have pts avoid exposure to extreme temps).	• **Retinal pigmentation** (thioridazine) • **Neuroleptic Malignant Syndrome FEVER, muscle rigidity,** seizures, sedation, autonomic instability, prolong QT. Tx-ICU, adm **dantrolene** (muscle relaxant) or **bromocriptine** (dopamine agonist).
8) Atypical Antipsychotics		9) Major Depression
Clozapine, quetiapine, olanzapine, ziprasidone, risperidone, aripiprazole (all block dopamine-D2 and 5-HT2 receptors). Tx: **1st-line schizophrenia (esp NEG symps)** due fewer EPS and anticholinergics. **Clozapine** for severe pts and **tardive dyskinesia**.	AE: **HTN, ↑WEIGHT, diabetes mellitus, hyperprolactinemia,** dyslipidemia, sedation, prolonged QT. **Clozapine** (2nd-line) for pts not responding to therapy, requires wkly **C**BC due to **agranulocytosis**.	Si/Sx- **>2WEEKS depressed** mood or anhedonia (loss of interest and/or pleasure) with **five or more of the following: SIG E CAPS.** Assoc- **propranolol** (most common med that can cause depression). Risk factor: chronic illness and stress.

Psychiatry

10) Major Depressive Disorder		
SIG E CAPS: **S- Sleep** (hypersomnia or insomnia) **I- Interest** (loss of interest) **G- Guilt** (feeling worthless) **E- ↓Energy** **C- ↓Concentration** **A- Appetite ↑or↓weight** **P- Psychomotor agitation** **S- Suicidal** ideations	Dx- **>2 WEEKS depression** with **+5 SIGECAPS.** All depressed pts should be screened for **suicidal ideations.** R/O **dysthymia (depression >2yrs),** bereavement, medical condition, **adjustment disorder (<3mos** of stressor), substance induced.	Tx- **antidepressants** (least six month period) **+ psychotherapy.** Refractory depression, use **electroconvulsive therapy (ECT).** **ECT is SAFE in pregnancy.** Can also be used in pregnant pts with psychotic depression. **Electroconvulsive therapy (ECT)** AE: retrograde and anterograde **amnesia.**

11) Major Depressive Disorder		12) Other Types of Depression
Subtypes of Depression: • **Atypical** ↑Weight, hypersomnia, rejection sensitivity. • **Psychotic features** Delusions and hallucinations. • **Seasonal** During the winter mos. • **Postpartum** More than **>1mos** postpartum.	**Clinical PEARL: Trichotillomania** Si/Sx- **pulls hair out,** resulting in alopecic patches (broken hair of varying length). Assoc- **depressive disorders,** OCD, borderline.	• **Dysthymia** Low level depression **>2 YEARS.** • **Adjustment Disorder** Depression within **<3 MONTHS of a stressor.** Tx- cognitive or psychodynamic psychotherapy. • **Bereavement Grief** for **1 MONTH- 1 YEAR.**

258

Psychiatry

13) Bereavement (grief)	14) Bipolar Disorders	
Normal reaction to the **loss of a loved one.** Si/Sx- similar to major depression that lasts several **MONTHS,** but **<1 YEAR,** with no psychotic features. Dx- 1mos- 1yr of grief. Tx- **psychotherapy.** If bereaved pt have **>2wks depression after major event** continue psychotherapy and start trial **antidepressants (SSRIs).**	• **Bipolar I** At least **one MANIC episode** or mixed episode. • **Bipolar II** At least one **major DEPRESSIVE episode** (MDE) and hypomanic episode.	Si/Sx- mania, **DIGFAST:** • **D- Distractibility** • **I- Insomnia** (↓sleep) • **G- Grandiosity** • **F- Flight** of ideas • **A- Activity/agitation** • **S- Sexual** drive • **T- Talkativeness** Lifetime Risk: 1% general pop, 5-10% if 1st-degree relative, 70% if monozygotic twins.

15) Bipolar Disorders		
Dx- **manic >1WEEK** and **3+ DIGFAST.** If pt is diagnosed with bipolar disease check **beta-hCG, TFT, and creatinine** before starting therapy with **Lithium.** Tx- **first-line** agents for long-term maintenance; **LITHIUM, lamotrigine, olanzapine, or quetiapine.**	Tx **Valproic acid, carbamazepine** 2nd-line agents (both are good alternatives for pts with renal disease that cannot be on lithium). Pt in acute **MANIC** episode that is **extremely agitated** and psychotic should be treated with **HALOPERIDOL** immediately (antipsychotic).	Tx For an **acute manic** episode **LITHIUM** should be continued for **one year** and if pt has **no relapses,** pt can be gradually **taper off** (tapered due to risk of suicide and relapse). **Lithium** AE: **diabetes insipidus** (C/I in kidney disease), hypothyroidism, Ebstein's anomaly.

Psychiatry

16) Other Types of Bipolar Diseases	17) SSRIs Antidepressants	
• **Rapid cycling** Four or more episodes (MDE, manic, mixed, or hypomanic) in **1 YEAR.** • **Cyclothymic** Chronic and less severe bipolar disorder that is for **>2 YEARS.**	Fluoxetine, paroxetine, **sertraline, citalopram, escitalopram, fluvoxamine.** Tx- **depression, anxiety.** Antidepressants can take up to **4-6wks** before pts will have symp relief.	AE- **sexual dysfunction** (impotence, delayed ejaculation, ↓libido), **GI distress, agitation,** insomnia, tremors. Comp: **Serotonin Syndrome** Cx- SSRI with MAOI. Si/Sx- **FEVER, myoclonus,** mental status changes.
18) Atypicals Antidepressants		19) TCAs Antidepressants
Bupropion, venlafaxine, mirtazapine, trazodone. Tx- **depression,** anxiety, chronic pain. **Bupropion** for **smoking cessation** and ↓ **sexual dysfunction.**	• **Bupropion** AE: ↑seizure (bulimia nervosa), ↓sexual dysfunction. • **Venlafaxine** AE: HTN. • **Mirtazapine** AE: ↑weight, sedation. • **Trazodone** AE: **priapism** (also prazosin can cause priapism), sedating.	Nor**triptyline,** ami**triptyline,** des**ipramine,** im**ipramine.** Tx- depression, anxiety, chronic pain, **migraine HA, enuresis.** AE- LETHAL overdose **arrhythmias (long QRS),** hyperthermia, dilated pupils, intestinal ileus, seizures, **hypotension.** Monitor in ICU for 3–4 days.

Psychiatry

20) TCAs Antidepressants	21) Anti-cholinergic Toxicity	22) Organophosphate
AE: **anticholinergic effects of TCAs** are dry mouth, blurred vision, urinary retention, sedation, constipation, dizziness. Tx- **sodium bicarbonate** shorten QRS, improves BP, and also **prevents arrhythmia.** **Clinical PEARL: Enuresis** Si/Sx- recurrent, involuntary voiding of urine in bed >5yo. Tx- **desmopressin** (1st-line), imi**pramine** (TCA, 2nd-line).	Cx- **diphenhydramine** (benadryl), TCAs, antipsychotics. AE: flushing, **dry mucous** membranes, sweating, **pupillary dilation, urinary retention,** and delirium. "**Red** as a beet, **dry** as a bone, **hot** as a hare, **blind** as a bat, **mad** as a hatter, and **full** as a flask." Tx-**physostigmine, neostigmine** (acetylcholinesterase inhibitor=> ↑acetylcholine).	**Organophosphate poisoning;** inhibits acetylcholinesterase=> ↑ **cholinergic excess.** Cx- **pesticides,** physostigmine, neostigmine, organophosphate poisoning. Si/Sx- bradycardia, miosis, rhonchi, muscle fasciculations, **"salivation, urination, lacrimation, and defecation."** Tx- **atropine** (immediately). Of equal importance remove all clothing and wash the body.

Psychiatry

23) MAOIs Antidepressants	24) Lithium Mood Stabilizers	25) Carbamazepine Mood Stabilizers
Phenelzine, Selegiline Tranylcypromine. Tx- **atypical** depression. AE- **sexual** dysfunction, orthostatic hypotension (drop systolic ↓BP >20), ↑weight, HTN crisis. **"Hypertensive CRISIS"** MAOIs (phenelzine, tranylcypromine, or selegiline) with **TYRAMINE** foods (cheese, red wine).	Tx- **mood stabilizer** (1st-line), **bipolar** prophylaxis**, acute mania.** AE- thirst, polyuria, **diabetes insipidus (DI)**, tremor, ↑weight, hypothyroidism, **tetratogenicity.** **Narrow therapeutic window, avoid in** renal disease. **Lithium toxicity >1.5mEq/L** Ataxia, delirium, dysarthria, renal failure.	Tx- **mood stabilizer** (2nd line), anticonvulsant, **trigeminal neuralgia.** AE- nausea, leukopenia, AV block, **aplastic anemia** (monitor CBC biwkly), **Stevens-Johnson syndrome.**
26) Valproic Acid Mood Stabilizers	27) Lamotrigine Mood Stabilizers	28) DSM-IV
Tx- **bipolar, anticonvulsant.** AE- tremor, sedation, alopecia, ↑weight, GI upset; nausea, vomiting, pancreatitis, thrombocytopenia. Comp- life threatening **hepatotoxicity, agranulocytosis.**	Tx- mood stabilizer (2nd line), **anticonvulsant.** AE- **blurred vision,** GI distress; nausea, vomiting, **Stevens-Johnson syndrome** (↑dose slowly to monitor for rash).	• **Axis I-** psychiatric disease • **Axis II-** MR and personality disorders • **Axis III-** physical and medical problems • **Axis IV-** social and environmental issues • **Axis V-** global assessment of function (GAF) 1-nonfunctional, 100-highly functional.

Psychiatry

29) Id, Ego and Super ego	30) Defense Mechanisms	
• **Id**: drives, insticts, sex and aggression (at birth). • **Ego**: **defense mechanisms**, judgment (shortly after birth). • **Super ego**: conscience (form during latency period)	• **Acting out** Behavioral outbursts. • **Altruism** Serving others to reduce own guilt. • **Blocking** Temporary block in thinking.	• **Displacement** Emotion shifting of unacceptable feelings from one onto another "safer." • **Denial** Avoid because it is too painful.
31) Defense Mechanisms		
• **Introgection** External world is part of self (I do what you do). • **Intellectualization** Excessive use of intellectual processes to avoid experience.	• **Isolation** Separation of an idea to avoid the affects (matter of fact). • **Humor** To avoid feeling personal discomfort.	• **Projection** Attributing own wish on someone else. • **Rationalization** Explanations to justify the unacceptable.
32) Defense Mechanisms		
• **Reaction formation** Unacceptable impulse transformed into opposite (acceptable). • **Regression** Return to earlier stage of development.	• **Splitting** All good or all bad (assoc- boarderline). • **Sublimation** Impulse gratification with unacceptable into acceptable.	• **Suppression** Consciously forgetting (abuse forgotten). • **Undoing**- acting out the reverse of unexceptable behavior.

Psychiatry

33) Personality Cluster A "WEIRD"	34) Cluster B "WILD"	
• **Paranoid** Si/Sx-distrustful, suspicious. • **SchizOID** Si/Sx- **avOID,** isolated, detached, **loners,** with restricted emotion. • **Schizotypal** Si/Sx- **ODD behavior** and appearance, with **"magical thinking."** Tx- **be clear, honest, and noncontrolling** (pts distrust psychiatrist).	• **Borderline** Si/Sx- **unstable** mood, unstable relationships, **"splitting"** (pt see individuals as all good, or all bad), poor self-image, **self-harm (cutting),** suicidal. • **Histrionic** Si/Sx- **attention seeking, sexually provocative,** excessively emotional.	• **Narcissistic** Si/Sx- entitlement, **grandiose of self,** lack empathy, need admiration. • **Antisocial** (Adult) Si/Sx- violate LAW and RIGHTS of others. (Child- **Conduct** dz). Tx- be firm, fair, and **consistent.**
35) Cluster C "WORRIED"		36) Generalized Anxiety
• **Obsessive Compulsive Personality Disorder (OCPD)** Si/Sx- preoccupied with control, perfectionism, order, and can be inflexible. **OCPD** pts **do not** recognize behavior as a problem. (OCD does recognize behavior as a problem).	• **Avoidant** Si/Sx- **fear** of being **disliked** or ridiculed, **rejection sensitive.** • **Dependent** Si/Sx- submissive and **CLINGY, feels helpless,** difficulty making decisions. Tx- do not push pts into decisions.	Si/Sx- **>6 MONTHS of excessive ANXIETY** and worry about events or activities in life. Pts often complain of **muscle tension,** easy fatigability, **restlessness,** poor concentration, **irritability,** and impaired sleep.

Psychiatry

37) Generalized Anxiety	38) Meds for Anxiety	
Dx- clinically. Tx- psychotherapy, lifestyle. **BUSPIRONE (1st-line)**, SSRIs, venlafaxine (2nd-line). • **Buspirone** for general anxiety. • **Propranolol** (beta-blockers) for performance anxiety. • **Benzos (alprazolam)** for immediate symp relief, needs to be **taper** as soon as pt is on long-term treatment.	• **SSRIs** fluoxetine, sertraline, paroxetine, citalopram, escitalopram, fluvoxamine. Tx- anxiety, OCD, PTSD, depression. AE- nausea, GI upset, agitation. • **Buspirone** Tx- **general anxiety**, OCD, PTSD, **smoking cessation.** AE- **no tolerance,** ↑risk of seizures (C/I in bulimia nervosa).	• **Beta-blockers** Tx- **PERFORMANCE anxiety**, PTSD. AE- bradycardia, hypotension. • **Benzodiazepines** Tx- acute anxiety, insomnia, **alcohol withdrawal**, muscle spasm, night terrors, sleepwalking. AE- tolerance, confusion, ↓quality of sleep. • **Flumazenil** Tx- benzo overdose.
39) Obsessive Compulsive Disease		
Low **SEROTONIN** in the brain, associated with impulsivity. Si/Sx **Obsessions**; persistent, unwanted thoughts=> distress and anxiety. **Compulsions**; repeated behaviors to ↓anxiety from obsessions. Pts **recognize behavior as excessive.**	Dx- clinical Tx- **SSRIs** (first-line); **paroxetine, fluvoxamine, fluoxetine. Cognitive-behavioral therapy** (CBT). Clomipramine (TCAs, 2nd-line).	• **OCD**- recognize behavior as a problem. • **OCPD**- "DO NOT" recognize behavior as a problem.

Psychiatry

40) PANIC Disorder

Si/Sx- unexpected, **recurrent "PANIC ATTACKS"** that peak within 10mins of **abrupt intense FEAR.**

Pts may have **palpitations,** tachypnea, chest pain, diaphoresis, nausea, trembling, dizziness. Pts feel that they may be **going crazy** and have a intense **fear of dying.**

Assoc- **agoraphobia** (fear of public places, or large crowds), **depression,** generalized anxiety, and substance abuse.

Dx- clinical, **>1 MONTH of panic attacks, with four** following symps: palpitations, chest pain, tachypnea, diaphoresis, nausea, trembling, dizziness.

Tx- **SSRI (1st-line),** CBT, TCAs.

In **acute panic attacks** give short term **benzodiazepines; alprazolam** (xanax) or cloazepam. Also start **long-term SSRI** at same time.

Once symps are controlled **taper benzo** and continue long term **SSRIs.**

41) Phobias

42) Post Traumatic Stress Disorder

Si/Sx- performance or social phobia with fear of embarrassment.

• **Specific phobias**
Fear of heights, animals, the dark, or fear of public places (agoraphobia).

Dx- clinical
Tx- **CBT** (cognitive behavioral therapy).

• **Social phobias**
Tx- **assertiveness training** (type of CBT) and **SSRIs (1st-line),** benzoziazepines (alprazolam), beta-blocker.

• **Performance**
Tx-**beta-blocker** (propranolol).

Si/Sx- **>1 MONTH** of having feelings of **survivor guilt, flashbacks,** intrusive memories.

Pts may have exaggerated reactions to triggers, nightmares, emotional numbing, amnesia, detachment, and/or depression.

Psychiatry

43) Post Traumatic Stress Disorder		
Dx- clinical, >1 MONTH of reexperiencing life-threatening traumatic events that leads to significant distress or impairment.	Tx- SSRI (first line); sertraline. Buspirone, TCAs, and MAOIs may also be helpful. Pts will benefit from psychotherapy and support groups.	Tx Short term beta-blockers and alpha2-agonists (clonidine) for anxiety. Avoid benzo because of risk of substance abuse.

44) Delirium vs Dementia		45) Dementia
DELIRIUM Si/Sx • Impaired attention • ACUTE onset • Fluctuating hr-to-hr • CLOUDED consciousness • Present of hallucinations • REVERSIBLE	**DEMENTIA** Si/Sx • Alert attention • GRADUAL onset • Progressive course • INTACT consciousness • Hallucinations in 30% • IRReversible	Cx- Alzheimer's (>50%), multi-infarct dementia (stepwise deterioration) stroke, trauma, Parkinson's, Huntington's, Wilson's disease, infx, neoplasia. Si/Sx- impairment in cognitive function with global deficits, but level of consciousness is stable.

46) Dementia		47) Delirium
Si/Sx-memory impairment with at least one or more of 5A's: • Amnesia • Aphasia (language) • Apraxia (motor) • Agnosia (recognize) • Abstract (planning) • Aggression (behavior) Dx- MMSE, r/o other causes; HIV, RPR, B12/folate def, U/A, head CT or MRI.	Tx- rigid DAILY structure with environmental cues. Cholinesterase inhibitors; donepezil, rivastigmine, or galantamine. Can also use low dose antipsychotics, but should avoid benzos (because can cause confusion).	Cx- ETOH, meds, infx, withdrawal, hypoxia, ICU psychosis, trauma. Si/Sx- WAXING and WANING of consciousness with short-term memory loss and disturbances; delusions, illusions, hallucinations.

Psychiatry

48) Delirium	49) Autism Spectrum	
Dx- check vitals, pulse oximetry, meds, infxs, U/A; "**think UTI in elderly**," identify underling cause. Tx- **underlying cause,** normalize fluids and electrolytes, low dose antipsychotics (**haloperidol**) for agitation.	Assoc- **fragile X syndrome, tuberous sclerosis.** Si/Sx- impaired **social** interaction and **communication** before the age of **<3yrs old.** Pts may lack social smile, eye contact, and/or lack interest in relationships. There may be restricted interests, preoccupation with objects.	Si/Sx • **Social** impairments • **Interaction** impairments • **Communication** restricted • **Interests** limited • **Repetitive** behavior Dx- clinical Tx: **behavioral management,** counseling with support for family.
50) Attention Deficit Hyperactivity		
Attention Deficit Hyperactivity Disorder (**ADHD**) Si/Sx- symps **before 7 years old** for **>6mos in two settings** (home and school, daycare): Poor attention span, **easily distracted,** hyperactivity, impulsivity, **fidgets,** and may continuously interrupts others.	Dx- clinical; **symps before 7 YEARS OLD in two settings.** Tx- behavior modification, **methylphenidate (Ritalin),** alpha 2-agonist (**clonidine**), antidepressants (SSRIs, nortriptyline, bupropion).	**Methylphenidate** AE: ↓appetite (↓weight), irritability, nervousness, insomnia, abd pain. **Clinical PEARL: Selective Mutism** Verbal and talkative in one setting but refuse to speak in another setting.

Psychiatry

51) Developmental Disorders	52) Disruptive Behavioral	53) Mental Retardation (MR)
• **Asperger's Syndrome** Si/Sx- **"autism-like,"** without language or cognitive delays. • **Rett's Disorder** Si/Sx-neurodegenerative disorder in **FEMALE after 5mos of normal development** (regression at 5mos). • **Childhood Disintegrative Disorder** Si/Sx- developmental **REGRESSION after 2yrs old.**	• **Oppositional Defiant Disorder** Si/Sx- defiant behavior **toward authority for >6 MONTHS** (may progress to conduct disorder). • Conduct Disorder Si/Sx- **violates RIGHTS of others,** nonaggressive (stealing, lie) or aggressive (robbery, rap). • Conduct- Child • Antisocial- Adults Tx: individual and family therapy.	Cx- chrom abn, teratogens, infxs, fetal alcohol syndrome (#1 **avoidable** cause of MR). • **Mild (IQ 50–70,** most cases) • Moderate (IQ 35–49) • Severe (IQ 20–34) • Profound (IQ <20) Tx- **therapy** for language, physical, social skills.
54) Tourette's Syndrome		
Assoc- **ADHD, OCD, learning disorders.** Si/Sx- multiple motor, vocal **TICS many times a day for >1year.**	Si/Sx- pts may have grimacing, blinking, grunting, and/or **coprolalia** (repetition of obscene words). Dx- clinical, symps prior to **18 years old for >1year.**	Tx- behavioral therapy, **haloperidol, PIMOZIDE** (dopamine antagonist), clonidine. Stimulants can worsen symps.

Psychiatry

55) Alcoholism

Si/Sx- look for signs of liver dz and ask **CAGE questionnaire:** **C- Cut** down **A- Annoyed** by criticism **G- Guilty** about drinking **E- Eye** opener	Comp: • **Delirium Tremens (DT's)** • **Mallory-weiss tears** • **Boerhaave syndrome** (rupture of esophagus) • **Korsakoff psychosis** • **Wernicke's encephalopathy** (AMS, ataxia, nystagmus)**.**	Pts can also get ulcers, **varices,** pancreatitis, gastritis, liver disease, and rhabdomyolysis. Dx- clinical, **CAGE questionnaire.** ↑LFTs (**AST**>ALT) "To**AST**ed." MCV >100 (folate def). Monitor pts for withdrawal symps.

56) Alcoholism

Tx- **folic acid,** multivitamins, **thiamine** (thiamine before glucose) to prevent **Wernicke's encephalopathy**. Give **benzodiazepine taper** for withdrawal symptoms. Possibly **disulfiram, or naltrexone** to help with dependence.	**Alcoholic Anonymous** for long-term treatment program. • **Intoxication** Si/Sx- disihibition, **slurred speech, ataxia,** impaired judgment (similar to benzo intoxication). Tx- **thiamine, glucose.**	• **Withdrawal** Si/Sx- **DTs** **"delirium tremens"** (fever, HTN, tachy, hallucination, disorientation), malaise, and possibly seizures. Tx-**benzodiazepine taper,** add haloperidol for hallucinations.

Psychiatry

57) Abused Drugs and Dependence		
Substance Abuse 1+ of the following: • Lack responsibilities • Legal problems • Hazardous situations • Continue to use despite problems	**Substance Dependence** 3+ of following: • Withdrawals • Tolerance • ↑Amounts used • Failure to cut down • ↑Time spent obtaining and using drugs • Continue despite problems	**Clinical PEARL:** **Pathologic Gambling** Preoccupation with gambling leading to financial instability. Pts are dishonest and evasive about gambling. Risk- **pramipexole** (dopamine agonists) used for treating parkinson's.
58) Amphetamine Intoxication	**59) Amphetamine Withdrawal**	**60) Opioids Intoxication**
Amphetamine and Cocaine **Intoxication** Si/Sx- **"DILATION"** **pupil**, tachycardia, agitation, euphoria, **cocaine chest pain,** HTN, psychosis. Erythema of tubinates and **nasalseptum** (cocaine). Risk- STEMI (cocaine). Dx- urine drug screen. Tx- **haloperidol** for severe agitation. Cocaine-related cardiac ischemia give **benzodiazepines, nitrates, and aspirin.**	Si/Sx- anxiety, **stomach cramps,** HA, lethargy, **"COCAINE BUGS,"** depression, anhedonia, cravings, **suicidal ideations.** **Clinical PEARL:** **Marijuana abuse** Si/Sx- euphoria, anxiety, dry mouth, tachy, ↑appetite, **conjunctival injection.**	**Opioids;** morphine, heroin. Si/Sx- **euphoria,** **"PINPOINT"** pupils; pupil contraction (miosis), bradycardia, hypotension, **CNS and** **resp depression.** Dx- urine drug screen. Tx- **naloxone/** **naltrexone,** long-term **methadone.**

Psychiatry

61) Opioids Withdrawal	62) PCP Intoxication	63) PCP Withdrawal
Opioids; morphine, heroin. Si/Sx- **rhinorrhea, "YAWNING,"** lacrimation, nausea, vomiting, **abd pain,** diarrhea, restlessness, **arthralgias, myalgias,** insomnia, anorexia, fever, DILATED pupils, piloerection, no seizures. Tx- **methadone.**	**Phencyclidine Hydrochloride (PCP)** Si/Sx- **VIOLENCE, assaultiveness,** belligerence, **VERTICAL** or horizontal **nystagmus.** Tx- **benzos or haloperidol.**	**Phencyclidine Hydrochloride (PCP)** Si/Sx Sudden **random violence,** due to recurrence of intoxication from GI reabsorption.
64) LSD Intoxication	**65) Benzodiazepines Intoxication**	**66)Benzodiazepines Withdrawal**
Lysergic Acid Diethylamide (LSD) Si/Sx- **HTN, visual** hallucinations, **DILATION pupils, "FLASHBACKS."** Dx- urine drug screen. Tx- counseling, benzos for anxiety, antipsychotics for psychotic symps.	Si/Sx **AMNESIA, ataxia,** mild respiratory depression, somnolence. Dx- urine drug screen.	Si/Sx- **rebound anxiety,** insomnia, tremor, tachycardia, HTN, **seizures, AMS.** **Abrupt cessation** is assoc with significant withdrawal symptoms.
67) Barbiturates	**68) Nicotine**	**69) Caffeine**
• **Intoxication** Si/Sx- respiratory depression. • **Withdrawal** Si/Sx- life-threatening **cardiovascular collapse,** delirium, anxiety, seizures.	• **Intoxication** Si/Sx- restlessness, anxiety, insomnia, arrhythmias. • **Withdrawal** Si/Sx- HA, anxiety, cravings, irritability, weight gain, insomnia, difficulty concentrating.	• **Intoxication** Si/Sx- restlessness, **diuresis,** arrhythmias, insomnia, psychomotor agitation. • **Withdrawal** Si/Sx- lethargy, **HA,** weight gain, cravings, irritability.

Psychiatry

70) Gender Identity Disorder		
Si/Sx- **cross-gender identification** and persistent discomfort with one's assigned sex or gender.	Assoc- substance abuse, depression, anxiety, and personality disorders. Tx- supportive psychotherapy, possibly sex-reassignment surgery.	**Clinical PEARL: Reaction Formation** Transformation of unwanted thoughts or feeling into opposite. Ex- homosexual man tries to date women.

71) Paraphilias		
More than **6mos** of unusual sexual fantasies, and/or urges. • **Fetishism** Using nonliving objects for sexual arousal. • **Transvestic fetishism** Cross-dressing for sexual arousal.	• **Voyeurism** Observing person unclothing or having sex. • **Exhibitionism** Arousal from exposing one's genitals to stranger. • **Frotteurism** Rubbing one's genitalia against nonconsenting person.	• **Sexual sadism** Sexual arousal from **inflicting PAIN** on sexual partner. • **Sexual masochism** Sexual **arousal from being hurt**, humiliated. • **Pedophilia** Urge to have sex with children.

Psychiatry

72) Anorexia Nervosa

Assoc- gymnastics, runners, models. Si/Sx- **refusal to maintain NORMAL body weight**, due to fear of weight gain, **amenorrhea,** and perceives self as fat. **Fasting, binge/purge** through vomiting laxatives, diuretics, and/or excessive exercise.	Dx- **psychiatric evaluation,** measure height and weight. If severe order CBC, electrolytes, and possibly ECG. Tx- **monitor weight gain,** individual and family **psychotherapy**. **Hospitalize** if severe; **BMI <18.5, bradycardia,** starvation, dehydration, abn electrolytes, or suicidal ideations.	Tx Can induce ovulation with **pulsatile GnRH therapy.** Comp- **osteoporosis,** estrogen deficiency, prolonged QT euthyroid sick syndrome. Anorexic pts that do become pregnant have risk of IUGR and being small for GA.

73) Bulimia Nervosa

Assoc- mood disorders, low self-esteem, OCD. Si/Sx- **2–3 times weekly of binge and purging** (surreptitious vomiting) or fasting. Pts have **NORMAL weight** or might be overweight with **normal menses.** Pt may have **dental enamel erosions,** scars on dorsal of hand, and/or **enlarged parotid gland.**	Dx- psychiatric evaluation. Surreptitious vomiting may show labs of serum ↑HCO3- and loss of H+, K+, Cl-. Tx- psychotherapy focused on **behavior modification,** possibly antidepressants.	Tx Correct electrolyte losses of K+, H+, Cl- with **potasium chloride.** **Clinical PEARL: Kleptomaina** Si/Sx- inability to resist the **impulse to steal**. Assoc- **bulimia nervosa.**

Psychiatry

74) Insomnia	75) Hypersomnia	76) Narcolepsy
Si/Sx- disturbance in normal rhythm of sleep with **difficulty initiating or maintaining sleep.** Dx- clinical Tx- **sleep schedule,** limit caffeine, **avoid naps,** relaxation techs. Tx-Pharmacotherapy is 2nd line with **diphenhydramine** (Benadryl), trazodone, zolpidem (ambien).	Si/Sx- excessive **DAYTIME SLEEPINESS** for **>1 month.** Dx- clinical, **>1mos** daytime sleepiness. Tx- **amphetamines** (stimulants, 1st-line), some pts may benifit from SSRI (antidepressants).	Si/Sx- excessive **DAYTIME SOMNOLENCE** for **>3 months**. Pts have ↓REM, **sleep attacks, cataplexy** (loss muscle tone), **sleep paralysis** upon waking in the morning. • **HypnopoMpic** (**M**orning hallucinations) • **HypnaGOgic** (**GO**ing to bed hallucinations)
77) Narcolepsy	**78) Sleep Apnea**	
Dx- clinical, **>3 MONTHS** of daytime sleepiness with **sleep attacks** (classic). Tx- **scheduled daily naps** + stimulants; **methylphenidate, modafinil.** Can use SSRIs for cataplexy.	Si/Sx- **disturbances in BREATHING** while sleeping=> leading to excessive daytime somnolence. • **Obstructive Sleep Apnea (OSA)** (most common) Cx- **OBESITY**, tonsillar hypertrophy (child), hypothyroidism Si/Sx- **obese, male,** with obstruction of airway that leads to **SNORING** and lack of airflow.	• **Central Sleep Apnea (CSA)** Si/Sx- airway and resp cease, repeated awakening, **morning HA**. Dx- **Polysomnography** (sleep study) shows ↑arousals, ↓O2 saturation. Tx **OSA**- ↓**weight, CPAP CSA**- mechanical ventilation (BPAP).

Psychiatry

79) Sexual Dysfunction		80) Somatization
Cx- biological or psychological. Si/Sx- problems in sexual desire, arousal, orgasim, or pain with sexual intercourse. Dx- determine if it is **biological** and/or **psychological** factors. Morning erection r/o biological cause.	Tx **Psychotherapeutic** strategies for psychological factors. **Sildenafil** (Viagra) or **bupropion** for biological factors. **Vaginismus** treat with Kegel exercises and dilators.	Si/Sx- **multiple** somatic complaints for several years of **4+ pain symps:** **GI (2), neuro (1), sexual/reproductive (1), and general pain.** Dx- clinical, with no medical explanation. Tx- regular appointments.

81) Hypochondriasis	82) Body Dysmorphic	83) Conversion Disorder
Si/Sx- **FEAR of having SEROUS DISEASE** despite medical reassurance for **>6mos.** Assoc- **emotional stress.** Dx- clinical. Tx- schedule regular appointments. **Clinical PEARL: Somatoform Pain Disorder** Si/Sx- **PAIN symps,** no medical findings. Tx- physical and behavioral therapy.	Si/Sx- **imagined body defect** (that looks normal in reality) that leads to distress. Assoc-depression, ↑plastic surgery. Tx- SSRIs may benefit.	"la belle indifference" Si/Sx- **intense emotion situation or STRESS** => that leads to deficit of motor or sensory; **blindness, paralysis,** in close relationship to the stressor (with no medical findings). Tx- resolves spontaneously.

Psychiatry

84) Factitious Vs Malingering	85) Sexual and Physical Abuse	
• **Factitious** (munchausen's syndrome): Fabricate symptoms **"sick role"** (primary gain) • **Malingering: M**oney (secondary gain) financial, housing, or narcotics.	Si/Sx- **unexplained injuries** with delayed medical treatment. Pts may have frequent ER visits, avoid eye contact, and may appear afraid. Assoc- low SES, substance abusers, marital discord, pregnancy. Dx- clinical In children- look for genital or anal trauma, and check for STDs.	Tx- **assessment of pts safety.** Provide medical care, counseling, support services, and **DOCUMENTATION!** **Clinical PEARL: Vaginismus** (involuntary muscle contraction of outer third of vagina). Cx- sexual trauma, emotional abuse, psychosexual conflicts.
86) Suicidality Risks	**87) Suicidality**	
SAD PERSONS: **S- Sex** (male) **A- Age** (older) **D- Depression** **P- Previous attempt** (greatest risk factor) **E- Ethanol**/substance **R- Rational** lacking **S- Sickness** (chronic) **O- Organized** plan **N- No** spouse **S- Social** support lacking	Si/Sx- depressed mood with hx +/- ethanol and/or substance abuse. Pt may have **recent stressor,** FH of suicide, and possibly **adm to a psychiatric institution.**	Dx- **psychiatric evaluation, FH, previous attempts** (greatest risk factor), hopelessness. Ask if pt has **any suicidal ideations,** or plan. Tx- emergent inpatient **hospitalization** against their will if endorses suicidality.

17 CHAPTER
PULMONARY

Pulmonary		
1) COPD		
Chronic Obstructive Pulmonary Disease (COPD); **bronchitis** or **emphysema** => ↓lung function and airway obstruction. Cx- chronic bronchitis, emphaysema. Si/Sx- dyspnea (SOB), cyanosis, cough, tachypnea. **New clubbing** in pt with COPD often indicates **lung cancer**.	Dx- CXR shows hyperinflated lungs, flat diaphragm, **"Bullae-Blebs."** ↓**FEV1/FVC** (diagnostic), ↑TLC, ↓**DLco** in emphysema (normal DLco in asthma). ABGs shows hypoxemia with **resp acidosis (↑Pco2).** ↓**Mortality**- home O2, smoking cessation (tx bupropion).	Comp • Try to avoid giving COPD pts high conc O_2 may **suppress resp drive.** • **Sedatives** should also be avoided because they can exacerbate hypoventilation. • **Carbon dioxide retention** can cause confusion, somnolence, seizures, coma. Tx- **NIPPV** is an excellent option for pts with COPD **exacerbation.**
2) COPD	**3) Chronic Bronchitis**	
Tx- **COPD:** **C- Corticosteroids** **O- Oxygen** **P- Prevention stop smoking** (tx bupropion), pneumococcal (1dose) and **influenza** (yrly) vaccines. **D- Dilators** beta-agonist; **albuterol**, anticholinergics; ipra**tropium**, tio**tropium.**	Cx- SMOKING. Si/Sx **COUGH >3 months for more than 2 years.** Cyanosis, mild dyspnea, **BARREL chest,** ↓breath sounds, use of accessory chest muscles, JVD, hypercarbia, hypoxia.	Dx- **CXR** shows hyperinflated lungs, **FLAT** diaphragm. ↓**FEV1/FVC,** ↑TLC. ABG- hypoxemia with resp acidosis (↑Pco2) Tx- corticosteroids, oxygen, prevention, dilators (albuterol, ipra**tropium,** tio**tropium**).

Pulmonary

4) Emphysema		
Si/Sx- dyspnea (SOB), **PURSED lips,** ↓breath sounds, hypercarbia, hypoxia, **THIN appearance.** Cx • **Smoking** (Centrilobular) • **Alpha-1 antitrypsin deficiency;** accumulation of alpha-1 antitrypsin in hepatocytes. Histology granules stain with **PAS** (periodic acid-Schiff).	Dx- CXR hyperinflated lungs, **Bullae-Blebs** (pathognomonic for emphysema), **↓FEV1/FVC,** ↑TLC, **↓DLco.** ABG- hypoxemia with resp acidosis (↑Pco2).	Tx- corticosteroids, oxygen, prevention, dilators (albuterol, ipra**tropium,** tio**tropium**) **Improve survival of COPD-** smoking cessation, and supplemental O2.

5) Asthma		
REVERSIBLE airway obstruction from bronchial **inflam, hyperreactivity, MUCOUS plugging,** and smooth muscle **hypertrophy.** Si/Sx- cough, accessory muscles use, ↑**expiratory duration,** episodic **WHEEZING,** worse at night and in the morning, and possible **pulsus paradoxus** (systolic ↓BP >10 on inspiration).	Dx- CXR shows hyperinflation. R/O GERD (asthma-like symps of wheezing with **new hoarseness in the morning**). **Clinical PEARL: Pulsus Paradoxus** (systolic ↓**BP >10 on inspiration**) Cx- severe asthma, cardiac tamponade, tension pneumothorax.	Dx • **ABGs-**mild hypoxia (↓O2) and **resp alkalosis.** • Spirometry/PFTs **↓FEV1/FVC,** ↑RV, ↑TLC, **normal Pco2.** • **Methacholine challenge** (use when PFT are normal and still want to r/o asthma).

Pulmonary

6) Asthma	7) Types of Asthma	
Tx-**ASTHMA** **A- Albuterol** **S- Steroid** inhaled or oral **T- Theophylline** (rare) **H- Humidified O₂** **M- Magnesium** (for severe exacerbations) **A- Anticholinergics** **Intubation** if PCO2>50, or PO2<50. Also, normalization of ABG is an **ominous sign** of impending resp failure.	• **Mild intermittent:** less than <2 days/wk, less than <2 nights/mos Tx- PRN **albuterol** • **Mild persistent:** more than >2/wk, more than >2 night/mos Tx- albuterol + LOW **inhaled corticosteroids** **(flunisolide).**	• **Moderate persistent:** DAILY, >1night/wk. Tx- albuterol, low inhaled corticosteroids, and **salmeterol.** • **Severe persistent:** frequent Tx- albuterol, salmeterol, and **HIGH inhaled** **corticosteroids** or PO corticosteroids.

8) Asthma Medications		
• **Albuterol** (beta 2-agonists) **short** acting, relax bronchial smooth muscle. AE- hypokalemia (drive potassium into cells), muscle weakness, arrhythmias, abn EKG. • **Salmeterol** (beta 2-agonists) **long** acting prophylaxis. • **Beclomethasone,** **prednisone** Inhibits the synthesis of cytokines. **Inhaled** **corticosteroids** 1st-line for long-term control.	• **Ipratropium** (muscarinic antagonists) Blocks muscarinic receptors, preventing bronchoconstriction. • **Theophylline** Bronchodilation. AE- neuro**toxicity** and cardio**toxicity**, SVT, tremor, hypotension, seizures, abd pain. Has a **narrow** **therapeutic index**.	• **Cromolyn** Prevent release of **mast cells**. Tx- **asthma** **prophylaxis,** not for acute attacks. Used for **EXERCISE induced** asthma bronchospasms. • **Antileukotrienes** (monte**lukast,** zafir**lukast, zileuton**) Blocks leukotrienes. **Clinical PEARL:** **Inhaled** **Corticosteroids** AE: oropharyngeal **THRUSH** (oral candidiasis).

Pulmonary

9) Bronchiectasis		10) Restrictive Lung Disease
Infx and inflam in the bronchi and bronchioles => leading to **permanent FIBROSIS** and **dilation** of the bronchi. Si/Sx- chronic cough, rales, wheeze, rhonchi, **frequent yellow/green sputum,** mucus, **hemoptysis**, with hx of **↑ pulm infxs.**	Dx- CXR **tram lines,** honeycombing. **CT scan** will show **DILATED airway.** Spirometry shows **↓ FEV1/FVC.** Tx- abxs, inhale corticosteroids. If severe lobectomy or lung transplant.	Loss of compliance => ↑ stiffness, ↓ expansion Si/Sx- dyspnea, cyanosis. Dx- ↓ TLC, ↓ FVC, **Normal FEV1/FVC.** Tx- supportive, avoid causative agents, corticosteroids, anti-inflam agents.
11) Interstitial Lung Disease		
Inflam and fibrosis of interalveolar septum. Cx- pneumoconiosis, vascular disease, granulomatous disease, idiopathic interstitial pneumonia, drugs.	Drugs; **Busulfan, bleomycin, nitrofurantoin, amiodarone (foamy changes** in lamellar inclusions), **radiation.** Si/Sx- nonproductive cough, **"velcro-like crackles,"** dyspnea on exercision, cyanosis.	Dx- CXR may show **ground-glass pattern** with a **"honeycomb"** pattern. **Normal FEV1/FVC, ↓ TLC, ↓ FVC, ↓ DLco.** Tx- supportive, **corticosteroids**.

Pulmonary

12) Sarcoidosis

Multisystem disease of unknown etiology. Assoc- african american (AA), females, **erythema nodosum,** violaceous skin plaques.	Si/Sx- fever, malaise, dyspnea, cough, **erythema nodosum, arthritis, uveitis,** and **lymphadenopathy.** Dx- Labs; ↑**ACE, hypercalcemia.**	Dx- CXR shows **HILAR adenopathy** and diffuse interstitial infiltrates. Lymph node biopsy or lung biopsy; **NON-CASEATING granulomas.** Tx- **systemic corticosteroids**.

13) Hypersensitivity Pneumonitis

Risk factor: environmental exposure. Assoc- **farmers,** malt workers, **bagassosis,** air conditioners. Cx • **Farmer's Actinomycete** spores from MOLDY HAY. • **Bagassosis Actinomycete** spores from SUGARCANE	Cx • **Malt workers Aspergillus** clavatus in GRAIN. • **Air-conditioner lung Actinomycete** spores from air conditioner. • **Bird fanciers** Antigens from bird droppings, feathers.	Si/Sx- cough, dyspnea **several hours after exposure.** Dx- CXR may be normal or have nodular infiltates. Chronic cases show fibrosis in upper lobes. Tx- **avoid exposure,** corticosteroids.

14) Pneumoconiosis

• **Asbestosis** Cx- insulation, brake lining, construction, shipbuilding, plumber. Dx- CXR shows **calcified "Pleural plaque."** ↑Risk- **bronchogenic cancer,** mesothelioma (rare).	• **Coal Miners** Cx- coal mines. Dx- nodular opacities (<2cm) **upper lung.** Assoc- **TB** • **Berylliosis** Cx- high-tech, dyes, electronics, ceramics, **dental material**. Dx- **hilar adenopathy**. Tx- corticosteroids.	• **Silicosis** Cx-**silica,** glass, pottery Dx- nodular opacities (<2cm) **upper lung, "EGGSHELL"** calcifications. ↑Risk TB. Tx- avoid triggers, supportive therapy, supplemental O_2.

Pulmonary

15) Idiopathic Pulmonary Fibrosis		16) Hypoxemia
Si/Sx- non-productive cough with **exertional dyspnea**, and inspiratory crackles. Dx- CT shows **honeycombing** and patchy opacities. PFTs show **restrictive pattern**. Biopsy to confirm diagnosis.	Tx- **corticosteroids,** cyclophosphamide, or azathioprine. If severe lung transplant. **Cyclophosphamide** AE: hemorrhagic cystitis, bladder carcinoma. **Glucocorticoids** AE- **neutrophilia,** ↓eosinophils, ↓lymph.	↓Partial pressure of O_2 in blood. Cx- **V/Q mismatch,** diffusion impairment, R-to-L shunt, ↑altitude (low inspired O2). Si/Sx- cyanosis, tachypnea, SOB.
17) Hypoxemia		
Dx- **pulse oximetry** shows ↓HbO2 saturation. **CXR** to r/o atelectasis, ARDS, PE, and pneumonia. **ABG**; ↑**A-a gradient** (V/Q mismatch or shunt). ↑**Paco2**=> • **Hypoventilation** • **A-a gradient**	↑**A-a gradient:** • If corrects with O2 => **V/Q mismatch** (asthma, COPD, interstital lung disease). • If **does not** correct => **SHUNT** (asthma, alveolar collapse, COPD).	Tx- If pt is on a ventilator ↑**O_2 by PEEP** 5-15cmH20. If PEEP is too high, there is risk of **tension pneumothorax;** SOB, hypotension, tachycardia, unilateral absence breath sounds. If pts are hypercapnic possibly increase the min ventilation.

Pulmonary

18) ARDS		
Acute Respiratory Distress Syndrome (ARDS); endothelial injury=> **refractory hypoxemia**, pulmonary edema and ↓lung compliance. Cx- pneumonia, trauma, sepsis, aspiration. Si/Sx- dyspnea, cyanosis, tachypnea, labored breathing, rales +/- fever.	• **Phase I** (acute) **Respiratory alkalosis**. • **Phase II** (6–48hr) Hypocapnia, hyperventilation, **wide A-a gradient.** • **Phase III Acute resp failure**, dyspnea, rale, diffuse infiltrate CXR. • **Phase IV Severe hypoxemia**, respiratory and metabolic acidosis.	Dx- **CXR** shows bilateral pulm infiltrates. Capillary wedge pressure <18 mmHg (r/o cardiac). **PaO2/FiO2 <200mmHg** (classic for ARDS) Dx- **ARDS** **A- Acute** onset **R- Ratio PaO2/FiO2< 200 D- Diffuse** infiltrates **S- Swan-Ganz** wedge pressure < **18mmHg** (no cardiac origin)

19) ARDS	20) Pulmonary Hypertension	
Tx- underlying disease. **Use PEEP** (5-15) to recruit collapsed alveoli. Minimize injury from mech ventilation with **low tidal volume ventilation** (↓mortality). Goal **PaO2 >60** mmHg or **SaO2>90%** on **FiO2 <0.6 (<60%).** FiO2 should be kept at relatively non-toxic values <60%, if pO2 >60 than ↓PiO2.	Mean **pulmonary arterial pressure >25mmHg** (normal =15). Cx- COPD, PE, HF, CHD. Si/Sx- syncope, dyspnea on exertion, **JVD, split S2, S4,** parasternal heave.	Dx- **CXR** may show **large central pulmonary arteries**. ECG may show **RVH**, ECHO shows right ventricular overload. Tx- supplemental O_2, vasodilators, diuretics, anticoagulation.

Pulmonary

21) Pulmonary Thromboembolism		
Cx- **DVT** deep leg vein, above the knee (>90%). **VIRchow's triad:** **V- Vascular** trauma **I- ↑**coagulability **R- Reduce** flow, stasis Risk factors: **OCP,** prolonged immobility.	Si/Sx- hypoxia, **tachycardia, tachypnea.** Pt may also have hemoptysis, **↓ breath sounds, hypotension, JVD,** SOB, pleuritic chest pain upon **inspiration.** Dx • **CXR** normal, **hampton's hump,** or **westermark's sign.** May also show right ventricular dilation.	Dx • **ABG: resp alkalosis (↑pH, ↓pCO2, ↓pO2).** • **Right heart cath:** ↑right heart pressure, ↑pulm artery pressure, **normal PCWP.** • **ECG: tachycardia, S1Q3T3** (S wave lead I, Q & T wave in lead III) rare. May show sign of **RBBB.**
22) Pulmonary Thromboembolism		
Heparin should be immediately initiated in any pt with **high likelihood of PE and resp distress** before diagnostic test are done. **Clinical PEARL: Homocystinuria (AR) Cystathionine** synthase deficiency. Si/Sx- **thromboembolic** events, MR, **downward dislocation of lens** (ectopia lentis), **Marfan's** features (tall stature, long extremities, hyperlaxity of joints, arachnodactyly), **fair complexion, blue eyes** (phenylketonuria features).	Dx • **D- dimer** in low risk (r/o PE). • **U/S** lower extremity. • **Spiral CT scan** with IV contrast (most commonly used to confirm PE). • **V/Q scan** shows mismatch. • **Angiogram** (gold standard, rarely done).	**DVT prophylaxis:** All immobile pts give **SQ heparin,** with early ambulation. Tx- start **heparin** (LMWH SC) with **warfarin** (following **INR for goal of 2–3).** Stop heparin after 5-7days and continue warfarin for 3-6mos. Use **IVC filter** if anticoagulation is contraindicated. In severe cases, if pt is **unstable use thrombolysis** (massive PE, hypotension).

Pulmonary

23) Lung Nodules		24) Lung Cancer
Cx • Recent immigrant- **TB** • Southwest (California) **Coccidioidomycosis** • Ohio- **histoplasmosis** • Smoking- **lung CA** Si/Sx- asymp, chronic cough, dyspnea. More benign if <35yo, **<2cm nodule,** smooth margins, no change in size.	↑**Risk-** smoker, hx of malignancy, >45yo, **>2cm nodule,** irregular margins. Dx- **view old CXR** if possible, **serial CXR,** chest CT (to determine extent of disease). Tx- low risk pts follow with CXR or CT every 3mos for 1yr. **High risk biopsy** via bronchoscopy (central), FNA (peripheral).	Si/Sx- cough, chest pain, hemoptysis, dyspnea, **weight loss,** smoking hx. Recurrent pneumonias in same anatomic location. • **Horner's syndrome** (sympathetic trunk): **miosis** (constrict pupil), **ptosis** (drooping eye), **anhidrosis** (no sweat).
25) Lung Cancer	26) Lung Cancer Paraneoplastics	
• **Superior vena cava syndrome:** obstruction of SVC. Si/Sx- HA, dyspnea, edema of face and neck, **varices in mid-esophagus.** Tx- radiation therapy (palliative care). • **Pancoast syndrome** (brachial plexus) Si/Sx- shoulder pain radiating to arm causing pain, paresthesias, and weakness.	**Paraneoplastic Syndromes:** • **All lung cancers** Acanthosis nigricans (darker, thick, velvety skin in body folds), **dermatomyositis,** anemia, DIC, eosinophilia, thrombocytosis.	• **SCLC** **ACTH** (polypeptide hormone), **SIADH,** peripheral neuropathy, **Lambert-Eaton syndrome.** • **Squamous cell lung cancer** ↑**PTHrP** (parathyroid hormone related protein), **Hypercalcemia.**

Pulmonary

27) Lung Cancer

	Dx	Tx
Dx- **CXR** shows solitary pulmonary **nodule** then order: **Chest CT** Evaluate chest CT to see if nodule has benign features or is suspicious for malignancy. • If CT of nodule looks **BENIGN**=> **serial CT** for two years.	• If CT of nodule is suspicious for **malignancy**=> **biopsy**; **bronchoscopy** (central), **FNA** (peripheral). May also order a PET scan (r/o mets). **Thoracoscopic biopsy** can be done with conversion if malignant to **thoracotomy**. Lung metastasis: **bone, adrenals, brain.**	**SCLC: unresectable,** radiation and chemotherapy; **cisplatin,** etoposide, docetaxel or carboplatin with paclitaxel. **Cisplatin** AE: nephrotoxicity, tinnitus, hearing loss, electrolyte abn, neurotoxicity, nausea and vomiting. **NSCLC: surgical resection.**

28) Small Cell Lung Cancer	29) NON-Small Cell Lung Cancer	
Cx- smoking Dx- **bronchoscopy with biopsy** (centrally located lung nodule). Paraneoplastic syndrome: **SIADH, Cushing/ ACTH, Eaton-Lambert,** peripheral neuropathy, subacute cerebellar degeneration, metastases often. **S**quamous and **S**mall cell are from **S**moking and are **CENTRAL.**	• **Adenocarcinoma** Include; **bronchoalveolar** (not assoc with smoking). Assoc- **NON-smokers** Dx- peripheral location. • **Large cell** (neuroendocrine CA) least common, with poor prognosis.	• **Squamous cell carcinoma** Cx- smoking Dx- ↑**PTHrP** (parathyroid hormone related protein), **hypercalcemia,** central location.

Pulmonary

30) Pneumothorax		
Air collection in pleural space. • **Primary spontaneous pneumothorax** Cx- rupture of **BLEBS,** in **tall, thin young males.**	• **Secondary pneumothorax** Cx- **trauma,** COPD (dilated alveolar blebs), TB, **thoracentesis,** subclavian line placement (CXR to confirm proper placement of central line), PCP, pneumonia, positive-pressure ventilation.	Si/Sx- sudden onset of pleuritis pain, **sudden SOB,** ↓breath sounds, absent fremitus, and hyperresonance. Triad: **hypotension,** ↑**JVD, tracheal deviation** (think tension pneumothorax).

31) Pneumothorax		
• **Tension pneumothorax** Trauma => **air into pleural space** during inspiration and trapped during expiration. Tx- **needle thoracostomy.**	Dx- CXR shows **collapsed lung with retraction from chest wall** (seen on end-expiratory films).	Tx- supplemental O_2, **CHEST TUBE placement.** Tension pneumothorax **immediate needle** decompression with **needle thoracostomy** at 2nd intercostal space in midclavicular line.

Pulmonary

32) Pleural Effusion		
Accumulation of **fluid in pleural space.** Si/Sx- dyspnea, pleuritic chest pain, dullness to percussion, and ↓breath sounds.	• **TRANSUDATE** Cx- **cirrhosis, CHF,** nephrotic. Dx-↑**PCWP** or ↓oncotic pressure.	• **EXUDATE** Cx- pneumonia, **malignancy, PE,** pancreatitis, tuberculosis (↑lymphocytic leukocytosis). Dx-↑**pleural vascular permeability**.

33) Pleural Effusion		
Dx- CXR **costophrenic angle blunting. Thoracentesis for** new effusions **>1cm decubitus view.** **LIGHT's criteria** for **EXUDATE:** • pleural to serum **Protein >0.5** • pleural to serum **LDH >0.6** • **pleural fluid LDH >2/3** upper normal limit serum LDH.	Comp- thoracentesis has risk of causing a **hemothorax** (↓left ventricular preload). Tx- underlying condition, parapneumonic effusion and **empyema** require **chest tube drainage + abxs.**	↑**Risk** parapneumonic effusion complication with: • +**gram** stain/culture • **pH <7.2** and/or • **glucose <60** Tx- all parapneumonic effusions require chest tube drainage and abxs.

18 CHAPTER
RENAL

Renal

1) NephrITIS

Cx- postinfectious, IgA/berger's, Wegener's, Goodpasture's, Alport's. Si/Sx- oliguria, • **HTN** • **Edema** • **Proteinuria** **(<1.5g/day)** • **Hematuria** (cola urine) **Clinical PEARL:** **Dialysis and/or** **Renal Transplant** Most common cause of death is from **cardiovascular disease.**	Dx- U/A shows **hematuria, ↓GFR, ↑BUN and creatinine.** ANA, ANCA, anti-GBM antibody and complement should be measured, and possibly renal biopsy. Tx- salt and water restriction, diuretics. Possibly dialysis, **corticosteroids** to reduces inflammation.	**Clincal PEARL:** **Cyclosporine** (immunosuppressant) AE: **nephrotoxicity,** HTN, neurotoxicity, glucose intolerance, infxs, malignancy (SCC of skin), **GINGIVAL hypertrophy, hirsutism,** GI upset (anorexia, nausea, diarrhea)

2) IgA Nephropathy		3) Goodpasture's Syndrome
IgA Nephropathy (Berger's disease) is the most common nephrITIS disease. Si/Sx- **hematuria 1-2 DAYS post-URI viral infx,** or GI infxs. Assoc- **Henoch Schonlein Purpura** (IgA vasculitis; purple spots, joint pain, GI problems, glomerulonephritis).	Dx- **↑IgA** serum, normal C3, **IgA deposits in mesangium** on electron microscopy. Tx- **ACEIs (1st-line),** glucocorticoids.	Si/Sx- dyspnea, **pulmonary** hemoptysis, with **kidney** involvement. Dx- **LINEAR anti-GBM** deposits on immunofluorescence. CXR shows pulmonary infiltrates. Tx- **plasma exchange,** steroid. If severe **emergency PLASMAPHERESIS** (in order to minimize the extent of the kidney damage).

Renal

4) Wegener's Granulomatosis

Granulomatosis with polyangiitis (Wegener's) Si/Sx- **respiratory, sinus, and kidney** involvement, **hemoptysis.** Pt may also have **cutaneous lesions** (tender nodules, palpable purpura, ulcerations).	Dx- U/A shows **proteinuria** and hematuria. **+C-ANCA** due to antibodies against **proteinase- 3, ↑CRP.** Granulomatous inflammation on biopsy of upper airway lesions. Renal biopsy show **immunoglobulin deposits** on immuno-fluorescence.	Tx- comb of cyclophosphamide and **corticosteroids.** **Clinical PEARL: Churg-Strauss** (Wegener's like) Si/Sx- **ASTHMA, eosinophilia.** Dx- biopsy shows granulomas + eosinophila.

5) Alport's syndrome (X-linked) & 6) Postinfectious Glomerulonephritis

5) Alport's syndrome (X-linked)	6) Postinfectious Glomerulonephritis	
Si/Sx- Can't HEAR, can't SEE, can't PEE. triad: • **Deafness** • **Eye disorder;** lenticonus (bulging of lens capsule) • **Hematuria** Dx- **skin biopsy** shows monoclonal antibodies against **alpha-5 of type IV collagen.** Renal biopsy shows **GBM "SPLITTING"** on electron microscopy. Tx- progress to renal failure, transplant.	Cx- **Group A beta Strep (GAS).** Si/Sx **2–3 WEEKS post-URI** streptococcal infection, edema, oliguria, HTN, hematuria, **"cola-colored urine."** Dx ↓C3 in SERUM, ↑ASO titer.	Dx Immunofluorescence (IF) shows granular **C3 deposition,** diffuse pattern of glomerular infiltrations. Electron microscopy (EM) shows subepithelial hump; **"LUMPY- BUMPY."** Tx- **supportive,** most are **self-limiting.**

Renal

7) NephrOTIC

Cx- NSAIDs, IV drugs, HIV, obesity, tumor, DM, amyloidosis, HCV, SLE, lupus, bacterial endocarditis. Si/Sx- foamy urine • **Proteinuria (>3.5g/day)** • **Hypoalbuminemia** • **Hyperlipidemia** • **Edema**	Comp- **renal vein thrombosis** (most common complication), hypercoagulability, accelerated atherosclerosis. Dx- U/A shows **proteinuria >3.5g/day.** ↓Albumin <3g/dL, hyperlipidemia. Renal biopsy (definitive diagnosis).	Tx- protein and salt restriction, **ACEIs,** antihyperlipidemics. Prevention: **Pneumococcus vaccine** in high-risk pts for strep pneumoniae.

8) Membranous Nephropathy

Most common nephrOTIC in **ADULTS.** Assco- **Hepatitis B infection (HBV),** malaria, syphilis.	Si/Sx- hyperlipidemia, foamy urine, edema. Comp- **renal vein thrombosis.** Dx- U/A shows proteinuria (>3.5g/day). Labs show ↓albumin.	Dx- IM shows glomeruli enlarged, thick capillary walls, and BM. **IgG and C3** deposits on **GBM** giving a appearance of **SPIKE-and-DOME.** Tx- **prednisone.**

Renal

9) Focal Segmental Glomerulosclerosis	10) Renal Amyloidosis	
Assoc- **African Americans (AA)**, IV drugs/**Heroin, HIV/AIDS**, obesity, HTN. Si/Sx- hyperlipidemia, foamy urine, edema. Dx- U/A shows proteinuria (>3.5g/day), hematuria. Labs show ↓albumin. Biopsy shows **sclerosis capillary tufts.** Tx- **prednisone,** ACEIs/ARBs.	Assoc- **Multiple myeloma, rheumatoid arthritis (RA)**, TB. Si/Sx- hyperlipidemia, foamy urine, edema. Dx- U/A shows proteinuria (>3.5g/day). Labs show ↓albumin. AXR shows **enlarged kidneys, hepato-splenomegaly.**	Dx Electron microscopy (EM) shows **APPLE-GREEN** birefringence under **polarized light** with **CONGO-RED stain.** Tx- **prednisone** and melphalan. If severe pt may need BMT.
11) Membrano-Proliferative		
Persistent activation of **alternative complement pathway** (IgG antibodies against C3 convertase). Assoc- **SLE, HCV, Cryoglobulinemia,** subacute bacterial endocarditis. Si/Sx- hyperlipidemia, foamy urine, edema.	Dx- **↓C3 in serum,** U/A shows proteinuria (>3.5g/day). Labs show ↓albumin. IF microscopy is **positive for C3**. Biopsy shows dense deposits of **"TRAM-TRACK"** (double layer GBM). Tx- **corticosteroids.**	**Clinical PEARL: Mixed Essential Cryoglobulinemia** Si/Sx- **palpable purpura, proteinuria,** and **hematuria.** Assoc-**HCV**. Dx-↓**complement** in serum, **circulating cryoglobulins** (confirm), RBC casts. Also test for HCV.

Renal

12) Minimal Change Disease (MCD)		13) Lupus Nephritis
Most common nephrOTIC syndrome in **CHILDREN.** Assoc- **Hodgkin's Lymphoma,** NSAIDs. Si/Sx- **POST-VIRAL illness=>** leading to edema, proteinuria hypoalbuminemia, and hyperlipidemia.	Dx- normal C3 and C4 levels and **NORMAL appearance** on light microscopy and immunofluorescence. **Electron microscopy (EM)** will show "FUSION of FOOT" processes of **podocytes.** Tx- **corticosteroids (1st line),** good prognosis.	Cx- **SLE** Si/Sx- can show both nephrOTIC and nephrITIC; edema, proteinuria, hyperlipidemia. Dx- U/A shows proteinuria and RBC. Histology shows **mesangial proliferation; immune complex deposition.** Tx- **prednisone**
14) Diabetis Nephropathy		
Glomerular **hyperfiltration** => intraglomerular HTN => thickening of GBM. Cx- **microangiopathy** from poorly controlled DM. Assoc-**DM neuropathy** (charcot's joint; neurogenic arthropathy) and **retinopathy.**	**2 FORMS:** • **Diffuse** hyalinization. • **Nodular** glomerulosclerosis "Kimmelstiel Wilson lesions." Dx- thickened GBM; ↑mesangial matrix. Biopsy shows **Kimmelstiel-Wilson lesions** (classic).	Tx- **tight blood sugar control, ACEIs/ARBs.** **Clinical PEARL: ACEIs** Risk of **angioedema,** switch to **candesartan (ARB).** ARBs; losartan and valsartan also cause angioedema.
15) Renal Casts		
• **Hyaline casts** Cx- dehydration, volume depletion, PRE-Renal (↓perfusion). • **RBC casts** Cx- **NephrITIC** syndrome. • **Broad, WAXY casts** Cx-Chronic renal failure	• **WBC's, Eosinophis** Cx- allergic, atheroembolic. • **"Muddy-Brown Casts"** Cx- **Acute Tubular Necrosis** (ATN)	• **WBC's, WBC Casts** Cx- **Pyelonephritis,** POST-Renal, **analgesic nephropathy;** papillary necrosis, tubulointerstitial nephrtis (painless hematuria).

Renal

16) Acidosis pH<7.4		
Respiratory ACIDOSIS (↓ **pH,** ↑PCO2) **pH<7.4**, PCO2 >40 Cx- **hypo**ventilation; lung disease, **opioids, narcotics,** sedatives, weak respiratory muscles. Compensatory effort to ↑pH => kidney will ↑bicarbonate and ↓Cl. Tx- correct underlying disease, **fluid hydration,** if severe administer **bicarbonate.**	**When determining acid/base abn:** 1st look at **pH** to determine if it is **acidosis or alkalosis.** Next look at **PCO2**; if pH and PCO2 are **both up or both down** it is **METABOLIC.** If pH and PCO2 are opposite it is **respiratory.**	**Metabolic ACIDOSIS** (↓ **pH,** ↓PCO2) **pH<7.4**, PCO2<40 Cx • **Normal anion gap** Diarrhea, RTA, hyperchloremia, aldosterone deficiency, addison disease. • ↑**Anion gap** Lactic acidosis, **DKA** diabetic ketoacidosis (DM), renal failure, aspirin (salicylate) intoxication.

17) Acidosis pH<7.4	18) Aspirin Intoxication	
Winter's formula Used to calculate expected PCO2 during respiratory compensation for primary metabolic acidosis. PCO2 in labs should match: **PaCO2= 1.5 (HCO3-) + 8.** If it matches it is complete respiratory compensation.	Si/Sx- fever, **tinnitus** and tachypnea. Dx- mixed **respiratory alkalosis** and anion gap **metabolic acidosis.** Ex- pH 7.36, PaCO2 22, HCO3 12. What is acid-base abn?	Answer: **pH <7.4** mean acidosis. **PCO2<40** meaning respiratory alkalosis. **Low HCO3** mean metabolic acidosis. It is both; **resp alkalosis** and **metabolic acidosis.**

Renal

19) Alkalosis pH>7.4

Respiratory **ALKALOSIS** ($\uparrow$ pH, $\downarrow$PCO2) pH>7.4, PCO2<40 Cx- atelectasis, hyperventilation, aspirin intoxication.	Metabolic **ALKALOSIS** ($\uparrow$ pH, $\uparrow$PCO2) pH>7.4, PCO2>40 Cx- vomiting, diuretics, hyperaldosteronism, antacids.	**Clinical PEARL: Metabolic Alkalosis** from vomiting. Tx- IV normal saline (IV 0.9% NaCl) and potassium (K+).

20) Acute Renal Failure (ARF)

Abrupt $\downarrow$ renal function. Si/Sx- **uremia, oliguria,** fatigue, confusion, pericardial rub, asterixis (flapping tremor), HTN.	Dx- check electrolytes, U/A for RBCs, WBCs, Casts, and eosinophils. U/S r/o obstruction. **Pre-Renal: FeNa<1%, UNa<20,** urine specific gravity >1.020, **BUN/Cr >20.**	Tx- discontinue any offending meds, balance fluids and electrolytes. Dialyze if needed to prevent buildup of **K+.**

21) Acute Renal Failure (ARF)

• **PRE-Renal** ($\downarrow$perfusion) Cx-dehydration, loop diuretics ($\downarrow$K, metabolic alkalosis). Si/Sx- $\downarrow$**skin turgor,** thirst, **dry mucous membranes,** hypotension, tachycardia.	• **Intrinsic** (nepron unit) Assoc- **NSAIDs,** contrast media, or toxins. Si/Sx- **foamy urine (proteinuria)** and/or hematuria; tea-color urine.	• **POST-Renal** (obstruction) Cx- prostatic disease, nephrolithiasis, distended bladder. Si/Sx- flank pain.

Renal

22) RTA TYPE I (Distal)		
Distal RTA Type I; defect in **H+ secretion into urine**=> inability to acidify the urine to pH less than 5.3 (↑ **urine pH**). Inability to excrete H+ and reabsorb K+ => **acidemia** (↑H+ in body) and **hypokalemia** (↓K+ reabsorb).	Cx • **NEPHROLITHIASIS** • Hypercalciuria • **Cirrhosis** • Sjogren's • SLE • Sickle cell disease • Drugs (lithium amphotericin) Si/Sx- **acidosis,** weakness, myalgia, muscle cramps.	**Clinical PEARL: Screening labs for RTA** will show low bicarbonate, ↑Cl-, and normal anion gap metabolic acidosis. Dx- serum ↓K+, URINE ↑pH>5.3. Tx- **potassium citrate**.

23) RTA TYPE II (Proximal)		
Proximal RTA Type II; defect in **reabsorption HCO3-** in the proximal convoluted tubules (PCT) => **bicarbonate wasting** and acidemia.	Cx • **Multiple myeloma** • **Fanconi's syndrome** (phosphaturia=> osteomalacia or rickets due **phosphate wasting**) • Drugs, poisoning • Vit D deficiency • Amyloidosis Si/Sx- acidosis, weakness, myalgia, muscle cramps.	Dx- serum ↓K+ urine ↓pH<5.3. Tx- **potassium citrate**. **Clinical PEARL: Multiple Myeloma** Triad: **renal failure, hypercalcemia,** and **bone pain** in an elderly pt is multiple myeloma until proven otherwise.

24) RTA TYPE IV (Distal)		
Aldosterone deficiency => defect in Na/K exchange in distal convoluted tubules (DCT) => leading to ↓Na+, ↑H+, ↑Cl-, ↑K+. Si/Sx- metabolic acidosis (↓pH, ↓PCO2), weakness, myalgia, muscle cramps.	Cx • **Aldosterone** deficiency • **Diabetic nephropathy** (non-anion gap metabolic acidosis) • **Addison's** (adrenal) • Renal insufficiency • Sickle cell disease • Pseudo-hypoaldosteronism, • Drug; **ACEIs,** amiloride, **spironolactone,** heparin.	Dx- **SERUM ↑K+, ↑Cl, ↑H+, ↓Na, metabolic acidosis** (mild or normal anion gap), urine pH<5.3. Tx- **furosemide** (mineralocorticoid), NaHCO3. Comp- **hyperkalemia**.

Renal

25) Chronic Kidney Disease		
Cx- **DM, HTN,** PCKD, glomerulonephritis. Si/Sx- asymp, HTN, edema, anemia, nausea, vomiting, uremic pericarditis. Assoc- **acquired perforating dermatosis (Kyrle disease)**; pruritus, umbilicated papules with central keratotic crust that favor lower extremities.	Dx Fluid retention, **metabolic acidosis, azotemia** ($\uparrow$BUN/Cr), **hyperkalemia, anemia** ($\downarrow$erythropoietin). **NORMAL** PT, PTT, and platelet count, but **prolonged BT**.	Dx Normal platelet count, but with **platelet dysfunction**. Impaired Vit D production, $\uparrow$**PTH,** $\downarrow$**Ca,** $\uparrow$**Ph**.
26) Chronic Kidney Disease		**27) Urgent Dialysis Indications**
Tx- **fluid restriction, ACEIs/ARBs, erythropoietin** (when Hb<10g/dL), **calcitriol** (1,25-OH Vit D), **oral Ph binders**. **Erythropoietin** AE: **HTN,** HA, flu-like symps. Also, remember when replacing **erythropoietin** make sure there is adequate **iron stores** for RBC production.	Tx **DDAVP** (recruit factor VIII from endothelial storage sites). Possible **hemodialysis** or renal transplantation (transplant is preferred due to better survival rates). **Clinical PEARL:** **CT scan with contrast** in pts with renal disease **NON-IONIC contrast agents** are assoc with lower incidence of contrast-induced nephropathy.	**AEIOU:** **A- Acidosis** **E- Electrolyte** abnormalities ($\uparrow$**K+**) **I- Ingestions**; salicylates, ethylene glycol, methanol, barbiturates, lithium, theophylline. **O- Overload** of fluids **U- Uremic** symptoms (nausea, bleeding, pruitus, myoclonus, pericarditis, encephalopathy).

Renal

28) ↑ Anion Gap Metabolic Acidosis		29) Thiazides Diuretics
Anion Gap = (Na+) - (Cl- + HCO3-) "MUDPILES" M- Methanol U- Uremia D- DKA P- Paraldehyde I- Intoxication L- Lactic acidosis E- Ethylene glycol S- Salicylates Normal Anion Gap (8–12)	Clinical PEARL: Ethylene Glycol poisoning (anti-freeze) Dx- U/A shows calcium oxalate crystals; rectangular, ENVELOPE-shaped crystals.	HCTZ, chlorothiazide Mech- inhibit Na+/Cl- in distal convoluted tubule (DCT). Tx- HTN, Gout, nephrolithiasis. AE- hypercalcemia, H2O loss, ↓Na+, ↓K+, ↑glucose, ↑LDL, ↑cholesterol, ↑triglycerides, ↑uric acid, metabolic alkalosis, sulfa allergy.
30) Loop Agents Diuretics	31) K+ Sparing Agents Diuretics	32) Carbonic Anhydrase Inhibitors
Furosemide, torsemide, ethacrynic acid, bumetanide Mech: inhibit Na+/K+/2Cl- ascending loop of Henle. Tx- HTN, hypercalcemia, hyperparathyroidism. "Loops LOSE Calcium" AE- hypocalcemia, ototoxicity (hearing loss, tinnitus), H2O loss, metabolic alkalosis, ↓K+, sulfa allergy (except ethacrynic acid).	Spironolactone, triamterene, amiloride Mech: collecting tubule • Aldosterone receptor antagonist (spironolactone). • Block Na+ channel (triamterene, amiloride) Tx- HTN, CHF, hypokalemia, hyperaldosteronism. AE- metabolic acidosis, hyperkalemia, gynecomastia (with spironolactone only).	Acetazolamide Mech- inhibit carbonic anhydrase=> block Na+/H+, ↑H+ reabsorption in proximal convoluted tubule (PCT). Tx- glaucoma, epilepsy, ↓cerebrospinal fluid in intracranial HTN, CHF. AE- metabolic acidosis, sulfa allergy.

Renal

33) Osmotic Agents Diuretic		34) Meds cause Hyperkalemia
Mannitol, Urea Mech-↑**tubular fluid osmolarity** (entire tubule) Tx- glaucoma, ↓intracranial pressure in head trauma. AE- **pulmonary edema** in CHF and **anuria** (no passage of urine).	**Clinical PEARL: Diuretic Abuse** Assoc- eating disorders Si/Sx- dehydration, weight loss, orthostatic hypotension. Dx- hypokalemia and hyponatremia. Serum ↓K+, ↓Na. Urine ↑K, ↑Na.	• **Beta-Blockers** • **ACEI/ARBs** • **K-sparing** • **Digitalis** • **Heparin** • **Cyclosporine** • **NSAIDs** • **Succinylcholine**
35) Nephrolithiasis		
Calcium oxalate most common renal stone (70-90%). Risk factors: ↓fluid intake, FH, **hyperparathyroidism,** gout, Type I RTA, meds; allopurinol, **loop diuretics,** chemotherapy. Si/Sx- acute severe, **colicky FLANK pain that radiates to testes or vulva**, with possibly nausea and vomiting.	Dx- **U/A** may show microscopic hematuria. **KUB** identifies **radiOpaque**, but can miss radioUcent. **Noncontrast Spiral CT of abd and pelvis** (gold standard), **U/S scan** is used to r/o obstruction and is also used in **pregnancy**.	Tx- **HYDRATION (fluid intake >2L/day) and analgesia** (1st-line). Stones that are <5mm can pass spontaneously. **ESWL** (Extracorporeal Shock-Wave Lithotripsy) if <3cm. **Dietary recommendations**: • ↓diet **protein, oxalate** • ↓**Na intake** • ↑**fluid intake** • ↑**dietary calcium**

Renal

36) Calcium Nephrolithiasis		37) Cystine Nephrolithiasis
Calcium oxalate (most common), **calcium phosphate**. Cx- hypercalciuria, **hyperparathyroidism,** idiopathic. Dx- KUB x-ray (kidneys, ureters, and bladder) shows **radiOpaque** kidney stones.	Tx- **hydration and analgesia** (1st-line). Recurrent hypercalciuric use **thiazide diuretic.** **Clinical PEARL: Familial Hypocalciuric Hypercalcemia (FHH)** Dx- ↑ **serum calcium,** ↓ **urine calcium,** normal PTH. (Primary hyperparathyroidism has both ↑Calcium in serum and urine).	Renal transport defect with **amino acids**: **COLA** Cystine, Ornithine Lysine, Arginine Si/Sx- recurrent kidney stones from childhood and +FH of stones. Dx- U/A shows **"HEXAGONAL"** crystals, KUB shows radiOpaque. Urinary **cyanide nitroprusside test** (↑ cystine levels, confirm). Tx- hydration, sodium restriction, **alkalinization of urine,** penicillamine.
38) Uric Acid Nephrolithiasis		**39) Struvite Nephrolithiasis**
URIC ACID kidney stones. Assoc- **gout,** xanthine oxidase deficiency, **chemotherapy** (↑ purine turnover). Dx- **U/A** shows ↑WBC, ↑RBC, **ACIDIC urine, NEEDLE-shaped crystals.** KUB shows no abnormalities because radio**lucent**.	Dx- **CT scan** or IV pyelography shows Radio**LUCENT stone** (transparent). Tx- hydration, oral **potassium bicarbonate or potassium citrate (1st-line)** soluble in alkaline urine of pH>6.5. Can also use allopurinol, **purine restriction** diet.	• **Struvite** (Mg-NH4-PO4) Cx- **Proteus** (urease-producing organisms), pseudomonas. Dx- **STAGHORN calculi,** radiOpaque, ↑ **pH ALKALINE urine** (same as RTA Type I). Tx- **hydration,** treat UTI, surgery for **staghorn stones.**

Renal

40) Hypernatremia (Na>145)		
Cx- usually from "WATER LOSS;" 6 D's • Dehydration • Diuresis • Diarrhea • Docs (iatrogenic) • Diabetes Insipidus • Disease (kidney, sickle cell)	Si/Sx- ↑thirst, oliguria (↓urine), weakness, doughy skin, AMS. Risk- orthostatic syncope. Dx- ↑BUN/Cr is useful indicator of dehydration. • Water loss- central or nephrogenic DI (large vol dilute urine).	Dx • Hypotonic fluid loss diarrhea, diuretics, DKA, ↓intake, burn, mannitol. •↑Na from ↑aldosterone. Tx- replace with oral water (IV 0.9% saline). Mild cases give D5W; gradually over 48–72hr (<0.5mEq/L/hr) to prevent cerebral EDEMA.
41) Hyponatremia (Na<135)		
Hypotonic Hyponatremia: • HyperVOLemic hyponatremia Cx- look for cause from "nephrOSIS, cirrhOSIS, or cardiOSIS." • EuVOLemic Cx- SIADH (most common) psychogenic polydipsia, renal failure. • HypoVOLemic Cx- diuretics (thiazides), DKA, bleeding, GI loss; diarrhea, vomiting (both can lead to ↑ADH to absorb more water).	Si/Sx- asymp, confusion, muscle cramps, lethargy, AMS. Dx- check serum and urine osmolality. Most are low serum osmolality <280mEq/L. Tx- normal saline (crystalloid; 0.9% NaCl) is best replacement of fluids.	Tx Use hypertonic (3%) saline if severe symptomatic pt, no more than 0.5 to 1mEqu/L/hr. Correct Na over >72hrs to prevent central pontine myelinolysis (risk of locked-in syndrome; can only move eyes, from rapid correction hyponatremia).

Renal

42) HyperVOLemic Hyponatremia	43) EuVOLemic Hyponatremia	44) HypoVOLemic Hyponatremia
"TOO much fluid" Cx- **cirrhosis, CHF,** nephritic syndrome, renal failure, secondary and tertiary adrenal insufficiency, hypothyroidism. Tx- **water restriction,** diuretics.	"**Normal** fluid volume" Cx- **SIADH, psychogenic polydipsia,** renal failure, drugs, oxytocin. Tx- **water restriction**. **Clinical PEARL: SIADH** Labs: ↓serum osmolality, ↑urine osmolality, **↑urine sodium (UNa>30)**	"**LOW** fluid volume" Cx- dehydration, diarrhea, vomiting, diuretics (esp **thiazides**), primary adrenal insufficiency bleeding, DKA. Tx- **normal saline** (IV **crystalloid; 0.9% NaCl**) to replace volume loss.
45) Hyperkalemia (K > 5)		
Cx • **↓Excretion:** Renal insufficiency, hypoaldosteronism, **Type IV RTA,** drugs; **spironolactone, ACEIs, NSAIDs.** • **Cellular Shifts:** Tissue injury (rhabdomyolysis), cell lysis, **acidosis,** exercise, drugs; **succinylcholine,** digitalis, arginine, beta-blockers, insulin deficiency. • **Spurious:** Hemolysis from **blood sample**.	Si/Sx- **weakness, paresthesias,** tingling, numbness, intestinal colic, areflexia. Dx- repeat blood draw, review medications. ECG; **tall, peaked T waves, wide QRS, sine waves** (risk of V-Fib, cardiac arrest).	Tx- "**C BIG K**" **C- Calcium gluconate** (**C**ardiac stabilization) **B- Bicarbonate** **B- Beta-2 agonist** (albuterol) **I- Insulin** **G- Glucose** (all shift K into cell) **K- Kayexalate** (remove K+ from body) Also, sodium polystyrene sulfonate, diuretics, and dialysis remove K+ from the body.

Renal		
46) Hypercalcemia (Ca>10.2)		
Cx- most common **Hyperparathyroidism**. **CHIMPANZES:** C- Calcium H- Hyperthyroidism I- Immobility M-Malignancy P- Paget's Disease A- Acromegaly N- Neoplasm Z- Zollinger-Ellison E- Excess Vit A, Vit D S- Sarcoidosis	Si/Sx • **Bones** (bone pain, fractures, osteopenia) • **Stones** (kidney stones) • **Abdominal groans** (constipation, intestinal colic) • **Psychiatric Overtones** (weakness, AMS)	Dx- **calcium** total/ionized, **PTH**, phosphate, PTHrP, Vit D, albumin, ECG may show **SHORT QT**. Tx-**hydration (0.9% saline infusion), furosemide, "Loops Lose Ca."** (Ca excretion), avoid thiazides. Pts with hypercalcemia due to malignancy should be given **bisphosphonates; zoledronic acid** (1st-line).
47) Hypocalcemia (Ca<8.2)		
Cx • **POST-SURGICAL thyroidectomy** (hypoparathyroidism; ↓PTH, ↓Ca, ↑Ph) • **Hypomagnesaemia** • **Malnutrition** • **Acute pancreatitis** • **Vit D deficiency** • **DiGeorge's** syndrome (**tetany** shortly after birth, **absence of thymic**) • **Post-surgery** (postop ↓calcium).	Si/Sx- **"PINS and NEEDLES"** sensation around mouth, feet, and hands. Pt also have **muscle cramps, TETANY, abdominal muscle cramps,** dyspnea, hyperactive deep tendon reflexes. • **Chvostek's sign** (facial spasm). • **Trousseau's sign** (carpal spasm, after placing BP cuff on arm causing arterial occlusion).	Dx- check Ca, PTH, Mg, and albumin levels. ECG may show a **prolonged QT.** Tx- Mg, **Calcium** supplements. **Clinical PEARL:** **↑pH (resp alkalosis)** =>↑Ca bound to albumin =>↓ionized calcium (active form) result in **hypocalcemia.**

Renal

48) Hypocalcemia (Ca<8.2)

Calcium correction for hypoalbuminemia: **Hypoalbuminemia** can have **low total plasma calcium,** but normal ionized Ca, so no symps.	For every $\downarrow$1g/dL **albumin** will $\downarrow$**calcium** 0.8mg/dL. **Corrected Ca= total Ca + 0.8 (4- albumin)**	Ex. pt appears to have hypocalcemia of Ca 8 and Albumin 2. **Corrected Ca= 8 + 0.8(4-2) = 9mg/dL** Serum Ca is 9, and is normal.

49) (Mg <1.5) Hypomagnesaemia

Cx- **alcoholics** (most common). • $\uparrow$**loss- diarrhea, vomiting,** diuretics, DKA, pancreatitis. • $\downarrow$**intake-** malnutrition, malabsorption.	Assoc- **hypocalcaemia, hypokalemia.** Si/Sx- GI upset, nausea, vomiting, muscle cramps, weakness. Dx- labs; $\downarrow$Mg, $\downarrow$Ca, and/or $\downarrow$K+ levels.	Dx- ECG **prolonged PR and QT** intervals. Tx- **Mg supplements.** Hypokalemia and hypocalcemia will not correct without normal Mg levels.

50) Polycystic Kidney Disease (PCKD)

Defect in epithelial cell differentiation => **cystic dilation** in renal tubules, as well as cysts in spleen, liver, and pancreas. • **ADPKD- AD**ults, $\uparrow$risk of **cerebral aneurysm.** • **ARPKD- child,** $\uparrow$risk liver fibrosis, portal **HTN.** Assoc- ADPKD1, ADPKD2.	Si/Sx- intermittent flank pain, **hematuria, HTN,** large **palpable** kidneys. Pts have recurrent **bilateral flank pain, UTI,** and nephrolithiasis. Pts may also have hepatic cysts and **cerebral BERRY aneurysms** (subarachnoid). Dx- **U/S scan (1st-line)** or CT scan shows multiple bilateral cysts.	Tx- manage UTIs and control BP with **ACEIs** to decrease rate of ESRD. **Clinical PEARL: Simple Renal Cysts** DX- **CT scan** shows **thin walls,** with no solid component, no enhancement. Tx- **reassurance,** almost always benign and do not require further evaluation.

Renal

51) Vesicoureteral Reflux (VUR)		
Retrograde of urine from bladder to ureters and kidney. • **Mild Reflux** (grade I–II) No ureteral or renal pelvic dilation. Tx- resolves spont. • **Moderate to Severe** (Grade III–V) Ureteral **dilation** and may have **caliceal blunting.** Si/Sx- **recurrent UTIs** in childhood.	Dx- **voiding cystourethrogram (VCUG)** to **detect abnormal** ureteral insertion sites and grade reflux. Tx- mild reflux give daily prophylactic **amoxicillin** if **<2mos old**, otherwise **nitrofurantoin or TMP-SMX** until resolves. Surgery for persistent high-grade (III-V) reflux.	**Clinical PEARL: Posterior Urethral Valves (PUV)** Si/Sx- distended palpable bladder and abnormally low urine or **anuria in first 24hrs of life,** in male neonate. Dx- **voiding cystourethrogram (VCUG).** Tx- catheter.
52) Hydronephrosis		**53) Hydrocele**
Dilation renal calyces from obstruction of urinary tract. Cx- **BPH, tumors, renal calculi, megaureter** (dilation of distal ureter without evidence of obstruction, M>F). Si/Sx- **asymp,** ↓urine, abd pain, **FLANK back pain**, UTIs.	Dx- ↑BUN/Cr. **U/S** or CT scan detect dilation of renal calyces and/or ureter. Tx- surgically correct, **sound wave lithotripsy** if calculi causing obstruction, or ureteral stent. **Foley or suprapubic catheter** for lower urinary tract obstruction.	Remnant of **processus vaginalis**. Si/Sx- asymp, **painless scrotal swelling.** Dx- **U/S scan** shows that the scrotum **transilluminates.** Tx- **none,** disappears spont by 12mos old. If hydrocele does not resolve, then remove to avoid risk of inguinal hernia.

Renal

54) V-Varicocele "V-Vormy"

Dilation **paminiform venous plexus, "Bag of WORMS."** Assoc- renal cell carcinoma. Si/Sx- asymp, vague aching scrotal pain, but mainly painless scrotal swelling.	Dx- **U/S DOES NOT Transilluminate** (more common to be on the **L>R**). **Abd CT** scan to r/o **renal cell carcinoma.**	Tx- varicocelectomy, ligation, or embolization. **Clinical PEARL:** **Renal Cell Carcinoma** Si/Sx- triad: • Flank pain • Hematuria • Palpable abdominal renal mass

55) Cryptorchidism

Failure of one or both **of testes to descend** into scrotum. Risk- **testicular malignancy.** Assoc: • **Infertility** • **Prematurity** • **Prader-Willi** • **Noonan syndrome** (hearing loss, low-set ears, MR, short stature, webbed neck).	Dx- **testes cannot be placed into scrotal sac** with gentle pressure. Tx- most spontaneously descend by 3mos. If testes do not descend **orchiopexy** by 6–12 mos. If found later **orchiectomy** to avoid risk of testicular cancer.	**Clinical PEARL:** **Prader-Willi** syndrome Deletion on **chrom 15.** Si/Sx- **obesity,** MR, hypogonadism, short stature, hypotonia, **almond-eyes, down-turned mouth,** small hands and feet.

56) Epididymitis

Infx of epididymis. Cx- **STDs; chlamydia, gonorrhea** in young. **E. Coli** in older men prostatitis. Can also be from reflux. Assoc- **>30yo.**	Si/Sx- painful scrotal swelling, tenderness, **POSITIVE Prehn's sign** (↓ **PAIN** with scrotal **elevation**).	Dx- U/A, culture for E. coli, gonorrhoeae, chlamydia. **U/S scan** shows ↑ blood **FLOW.** Tx- fluoroquinolones, tetracycline, NSAIDs.

Renal

57) Testicular Torsion		
Twisting of spermatic cord leading to ischemia. Si/Sx- nausea, vomiting, **LOSS cremasteric reflex.** Assoc- **<30yo.**	Si/Sx- intense, acute scrotal pain, **NEG Prehn's sign (PAIN continues with scrotal elevation).** Dx- U/S ↓ blood FLOW. If high suspicion proceed to surgery.	Tx- **attempt manual detorsion**. If attempt does not work immediate surgery to salvage testis (>6hrs ischemia). **Orchiopexy of both testes** to prevent future torsion.
58) Erectile Dysfunction		
Risk factors: **DM, HTN atherosclerosis**. Assoc: prostate cancer, meds; **beta-blockers, SSRIs, TCAs,** diuretics. Si/Sx **Nocturnal penile tumescence testing** for early morning erection. If pt **DOES NOT** have **early morning erection it is ORGANIC** (atherosclerosis, DM, HTN, meds).	Si/Sx If pt has early **morning erection** => it is **not a organic**. It is instead due to **nonorganic** cause like stress, relationship problems, and/or anxiety. Dx- check **testosterone**, gonadotropin, and prolactin levels. If ↑ **prolactin** can be from ↓ androgen activity. Tx **Psychotherapy** or sex therapy for nonorganic.	Tx Organic cause: • Silden**afil (Viagra),** tadal**afil (Cialis),** varden**afil (Levitra).** **C/I- sildenafil** with **nitrates** has risk of ↓BP and can lead to MI. • Possibly **penile prostheses** (vacuum device) if pts fail sildenafil therapy (phosphodiesterase type 5 inhibitor). • Hypogonadism tx with **testosterone.**

Renal

59) Benign Prostatic Hyperplasia (BPH)

Enlargement of prostate in **CENTRAL periurethral zone.**

Si/Sx- **weak stream,** bladder fullness, **hesitancy,** retention, UTIs, renal calculi, hydronephrosis.

Dx- **DRE;** uniform, rubbery, enlarged prostate. **U/A and UCx** to r/o infx and hematuria. **BUN/Cr** to r/o renal insufficiency. **Abd U/S** to r/o **urinary obstruction** or hydronephrosis.

Tx
• **Finasteride** (5-alpha reductase inhibitor) inhibits dihydrotestosterone.

• Terazo**sin** (alpha-blocker) relax smooth muscle of bladder neck and prostate.

Transurethral resection of prostate (TURP) for moderate to severe symp.

60) Prostate Cancer

Risk factors: advanced age, FH.

Si/Sx- asymp, **urinary retention, back pain** (bone mets).

Prevention- **men >50yo do annual DRE.**

Dx- DRE with **palpable nodules,** ↑**PSA** >4ng/mL **PSA screening** is also used in follow-up to screen for recurrence.

↑**PSA**- can be increased in prostatic CA, UTI, BPH, and prostatitis.

Dx
U/S guided transrectal biopsy (adenocarcinoma) with **GLEASON** histologic (for grading).

CXR and bone scan to look for mets that may show ↑bone density or osteoblastic activity.

Clinical PEARL: Acute Prostatitis Si/Sx- **urinary urgency,** dysuria, perineal pain and tenderness, **boggy prostate.** Dx- culture mid-stream urine sample. Tx-abx therapy.

Tx- **radical prostatectomy** and **radiation therapy.**

Tx- for metastatic disease give **GnRH agonist or flutamide and chemotherapy.**

Salvage therapy (when standard treatment fails) salvage radiation can help provide long-term control.

Bony metastases to the back can be treated with **radiation therapy** after orchiectomy has been done.

Renal

61) Testicular Cancer

Cx- **Germ cells** (95%). Assoc- 15–30yo. Risk factors: **Cryptorchidism,** Klinefelter's syndrome. Si/Sx- **PAINLESS, hard mass, large testes.** Dx- **testicular U/S** shows solid testicular mass=> **radical orchiectomy** (biopsy can be done after removal). CXR or CT of abd/pelvic to check for **mets.**	**Types:** • **Leydig cell tumors** ↑Testosterone, **↑ESTROGEN,** ↓LH, ↓FSH. • **Choriocarcinoma** ↑Beta-hCG • **Non-seminomatous** germ cell (yolk sac). ↑**AFP and** ↑**B-hCG**	Tx- **radical orchiectomy.** • **Seminomas** treat with chemotherapy and radiation. • **Nonseminomatous** germ cell tumors use platinum chemotherapy.

62) Renal Cell Carcinoma

Adenocarcinoma (90%) Risk factors: smoking, obesity, von Hippel-Lindau disease. **Clinical PEARL: von Hippel-Lindau** Si/Sx- cafe' au lait spots, pheochromocytoma, angiomatosis in retina with vision loss, hemangioblastomas (CNS tumors).	Si/Sx- **hematuria, flank pain, and palpable FLANK mass.** Pts may also have fever, anemia, and polycythemia (↑erythropoietin production). Dx- U/S and/or **CT shows renal mass** (complex cysts or solid tumor).	Tx- **surgical resection,** sorafenib, sunitinib (tyrosine kinase inhibitors) newer drug that ↓tumor angiogenesis and cell proliferation. Only 15-30% respond to radiation and chemotherapy.

Renal

63) Bladder Cancer

Transitional cell carcinoma (bladder mass).	Dx- **CYSTOSCOPY with biopsy** (gold standard, diagnostic).	Tx • **Carcinoma in situ** Tx-chemotherapy.
Risk- **SMOKING**, men, **cyclophosphamide, schistosomiasis,** aniline dyes.	**U/A** shows hematuria, **intravenous pyelogram (IVP)** to examine upper urinary tract**.**	• **Superficial CA** Tx- **transurethral resection** and chemotherapy.
Si/Sx- asymp, **gross hematuria,** urgency, dysuria.	MRI, CT, and bone scan to define invasion and mets.	• **Invasive without mets** Tx- **radical cystectomy** or radiotherapy (radiation therapy).
	There is **no screening** methods for bladder cancer.	• **Invasive cancer with distant metastases** Tx-chemotherapy alone.

19 CHAPTER
HISTORY AND PHYSICAL EXAM

History and Physical	
Identifying Data	Date_____Time_____Room_____ Name of informant (pt, relative)_____ Patient's name_____age____race____ sex M / F.
Chief Complaint	Reason seeking medical care and duration, symptoms_____
History Present Illness (HPI)	**SOCRATES** S- Sight____ O- Onset____C- Character (come/go) ____ R- Radiation____ A- Associated____ T- Timing____ E- Exacerbation____S- Severity (1–10)____ _____ _____ _____ _____ (Course of pt's illness: when it began, past illnesses, surgeries, and past diagnostic test)
Past Medical History (PMH)	O Surgeries_____ O Hospitalizations_____ O Medical problems: O Diabetes, O Hypertension, O Peptic Ulcer, O Asthma, O MI, O Cancer.
Medications	1._____ 2. _____ 3. _____ 4. _____ 5._____ 6. _____
Allergies	O NDKA
Family History	O Patient's disorder_____ _____ O Asthma, O CAD, O Heart Failure, O Cancer, O Tuberculosis, O Other
Social History	O Alcohol, O Smoking, O Drug usage_____ O Marital status_____ O Employment situation_____ O Level of education_____

History and Physical		
Review of Systems (ROS)	**General**	O Weight, O Appetite, O Fever, O Chills, O Fatigue, O Night sweats.
	Skin	O Rashes, O Skin discolorations.
	HEENT	O Headaches, O Dizziness, O Visual changes, O Tinnitus/Vertigo, O Hearing loss, O Nose bleeds, O Sinus diseases, O Throat pain.
	Resp	O Cough, O Shortness of breath, O Sputum (color).
	Cardio	O Chest pain, O Orthopnea, O Paroxysmal nocturnal dyspnea, O Dyspnea on exertion, O Edema, O Valvular disease.
	GI	O Dysphagia, O Abd pain, O Nausea, O Vomiting, O Hematemesis, O Diarrhea, O Constipation, O Melena, O Hematochezia.
	GU	O Dysuria, O Frequency, O Hesitancy, O Hematuria, O Discharge.
	Gyn	Gravida/para_____ O Abortions, Age of menarche_____ Last menstrual period_____ frequency_____ duration_____ O Menopause, O Dysmenorrhea, O Contraception, O Vaginal bleeding, O Vaginal discharge, O Breast masses.
	Endo	O Polyuria, O Polydipsia, O Skin or hair changes, O Heat intolerance.
	Ext	O Joint pain, O Swelling, O Arthritis, O Myalgias.
	Skin/ Lymph	O Easy bruising, O Lymphadenopathy.
	Neuro	O Weakness, O Seizures, O Memory changes, O Depression.

History and Physical		
Physical EXAM	General	O ill, O well, or O malnourished.
	Vital Signs	Temp_____, HR_____, Resp_____, BP_____, **O₂ Sat_____In_____ Outs_____** **Lines _____** (Foley, PICC line, Central line)
	Skin	O Rashes, O Scars, O Moles
	Lymph	O Cervical, O Supraclavicular, O Axillary, O Inguinal nodes Size_____, _____Tenderness.
	HEENT	O PERRLA, O EOMI, O Visual fields, O Funduscopy (papilledema, arteriovenous nicking, hemorrhages, exudates), O Scleral icterus, O Ptosis, O Tympanic membranes (dull, shiny, intact, bulging), O Mucus membrane moisture, O Oral lesions, O Dentition, O Pharynx, O Tonsils, O JVD at 45 degrees, O Thyromegaly, O Masses, O Bruits.
	Chest	O Equal expansion, O Normal breath sounds, O Rhonchi, O Crackles, O Rubs.
	Heart	O RRR, O S1, S2, O Gallops (S3, S4), O Murmurs (grade 1–6), O Pulses (0–2+).
	Abdomen	Contour (flat, scaphoid, obese, distended), O Scars, O Normal bowel sounds, O Bruits, O Tenderness, O Masses, O Hepatomegaly, O Splenomegaly, O Guarding, O Rebound, O Costovertebral angle tenderness (CVAT), O Suprapubic tenderness.

History and Physical		
Physical Exam	**Breast**	O Dimpling, O Tenderness, O Masses, O Nipple discharge, O Axillary masses.
	GU	O Inguinal masses, O Hernias, O Scrotum, O Vesticles, O Varicoceles.
	Pelvic	O Vaginal mucosa, O Cervical discharge, O Uterine size, O Masses, O Ovaries.
	Ext	O Joint swell, O Range motion, O Edema (1–4+), O Cyanosis, O Clubbing, O Pulses.
	Rectal	O Sphincter tone, O Masses, O Fissures, O Prostate (nodules, tenderness, size).
	Neuro	O AOX____, O Normal gait, O Strength (graded 0–5), O Touch sensation, O Pressure, O Pain, O Deep tendon reflexes (graded 0–4+), O Romberg test.
	CN Exam	O **I:** Smell. O **II:** Vision and visual fields. O **III, IV, VI:** Pupil light, EOMI, ptosis. O **V:** Facial sensation, open jaw against, corneal reflex. O **VII:** Close eyes, smile, show teeth. O **VIII:** Hears watch tic, Weber test, Rinne test. O **IX, X:** Palette midline "ah," speech. O **XI:** Shoulder shrug, turns head against resistance. O **XII:** Tongue in midline.

History and Physical		
Labs	Basic Chem	O **CBC**, O **BMP** (Basic metabolic panel), O **LFTs** (Liver function tests).
	Cardio	O ECG, O **Echo EF%**, O CKMB, O Trop I.
	Radiology	O **CXR**, O Abd/PelvXR, O **CT**, O MRI.
	Pulmonary	O **ABG**, O **O₂ Sat**, O Bronchoscopy.
	ID	O **AFB (Acid Fast Bacillus)**, O **BCx**, O **UCx**, O **WoundCx**, O **SputumCx**, O **LineCx**.
	Lines	O **Foley catheter**, O **PICC lines**, O **Central lines.**

Assessment	Patient is a _____year-old, _____(race), M / F
	_____
	_____
	_____
	(Discuss different diagnoses and give reasons to support working diagnosis and reasons for excluding other diagnoses.)

Plan
LAID:
O L-Labs
O A-Ambulation
O I-IV fluid
O D-Diet

Problem	Plan (including testing, laboratory studies, medications, and antibiotics)
1	
2	
3	
4	
5	
6	
7	
8	
9	
10	

20 CHAPTER
SOAP CHECKLIST

SOAP Checklist	
Date/ Time	Room_____ Patient's name_____ age_____ race_____sex M / F
OE (overnight event)	
S- Subjective (pain, urine, bowel movement, ambulation)	**PAIN: "SOCRATES"** **S**-Sight_____ **O**-Onset_____ **C**-Character (come/go) _____ **R**-Radiation_____ **A**-Associated_____ **T**-Timing_____ **E**-Exacerbation_____ **S**-Severity (1–10)_____**Urine**_____ **Bowel movement**_____**Ambulation**_____ **General:** O Fever, O Chills, O Fatigue, O Night sweats, O Headaches, O Cough, O SOB, O Chest pain, O Edema **GI:** O Dysphagia, O Abd pain, O Nausea, O Vomiting, O Hematemesis, O Diarrhea, O Constipation, O Melena (black stool), O Hematochezia (bright red-blood rectum). **GU:** O Dysuria, O Frequency, O Hesitancy, O Hematuria, O Discharge. **Ext:** O Joint pain, O Swelling, O Arthritis, O Myalgias.
O- Objective	General: O ill, O well, or O malnourished. Vital Signs: Temp_____, HR_____, Resp_____, BP_____. Skin: O Rashes, O Scars, O Moles. Lymph: O Cervical, O Supraclavicular, O Axillary, O Inguinal nodes Size_____, _____Tenderness.

SOAP Checklist		
O- Objective		
	HEENT	O PERRLA, O EOMI, O Visual fields. O Funduscopy (papilledema, arteriovenous nicking, hemorrhages, exudates), O Scleral icterus, O Ptosis, O Tympanic membranes (dull, shiny, intact, bulging), O Mucus membrane moisture, O Oral lesions, O Dentition, O Pharynx, O Tonsils, O JVD at a 45 degree, O Thyromegaly, O Masses, O Bruits, O Abdjugular reflux.
	Chest	O Equal expansion, O Normal breath sounds, O Rhonchi, O Crackles, O Rubs.
	Heart	O RRR, O S1, S2, O Gallops (S3, S4), O Murmurs (grade 1–6), O Pulses (0–2+).
	Abdomen	Contour (flat, scaphoid, obese, distended), O Scars, O Normal bowel sounds, O Bruits, O Tenderness, O Masses, O Hepatomegaly, O Splenomegaly, O Guarding, O Rebound, O Costovertebral angle tenderness (CVAT), O Suprapubic tenderness.
	Breast	O Dimpling, O Tenderness, O Masses, O Nipple discharge, O Axillary masses.
	GU	O Inguinal masses, O Hernias, O Scrotum, O Vesticles, O Varicoceles.

SOAP Checklist			
O- Objective	**Pelvic**	O Vaginal mucosa, O Cervical discharge, O Uterine size, O Masses, O Ovaries.	
	Ext	O Joint swell, O Range motion, O Edema (1-4+), O Cyanosis, O Clubbing, O Pulses	
	Rectal	O Sphincter tone, O Masses, O Fissures, O Prostate (nodules, tenderness, size).	
	Neuro	O AOX____, O Normal gait, O Strength (graded 0–5), O Touch sensation, O Pressure, O Pain, O Deep tendon reflexes (graded 0-4+), O Romberg test.	
	CN Exam	O **I:** Smell. O **II:** Vision, visual fields. O **III, IV, VI:** Pupil light, EOMI, ptosis. O **V:** Facial sensation, open jaw against, corneal reflex. O **VII:** Close eyes, smile, teeth. O **VIII:** Hears watch tic, Weber test, Rinne test. O **IX, X:** Palette midline "ah," speech. O **XI:** Shoulder shrug, turns head against resistance. O **XII:** Tongue in midline.	

SOAP Checklist

Labs	
A- Assessment	Patient is a ____ year-old, _____ (race), M / F _____ _____ (Discuss different diagnoses and give reasons to support working diagnosis, and reasons for excluding other diagnoses.)

P- Plan
LAID:
O L-Labs
O A-Ambulation
O I-IV fluid
O D-Diet

Problem	Plan (including testing, laboratory studies, medications, and antibiotics)
1	
2	
3	
4	

ABBREVIATIONS KEY

AA	Amyloid A Protein		ANC	Absolute Neutrophil Count
A-a	Alveolar-Arterial Gradient		APC	Activated Protein C
AAA	Abdominal Aortic Aneurysm		AR	Autosomal Recessive
			ARBs	Angiotensin II Receptor Blockers
Ab	Antibody		ARDS	Acute Respiratory Distress Syndrome
ABeta	Amyloid Beta			
ABG	Arterial Blood Gas		ARF	Acute Renal Failure
ABI	Ankle-Brachial Index		AROM	Artificial Rupture Of Membranes
Abd	Abdomen			
Abn	Abnormal		ARPKD	Autosomal Recessive Polycystic Kidney Disease
ACA	Anterior Cerebral Artery			
Ach	Acetylcholine		AS	Aortic Stenosis
Accel	Accelerations		ASD	Atrial Septal Defect
ACEI	Angiotensin Converting Enzyme Inhibitor		ASA	Aspirin
			Asymp	Asymptomatic
Accum	Accumulation		ATN	Acute Tubular Necrosis
ACTH	Adrenocorticotropic Hormone		AV Block	Atrioventricular Block
			AVN	Avascular Necrosis
ACTZ	Hydrochlorothiazide		AVNRT	Atrioventricular Nodal Reentry Tachycardia
AD	Autosomal Dominant			
ADH	Antidiuretic Hormone		AVRT	Atrioventricular Reciprocating Tachycardia
ADHD	Attention-Deficit Hyperactivity Disorder			
Adm	Administration		AXR	Abdominal X-Ray
ADPKD	Autosomal Dominant Polycystic Kidney Disease		AZT	Zidovudine
			BCR-ABL	BCR gene chrom 9 joins ABL gene chrom 22
AE	Adverse Effects		BCx	Blood Culture
AF	Atrial Fibrillation		Benzo	Benzodiazepines
AFI	Amniotic Fluid Index		hCG	Human Chorionic Gonadotropin
AFP	Alpha-Fetoprotein			
Ag	Antigen		BBP	Biophysical Profile
AGC	Atypical Glandular Cells		BP	Blood Pressure
AI	Adrenal Insufficiency		BPH	Benign Prostatic Hyperplasia
AIDS	Acquired Immune Deficiency Syndrome		BPPV	Benign Paroxysmal Positional Vertigo
AlkPh	Alkaline Phosphatase			
AL	Amyloid Light Chain		BM	Bone Marrow
ALL	Acute Lymphoblastic Leukemia		BMD	Bone Mineral Density
			BMT	Bone Marrow Transplantation
ALS	Amyotrophic Lateral Sclerosis/ Lou Gehrig's Disease		BPH	Benign Prostatic Hyperplasia
AMD	Age-Macular Degeneration		Brady	Bradycardia
			BSA	Body Surface Area
AML	Acute Myeloid Leukemia		BUN	Blood Urea Nitrogen
AMS	Altered Mental Status		Ca	Calcium
Abxs	Antibiotics		CA	Cancer

CABG	Coronary Artery Bypass Graft	**CXR**	Chest Radiograph
CAD	Coronary Artery Disease	**D&C**	Dilation & Curettage
CAH	Congenital Adrenal Hyperplasia	**D&E**	Dilation & Evacuation
CBC	Complete Blood Count	**DCT**	Distal Convoluted Tubule
CBD	Common Bile Duct	**DDAVP**	Desmopressin
CBT	Cognitive Behavioral Therapy	**Def**	Deficiency
CCB	Calcium Channel Blockers	**DEXA**	Dual Energy X-ray Absorptionmetry
CD	Crohn's Disease	**DHEAS**	Dehydroepiandrosterone Sulfate
CEA	Carcinoembryonic Antigen	**DI**	Diabetes Insipidus
CF	Cystic Fibrosis	**DIC**	Disseminated Intravascular Coagulation
CGD	Chronic Granulomatous Disease	**DIP**	Distal Interphalangeal Joint
CHADS2	Congestive Heart Failure, Hypertension, Age, Diabetes Mellitus	**DKA**	Diabetic Ketoacidosis
CHF	Congestive Heart Failure	**DLco**	Diffusing Capacity for carbon monoxide
Chemo	Chemotherapy	**DM**	Diabetes Mellitus
Chrom	Chromosome	**DMD**	Duchenne Muscular Dystrophy
CI	Confidence Interval	**DRE**	Digital Rectal Examination
CINI, II, III	Cervical Intraepithelial Neoplasia	**DTaP**	Diphtheria Tetanus and Pertussis
CK	Creatine Kinase	**DTs**	Delirium Tremens
CK-MB	Creatine Kinase-MB Isoenzyme	**DVT**	Deep Venous Thrombosis
CLL	Chronic Lymphocytic Leukemia	**Dz**	Disease
CML	Chronic Myelogenous Leukemia	**EBV**	Epstein Barr Virus
CMT	Cervical Motion Tenderness	**ECG**	Electrocardiogram
CMV	Cytomegalovirus	**ECT**	Electroconvulsive Therapy
CN	Cranial Nerves	**Echo**	Echocardiography
CNS	Central Nevous System	**EDTA**	Ethylene-diaminetetracetic acid
CO	Cardiac Output	**EF**	Ejection Fraction
Comp	Complications	**EFW**	Estimated Fetal Weight
COPD	Chronic Obstructive Pulmonary Disease	**EEG**	Electroencephalography
CPAP	Continuous Positive Airway Pressure	**EGD**	Esophagogastro-duodenoscopy
Cr	Creatinine	**EKG**	Electrocardiogram
CRL	Crown Rump Length	**EMG**	Electromyogram
CRP	C-reactive Protein	**ENT**	Ear Nose Throat
CSA	Central Sleep Apnea	**EOM**	Extra-Orbital Muscles
CSF	Cerebrospinal Fluid	**EPS**	Extrapyramidal
CST	Contraction Stress Test	**ER**	Estrogen Receptor
CT	Computed Tomography	**ERCP**	Endoscopic Retrograde Cholangio-Pancreatography
CVD	Cardiovascular Disease		
CVS	Chrionic Villus Sampling	**ESR**	Erythrocyte Sedimentation Rate
Cx	Cause		

ESRF	End Stage Renal Failure	**HIDA**	99Tc Heptato-
ETOH	Alcohol		iminodiacetic Acid
Ex	Example	**Hib**	H Influenzae Type b
Expo	Exposure	**HIV**	Human
F	Female		Immunodeficiency Virus
FAP	Familial Adenomatous	**HNPCC**	Hereditary Nonpolyposis
	Polyposis		Colorectal Cancer
FDP	Fibrin Degradation	**HONKS**	Hyperosmolar
	Products		Non-Ketotic Symdrome
FEV1/FVC	Tiffeneau index	**H&P**	History and Physical
FFP	Fresh Frozen Plasma	**HPV**	Human Papillomavirus
FH	Family History	**HRT**	Hormone Replacement
FHR	Fetal Heart Rate		Therapy
FHT	Fetal Heart Tracing	**HSV**	Herpes Simplex Virus
FM	Fine Motor	**HSIL**	High-Grade Squamous
FNA	Fine Needle Aspiration		Intraepithelial Lesions
FSH	Follicle Stimulating	**HTN**	Hypertension
	Hormone	**HUS**	Hemolytic Uremic
GA	Gestational Age		Syndrome
GAF	Global Assessment of	**Hx**	History
	Functioning	**IBD**	Irritable Bowel Disease
GAS	Group A Streptococcal	**ICP**	Intracranial Pressure
GBM	Glomerular Basement	**ICU**	Intensive Care Unit
	Membrane	**IGF-1**	Insulin-Like Growth
GBS	Group B Streptococci		Factor 1
Gen	Generation	**IMA**	Inferior Mesenteric
GERD	Gastroesophageal Relux		Artery
	Disease	**Inflam**	Inflammation
GH	Growth Hormone	**Inh**	Inhibit
GNR	Gram Negative Rods	**INH**	Isoniazid
GM	Gross Motor	**Infx**	Infection
HA	Headeache	**INR**	International
HAART	Highly Active		Normalized Ratio
	Antiretroviral	**IOP**	Intraocular Pressure
	Therapy	**IPV**	Inactivated Polioviurs
HbO2	Hemoglobin Oxygen	**ITP**	Idiopathic
	Saturation		Thrombocytopenic
HBV	Hepatitis B Virus	**IUD**	Intrauterine Device
HCV	Hepatitis C Virus	**IUFD**	Intrauterine Fetal
HCTZ	Hydrochlorothiazide		Demise
HDL	High Density	**IUGR**	Intrauterine Growth
	Lipoprotein		Restriction
HELLP	Hemolysis, Elevated	**IV**	Intravenous
	Liver enzymes	**IVC filter**	Inferior Vena Cava
	Low Platelet count		Filter
HepA	Hepatitis A	**IVIG**	Intravenous
			Immunoglobulin
		IVP	Intravenous Pyelogram
HER2	Human Epidermal		
	Growth Factor	**JIA**	Juvenile Idiopathic
	Receptor 2		Arthritis
HF	Heart Failure	**Jt**	Joint
HHV	Human Herpes Virus	**JVD**	Jugular Venous
			Distension

JVP	Jugular Venous Pressure	**MGUS**	Monoclonal Gammopathies of Unknown Significance
KADE	Fat-Soluble Vitamins K, A, D, and E		
KD	Kidney Disease	**MHA**	Microangiopathic Hemolytic Anemia
K+	Potassium		
KOH	Potassium Hydroxide	**MI**	Myocardial Infarction/Ischemia
KUB	Kidneys, Ureters, and Bladder Radiograph		
		MM	Multiple Myeloma
Lang	Language	**MMA**	Methylmalonic Acid
		MMR	Measles, Mumps, Rubella
LBBB	Left Bundle Branch Block		
LDH	Lactate Dehydrogenase	**MMSE**	Mini-Mental Status Exams
LDL	Low-Density Lipoprotein		
LES	Lower Esophageal Sphincter	**Mos**	Months
		MR	Mental Retardation
LFT	Liver Function Test	**MRA**	Magnetic Resonance Angiogram
LH	Luteinizing Hormone		
LLQ	Left Lower Quadrant	**MRI**	Magnetic Resonance Imaging
LMN	Lower Motor Neurons		
LMP	Last Menstrual Period	**MRSA**	Methicillin Resistant Staphylococcus Aureus
LOC	Loss of Consciousness		
LP	Lumbar Puncture	**MS**	Multiple Sclerosis
LUQ	Left Upper Quadrant	**MSAFP**	Maternal Serum Alpha-Fetoprotein
LR	Likelihood Ratio		
LRI	Lower Respiratory Infection	**Multi**	Multiparous
		Na	Sodium
LSD	Lysergic Acid Diethylamide	**Neg**	Negative
		NF1	Neurofibromatosis/ Von Recklinghausen's
LSE	Libman-Sacks Endocarditis		
		NG	Nasogastric Tube
LSIL	Low-Grade Squamous Intraepithelial Lesions	**NMS**	Neuroleptic Malignant Syndrome
Lymph	Lymphocytic	**NNRTI**	Non-Nucleoside Reverse Transcriptase Inhibitors
M	Male		
MAC	Mycobacterium Avium-Intracellulare	**NPH**	Neutral Protamine Hagedorn Insulin
MCA	Middle Cerebral Artery	**NPO**	Nil Per Os or NBM (nothing by mouth)
MCP	Metacarpophalangeal Joint		
		NRTI	Nucleoside Reverse Transcriptase Inhibitors
MCV	Mean Corpuscular Volume		
		NPV	Negative Predictive Value
MDE	Major Depressive Episode		
		NSAIDs	Non-Steroidal Anti-Inflammatory Drugs
Mech	Mechanism		
Meds	Medications	**NSCLC**	Non-Small Cell Lung Cancer
MEN I	Multiple Endocrine Neoplasia I		
		NST	Nonstress Test
MEN II	Multiple Endocrine Neoplasia II	**NSTEMI**	Non-ST Elevation Myocardial Infarction
Mets	Metastasis	**NTD**	Neural Tube Defects
Mg	Magnesium	**O&P**	Ova and parasites in stool
		O2	Oxygen

OCD	Obsessive Compulsive Disorder	**POC**	Products Of Conception
OCP	Oral Contraceptive Pills	**PPD**	Tuberculosis Skin Test
OGTT	Oral Glucose Tolerance Test	**PPROM**	Preterm Premature Rupture Of Membrane
OR	Odds Ratio	**PPV**	Positive Predictive Value
OSA	Obstructive Sleep Apnea	**PR**	Progesterone Receptor
PAD	Peripheral Artery Disease	**PUD**	Peptic Ulcer Disease
PAN	Polyarteritis Nodosa	**Pulm**	Pulmonary
PAPPA	Pregnancy Associated Plasma Protein-A	**Preg**	Pregnancy
		PreOp	Preoperational
PBC	Primary Biliary Cirrhosis	**Prim**	Primiparous
		PROM	Premature Rupture Of Membranes
PCA	Posterior Cerebral Artery	**PSC**	Primary Sclerosing Cholangitis
PCI	Percutaneous Coronary Intervention	**Pts**	Patients
PCKD	Polycystic Kidney Disease	**PT**	Prothrombin Time
Pco2	Partial Pressure of Carbon Dioxide	**PTSD**	Post-Traumatic Stress Disorder
PCOS	Polycystic Ovarian Syndrome	**PTT**	Partial Thromboplastin Time
PCP	Pneumocystis Jiroveci	**PVCs**	Premature Ventricular Contractions
PCR	Polymerase Chain Reaction	**PVR**	Peripheral Vascular Resistance
PCT	Proximal Convoluted Tubule	**RBBB**	Right Bundle Branch Block
PCV	Pneumococcal	**RA**	Rheumatoid Arthritis
PCWP	Pulmonary Capillary Wedge Pressure	**RAIU**	Radioactive Iodine Uptake
PDA	Patent Ductus Arteriosus	**RDS**	Respiratory Distress Syndrome
PEA	Pulseless Electrical Activity	**Recom**	Recommended
		Resp	Respirations
PE	Pulmonary Embolism	**RF**	Rheumatoid Factor
PEEP	Positive End Expiratory Pressure	**Rh**	Rhesus blood group system (D antigen)
PFTs	Pulmonary Function Tests	**RhoGAM**	Rho(D) Immune Globulin
Ph	Phosphate	**RIPE**	Rifampin, Isoniazid, Pyrazinamide, Ethambutol
Phil	Philadelphia Chromosome	**RLQ**	Right Lower Quadrant
PID	Pelvic Inflammatory Disease	**RMSF**	Rocky Mountain Spotted Fever
PIP	Proximal Interphalangeal Joint	**R/O**	Rule Out
		ROM	Range Of Motion
PKU	Phenylketonuria	**RPR**	Rapid Plasma Reagin
PMN	Polymorphonuclear Leukocytes	**RUQ**	Right Upper Quadrant
		RR	Relative Risk also Respiratory Rate
PNH	Paroxysmal Nocturnal Hemoglobinuria	**RTA**	Renal Tubular Acidosis
Po2	Partial Pressure of Oxygen	**RVH**	Right Ventricular Hypertrophy

S1Q3T3	S wave lead I, Q and T lead III	**TIA**	Transient Ischemic Attack
S1	First Heart Sound	**TIBC**	Total Iron Binding Capacity
S2	Second Heart Sound		
S3	Third Heart Sound	**TIMI Score**	Thrombolysis In Myocardial Infarction
S4	Fourth Heart Sound		
SAB	Spontaneous Abortion	**TLC**	Total Lung Capacity
SAGG	Serum-Ascites Albumin Gradient	**TOF**	Tetralogy of Fallot
		TM	Tympanic Membrane
SAH	Subarachnoid Hemorrhage	**tPA**	Tissue Plasminogen Activator
SBO	Small Bowel Obstruction	**TPN**	Parenteral Nutrition
SBP	Spontaneous Bacterial Peritonitis	**TRAP**	Tartrate-Resistant Acid Phosphatase
SCC	Squamous Cell Carcinoma	**Trim**	Trimester
		TropI	Troponin I
SCLC	Small Cell Lung Cancer	**TropT**	Troponin T
SCID	Severe Combined Immunodeficiency	**TSH**	Thyroid Stimulating Hormone
StoolCx	Stool Culture	**TTP**	Thrombotic Thrombocytopenic Purpura
SD	Standard Deviation		
Sen	Sensitivity		
SIADH	Syndrome of Inappropriate Antidiuretic Hormone	**TURP**	Transurethral Resection of Prostate
		Tx	Treatment
Si/Sx	Signs and Symptoms	**U/A**	Urine Analysis
SIRS	Systemic Inflammation Response Syndrome	**UA**	Unstable Angina
		UC	Ulcerative Colitis
SMA	Superior Mesenteric Artery	**UCx**	Urine Culture
		UMN	Upper Motor Neurons
Spec	Specificity	**URI**	Upper Respiratory Infection
Spont	Spontaneously		
SSRI	Selective Serotonin Reuptake Inhibitor	**U/S**	Ultrasound
		UTI	Urinary Tract Infection
STEMI	ST Elevation Myocardial Infarction	**VCUG**	Voiding Cystourethrogram
Staph	Staphylococcus Aureus	**VDRL**	Venereal Disease Research Laboratory Test (syphilis)
Strep	Streptococcus		
SJS	Stevens-Johnson Syndrome		
		Vfib	Ventricular Fibrillation
SLE	Systemic Lupus Erythematosus	**VINI, II, III**	Vulvar intraepithelial Neoplasia
SOB	Short of Breath	**Vit**	Vitamin
Stim	Stimulate	**Vol**	Volume
Symp	Symptoms	**V/Q**	Ventilation-Perfusion
Tachy	Tachycardia	**VSD**	Ventral Septal Defect
TAH/BSO	Total Abdominal Hysterectomy with Bilateral Salpingo-Oophorectomy	**VT**	Ventricular Tachycardia
		VUR	Vesicoureteral Reflux
		VZV	Varicella-Zoster Virus
TB	Tuberculosis		
TEN	Toxic Epidermal Necrolysis		
TFTs	Thyroid Function Tests		

WBC	White Blood Cells	**XR**	X-Linked Recessive
wk	Week	**yo**	Years old
w/o	Without	**yr**	Years

INDEX

Hyperestrogenism, 82
Hyperkalemia (K>5), 297, 298,
   299, 300, 303
   Medications that cause
   hyperkalemia, 300
Hypernatremia (Na>145), 302
Hyperosmolar non-ketotic symdrome
   (HONKS), 51
Hyperparathyroidism, 56, 300, 304
Hyperprolactinemia, 47, 53, 216, 257
Hypersegmented neutrophils, 86
Hypersensitivity pneumonitis, 282
Hypersensitivity reactions, 20, 35-36
Hypersomnia, 275
Hypertension, 12-13
Hypertensive crisis, 262
Hyperthermia, 44
Hyperthyroidism, 52
Hypertrophic cardiomyopathy, 19
Hypertrophic obstructive
   cardiomyopathy, 19
Hypnagogic, 275
Hypnopompic, 275
Hypocalcemia (Ca<8.2), 228, 304-305
   Corrected calcium, 305
Hypochondriasis, 276
Hypomagnesaemia (Mg<1.5), 304, 305
Hyponatremia (Na<135), 302-303
   Hypervolemic, 302
   Euvolemic, 302
   Hypovolemic, 302
Hyposthenuria, 90
Hypothermia, 257
Hypothyroidism, 53, 216
Hypovolemic shock, 41, 44
Hypoxanthine-guanine phosphoribosyl
   transferase (HPRT), 143
Hypoxemia, 283
Hysterectomy, 222
Hysterosalpingogram, 219

I

Ice test, 167
Id, 263
Idiopathic pulmonary fibrosis, 283
Idiopathic thrombocytopenic
   purpura (ITP), 102
Iduronate sulfatase deficiency, 231
IgA deficiency, 237
IgA nephropathy, 290
IgM cold agglutinin antibodies, 128
Ileus, 68
Imatinib, 94
Imipramine, 261

Imiquimod, 32
Immunization schedule, 254
   Preterm immunization, 254
Immunodeficiencies, 235
Imperforate anus, 249
Imperforate hymen, 211
Impetigo, 23
Implanon, 208
In vitro fertilization, 212
Incomplete/partial molar
   pregnancy, 202
Incontinence, 217-218
Incorrect dating, 184
India-ink stain, 118
Indirect coombs, 88
Indirect inguinal hernias, 73
Indomethacin, 228
Incentive spirometry, 204
Incidence, 57
Infantile GERD, 64
Infantile spasms, 156, 179
Infective endocarditis, 130
Inferior vena cava filter
   (IVC filter), 285
Infliximab, 71
Influenza, 108
Informed consent, 62
Inguinal hernias, 73
Inhaled corticosteroids, 280
Inhibition of P-450, 40
International normalized ratio
   (INR), 100, 285
Insomnia, 275
Insulin, 49, 303
Interferon-beta, 169
Interstitial cystitis, 124
Interstitial lung disease, 281
Intracerebral hemorrhage, 162-163
Intraductal papilloma, 206
Intrahepatic cholestasis of
   pregnancy, 79
Intranuclear ophthalmoplegia, 169
Intrauterine device (IUD), 208
Intrauterine fetal demise (IUFD), 194
Intrauterine growth
   restriction (IUGR), 201
Intravenous immunoglobulin
   (IVIG), 167, 168, 235,
   236, 238, 240
Intravenous pyelogram
   (IVP), 311
Intraventricular hemorrhage, 161
Intubation, 37, 280
Intussusception, 233, 240

ABOUT THE AUTHOR

Rachelle Doom, MD, is dedicated to excellence. She has earned four degrees while traveling throughout the world to work with nonprofit organizations. Her work has included serving the AIDS population of Africa, working with orphans, and building schools in El Salvador. Dr. Doom would like to give special thanks for all the support from; **Tom Doom, Lois Doom, Monique Vandenberg, Wendi Holland, Mekella Holland, Jaimee Holland, Doug Holland, Shannon Levine and Madhavi Boga**.

www.ingramcontent.com/pod-product-compliance
Lightning Source LLC
Chambersburg PA
CBHW051439170526
45166CB00001B/46